Current Treatment of Anorexia Nervosa and Bulimia

Editors:
Pauline S. Powers
Robert C. Fernandez
Tampa, Fla.

Karger Biobehavioral Medicine Series 4

Current Treatment of Anorexia Nervosa and Bulimia

9 figures and 34 tables, 1984

KARGER
Basel · München · Paris · London · New York · Tokyo · Sydney

Karger Biobehavioral Medicine Series

1 C.B. Scrignar: Stress Strategies. The Treatment of the Anxiety Disorders
X + 262 p., 12 fig., 8 tab., 1983. ISBN 3–8055–3605–4

2 Biobehavioral Bases of Coronary Heart Disease. T.M. Dembroski, T.H. Schmidt, G. Blümchen (eds.)
XVIII + 482 p., 100 fig., 51 tab., 1983. ISBN 3–8055–3629–1

3 W. Linden: Psychological Perspectives of Essential Hypertension. Etiology, Maintenance, and Treatment
X + 130 p., 5 fig., 6 tab., 1984. ISBN 3–8055–3662–3

National Library of Medicine, Cataloging in Publication
Current treatment of anorexia nervosa and bulimia
Editors, Pauline S. Powers, Robert C. Fernandez.–
Basel; New York: Karger, 1984 (Karger biobehavioral medicine series; v. 4)
Includes index.
1. Anorexia Nervosa – therapy 2. Hyperphagia – therapy
I. Powers, Pauline S. II. Fernandez, Robert C. III. Series
W1 KA821M v.4 [WM 175 C976]
ISBN 3–8055–3879–0

Drug Dosage

The authors and the publisher have exerted every effort to ensure that drug selection and dosage set forth in this text are in accord with current recommendations and practice at the time of publication. However, in view of ongoing research, changes in government regulations, and the constant flow of information relating to drug therapy and drug reactions, the reader is urged to check the package insert for each drug for any change in indications and dosage and for added warnings and precautions. This is particularly important when the recommended agent is a new and/or infrequently employed drug.

Printed in Switzerland by Thür AG Offsetdruck, Pratteln
ISBN 3–8055–3879–0

Contents

List of Contributors

Eubanks, Rebecca, Clinical Associate, Department of Psychiatry and Behavioral Medicine, University of South Florida College of Medicine, Tampa, Fla.

Fernandez, Robert C., Associate Chairperson and Director of Education, Department of Psychiatry and Behavioral Medicine, University of South Florida College of Medicine, Tampa, Fla.

Golloway, Glenn G., Associate Professor, Department of Psychiatry and Behavioral Medicine, University of South Florida College of Medicine, Tampa, Fla.

Halmi, Katherine A., Associate Professor of Psychiatry, Cornell University Medical College, The New York Hospital, Westchester Division, N.Y.

Knight, Judith C., Decatur Hospital, Decatur, Ga.

Litton, Susan C., Counseling Center, Georgia State University, Atlanta, Ga.

Maher, Michael S., Assistant Professor, Department of Psychiatry and Behavioral Medicine, University of South Florida College of Medicine, Tampa, Fla.

Miller, Sharon Glick, Assistant Professor, Department of Psychiatry and Behavioral Medicine, University of South Florida College of Medicine, Tampa, Fla.

Powers, Henry P., Clinical Instructor, Department of Psychiatry and Behavioral Medicine, University of South Florida College of Medicine, Tampa, Fla.

Powers, Pauline S., Associate Professor, Director, Division of Consultation/Liaison Psychiatry, Director, Eating Disorders Clinic, Department of Psychiatry and Behavioral Medicine, University of South Florida College of Medicine, Tampa, Fla.

Raj, Ashok B., Assistant Professor, Department of Psychiatry and Behavioral Medicine, University of South Florida College of Medicine, Tampa, Fla.

Roth, Deborah, Assistant Professor, Department of Psychiatry and Behavioral Medicine, University of South Florida College of Medicine, Tampa, Fla.

Root, Allen W., Professor and Associate Chairperson, Department of Pediatrics, University of South Florida College of Medicine, Tampa, Fla.

Shaw, Kailie, Assistant Professor, Associate Director of Education, Department of Psychiatry and Behavioral Medicine, University of South Florida College of Medicine, Tampa, Fla.

Yager, Joel, Professor and Director, Eating Disorders Clinic, UCLA Neuropsychiatric Institute, Department of Psychiatry and Biobehavioral Sciences, University of California, Los Angeles School of Medicine, Los Angeles, Calif.

Foreword

The history of mankind mirrors an ongoing search for sufficient food. As the social historian *Braundel* notes, 'Tell me what you eat and I'll tell you who you are'. The old German proverb 'der Mensch ist was er isst' (a man is what he eats) supports the notion that one's food is a designation of an individual's social status as well as his civilization or culture [1]. The spice routes promoted exploration of both the Western and Eastern hemispheres. European colonial migration was promoted by the search for dietary ingredients. It is a paradox that disorders such as anorexia nervosa or bulimia exist in a society where foodstuffs have never been more abundant.

It has been over 300 years since *Morton* first clinically described anorexia nervosa by outlining 'The nervous consumption caused by sadness and anxious cares' [2]. *Binswanger's* [3] elegant article on 'The Case of Ellen West' describes in brilliant detail the existential anguish of the anorexic as she poetically documents her dilemma:

> I'd like to die just as the birdling does
> That splits his throat in highest jubilation;
> And not to live as the worm on earth lives on,
> Becoming old and ugly, dull and dumb!
> No, feel for once how forces in me kindle,
> and wildly be consumed by my own fire.

This inherent dilemma, the fear of getting fat as well as being consumed by one's own 'fire', phenomenologically decribes many anorexics. Yet existential analysis and phenomenologic documentation of the anorexic's experience is only one element needed to fully comprehend such an eating disorder and to develop methods for treatment. Drs. *Powers and Fernandez* have thus integrated various conceptual models found within psychiatry. The role of biologic factors, as discussed by Dr. *Root;* psychological issues, noted by Dr. *Powers* in Chapter 2 and Drs. *Roth and Galloway* in Chapter 6; learned behaviors reviewed by Dr. *Halmi;* sociocultural implications discussed in terms of a small nuclear family culture and social system by Mrs. *Miller* all reflect various approaches to the problem of self-willed starvation or forced self-induced emesis. As *Lazare* [4] has suggested, these various models, whether biologic, psychological, behavioral or sociocultural, all complement one another to form the various answers to specific questions. The authors pose three basic questions which they most elegantly attempt to answer: What are the various definitions of anorexia nervosa and bulimia? What are the etiologic factors known in these conditions, and how might each of these entities be properly treated? Only by looking at the condition from multiple perspectives can such questions be answered. Further support to the integrated approach that Drs. *Powers and Fernandez* have developed in this volume is provided by the contribution of *McHugh and Slavney* [5] on the need to circumvent the brain-mind dysfunction. Recognition of the need to approach psychiatric entities as a dialectic allows the role of formal characteristics in viewing man as a biologic organism to complement functional explanations of the subjective human experience. When these two approaches are synthesized, various views may complement one another as opposed to conflicting views and as contradictory aspects. So it is with eating disorders. Biologic issues may in fact operate within the anorexic, but so do psychologic factors that may provide a threshold for the disease to occur. Until more specific etiologic factors are found, we must rely on a variety of empirical treatment approaches. These are beautifully described within the following pages. This book should be read by all physicians who treat eating disorders. As such entities are becoming increasingly common, it would seem appropriate for all psychiatric physicians and primary care practitioners to have such information available. Drs. *Powers and Fernandez* should be congratulated in providing such a lucid discussion of two vexing clinical problems.

Thomas N. Wise
Georgetown University Medical Center and
The Johns Hopkins Medical Institutions

References

1 Braundel, F.: The structures of everyday life, pp. 103–182 (Harper & Row, New York 1979).

2 Silverman, J.A.: Richard Morton, 1637–1698, limner of anorexia nervosa. J. Am. med. Ass. *250:* 2830–2832 (1983).

3 Binswanger, L.: The case of Ellen West; in May, Angel, Ellenberger, Existence, pp. 237–363 (Clarion, New York 1958).

4 Lazare, A.: Hidden conceptual models in clinical psychiatry. New Engl. J. Med. *288:* 345–351 (1973).

5 McHugh, P.R.; Slavney, P.: The perspectives of psychiatry (Johns Hopkins University, Baltimore 1983).

Preface

This book is designed to provide the clinician with information currently needed to permit comprehensive assessment and treatment of patients with anorexia nervosa and bulimia. Both conditions are increasing in incidence and prevalence and both are complex medical-psychiatric disorders. Expertise in diagnosis and treatment methods is needed by many medical specialists and mental health professionals. Although research findings are included and referenced throughout the book, our general goal is to provide a handbook for the clinician planning to treat patients with these eating disorders.

Throughout the book we have endeavored to stress the complex and diverse nature of the various etiological factors which converge to produce common symptoms. A theme woven throughout the chapters is the need to provide careful and comprehensive evaluation and to design an individualized treatment program that usually involves several modalities for the individual patient. This necessitates that the clinician possess a broad range of diagnostic and treatment skills and be able to work effectively as part of a multidisciplinary team.

We have used both American units of measure (pounds, calories, degrees Fahrenheit, inches and feet) as well as metric units of measure (kilograms, joules, degrees centigrade, centimeters and meters) to facilitate reading for both American and European audiences. Furthermore, since the majority of patients with eating disorders are female, many authors of the chapters in this book have used primarily the feminine pronouns, her and she.

The introduction briefly outlines the history of anorexia nervosa and bulimia, presents the diagnostic criteria and differential diagnostic considerations and reviews the known epidemiological data and prognostic factors. It also reviews the limited efforts to date as regards primary, secondary, and tertiary prevention and proposes the need for additional preventive measures. The remainder of the book is divided into four sections. In the first section the major treatment modalities including psychotherapy, pharmacotherapy, behavioral treatment and family therapy are presented. The second section elucidates certain conceptual models which are designed to aid the clinician in understanding the eating disorders including psychodynamic issues, cognitive disturbances, and the biological aspects of the eating disorders. The multidetermined nature of the conditions is highlighted by a chapter which proposes that the eating disorders are models for psychosomatic illness. The third section presents a review of the integrated treatment of anorexia nervosa and bulimia including the role of the nutritionist and medical consultant. A thorough synthesis of the results of studies utilizing psychological testing is presented. One chapter elucidates the therapeutic use of symptoms, signs and laboratory data resulting from abnormal eating practices and various purging behaviors. The final section is devoted to an in-depth study of the various group approaches for anorexia nervosa and bulimia. This section includes a critical review of well-known national self-help groups including their advantages and limitations and proposes an appropriate role for such groups in the treatment of these patients.

Pauline S. Powers
Robert C. Fernandez

To the memory of my father, Floyd Smith
Pauline S. Powers

To the memory of my father, C.G. Fernandez, MD,
and of my friend Joe A. Fernandez
Robert C. Fernandez

1 Introduction

Pauline S. Powers, Robert C. Fernandez

Anorexia nervosa and bulimia are complex psychosomatic disorders heavily influenced by cultural factors. In the last decade, both conditions appear to have increased in incidence and both have been the focus of intense scrutiny by a broad spectrum of investigators in the biological and behavioral sciences. In this chapter we will briefly review certain background information as a prelude to the comprehensive overview of treatment provided in subsequent chapters. This preliminary information will include a brief historical review, diagnostic issues, epidemiology, etiological and risk factors, significant cultural influences and prognosis. We will conclude with a discussion of the need to direct future efforts in the area of prevention.

History

Anorexia nervosa has probably occurred since at least the 4th century. *Lacey* [1] notes that one of the earliest references was that of St. Jerome writing to his protege Eustochium, a young well-bred girl; he wrote: 'Let your companions be women, pale and thin with fasting.' Her sister, Blessila, also under St. Jerome's tutelage, died of the regimen and may be the earliest recorded victim of the disorder. Princess Margaret of Hungary (born circa 1045 and died 1093) may have had anorexia nervosa [*Halmi, K.:* Grand rounds, University of South Florida, April 1983]. *Lacey* [1] also has reported the medieval Christian legend of St. Wilgefortis. She was of high social class (the daughter of the King of Portugal) and the legend holds that as a young woman she fasted and prayed to God to deprive her of her beauty in order to turn away male attention. After adopting a regime of prayer, asceticism and self-starvation, she began to grow hair on her face and body. In some countries she was adopted as the patron saint of women seeking to liberate themselves from men. Various forms of the legend appeared throughout Europe in the Middle Ages and may indicate that the condition was not rare at that time. *McLeod* [2] has postulated that some women who were believed to be witches in the Middle Ages may in fact have been anorectics: the seeming capacity to live without food coupled with restless energy may have been construed as evidence of evil possession.

The first clinical descriptions of the condition were written in the 1600s. Although conditions were alluded to that were probably anorexia nervosa in 1668 by *Hobbes* [3] and in 1669 by *Reynolds* [4], *Morton* [5] is usually credited with the first clinical description of anorexia nervosa in 1694. His initial vivid description is still clinically accurate. He describes an 18-year-old woman as follows:

'In the month of July she fell into a total suppression of her Monthly Courses from a multitude of Cares and Passions of her Mind ... From which time her Appetite began to abate and her Digestion to be bad; her flesh also began to be flaccid and loose, and her looks pale ... She was wont by her studying at Night, and continually pouring upon Books, to expose herself both Day and Night to the injuries of the Air ... I do not remember that I did ever in all my practice see one, that was conversant with the living, so much wasted with the greatest degree of a Consumption (like a Skeleton, only clad with Skin) yet there was no Fever but on the contrary a coldness of the whole Body ... only her Appetite was diminished, and her Digestion uneasy with Fainting Fits, which did frequently return upon her.'

Morton's patient refused the medication offered and died 3 months later. This patient was 1 of 2 with severe weight loss which he distinguished from others with tuberculosis; he labeled their condition as 'nervous consumption'.

That the condition was recognized in the mid-1800s is illustrated by the poem published in 1844 by a physician, *Hoffmann* [6] (fig. 1). In 1868 Sir *William Gull* [7] briefly described 'hysteric apepsia' and in 1874 he began using the term 'anorexia nervosa' and described factors he considered important in the development of the disorder including a 'morbid mental state' [8]. In 1873 *Lasègue* [9] independently described the disorder as 'anorexia hystérique'. He described the characteristic denial and cognitive distortions and body image disturbance particularly well:

'... An inexhaustable optimism, against which supplications and menaces alike are of no avail: "I do not suffer and must then be well ..." So often have I heard this phrase repeated by patients, that now it has come to represent for me a symptom – almost a sign ... The whole disease is summed in this intellectual perversion' [9, p. 151].

'The patient, when told that she cannot live upon an amount of food that would not support a young infant, replies that it furnishes sufficient nourishment for her, adding that she is neither changed nor thinner' [9, p. 150].

The condition was sufficiently common that a typical anorectic patient was described in 1908 in a textbook of medicine [10]. In 1914, *Simmonds* [11], a German pathologist, described a patient with cachexia who had pitu-

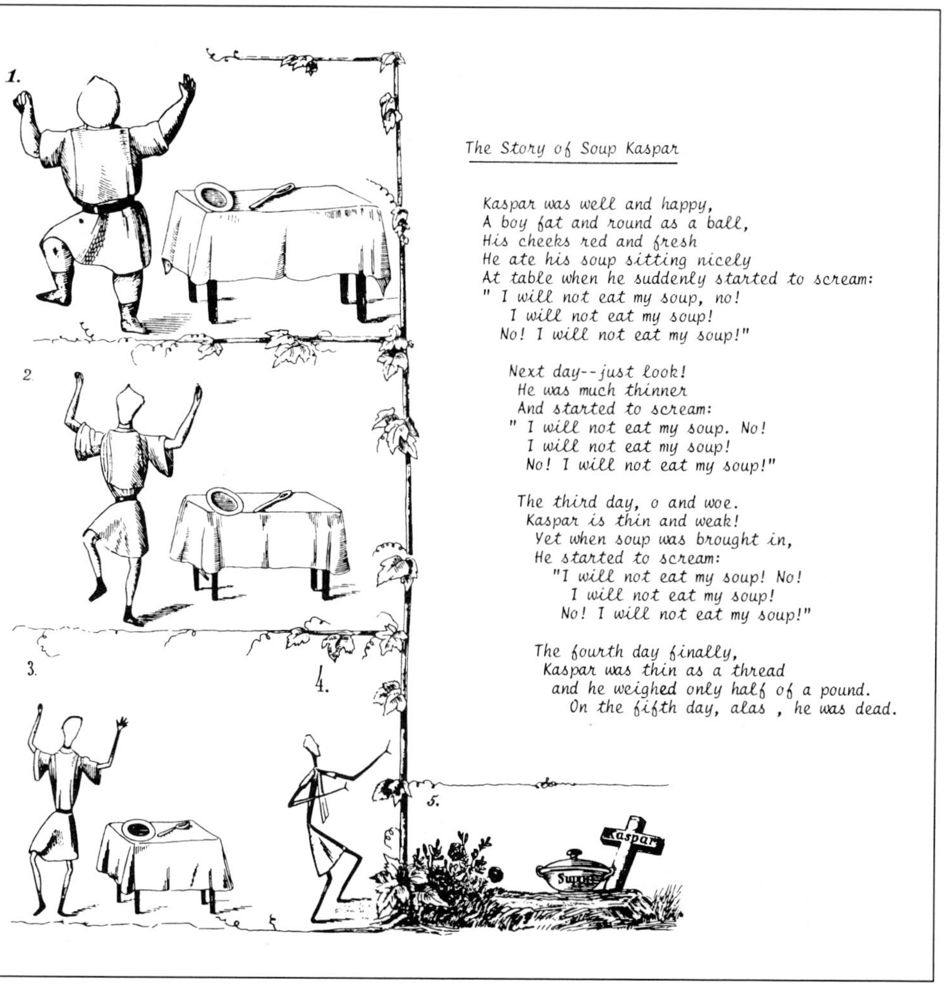

Fig. 1. 19th century poem by *Heinrich Hoffmann* [6], translated from the German by *Ursula Mahlendorf.* Reprinted, with permisson, from [62].

itary destruction at autopsy, and during the next 30 years there was confusion between pituitary insufficiency (Simmonds' disease) and anorexia nervosa. In the last 35–45 years the delineation of anorexia nervosa as a psychiatric disorder with significant biological ramifications has emerged from the studies of *Bruch* [12], *Crisp* [13], and others. *Minuchin* et al. [14] have added a family system dimension to the understanding of the disorder.

Bulimia is a term that has been used in two ways, as a symptom and as a syndrome. The symptom bulimia is a synonym for binge-eating. The diagnostic criteria for the syndrome bulimia are described later in this chapter. Binge-eating is probably a normal physiological response to starvation and has occurred throughout history whenever there were irregular food supplies. In early Roman times, food was relatively plentiful and binge-eating and purging were common. Vomitoria were described and *Seneca* [15] (a critical stoic philosopher who lived about 65 AD) wrote, 'Men eat to vomit and vomit to eat'. There have been sporadic reports in the medical literature of psychogenic vomiting, and in the last 50 years binge-eating and purging have been described as part of the anorexia nervosa syndrome. In the last 10 years, public and medical attention has focused on the syndrome bulimia as a disorder separate from anorexia nervosa.

Diagnostic Issues

Diagnosis of Anorexia Nervosa

According to the *Diagnostic and Statistical Manual* (DSM III) [16], anorexia nervosa is characterized by a weight loss of 25% of original body weight, an intense fear of becoming obese, disturbance of body image and refusal to maintain weight over a normal minimal weight for age and height (table I). This diagnostic scheme is essentially an amalgamation of *Bruch's* [12] criteria for primary anorexia nervosa and the criteria proposed by *Feighner* et al. [17] for research purposes. *Bruch's* [12] criteria are psychological ones and include body image disturbance, a decreased sense of internal awareness, and a paralyzing sense of ineffectiveness. The criteria used by *Feighner* et al. [17] are essentially a checklist of symptoms that are easily elicited but do not suggest guidelines for either understanding the psychopathogenesis of the condition or treating the disorder.

The DSM III criteria have been criticized on several grounds. First, amenorrhea (either primary or secondary) is not an inclusion criterion for female patients. Not only is amenorrhea an invariable part of the presenting picture in females [18], but restoration of menses may signal full psychobiological recovery. A second criticism of the criteria is that the term 'body image disturbance' is not defined and represents a nebulous concept. Some authors [19] contend that a small percentage of patients do not have a demonstrable disturbance in the perceptual aspect of body image (i.e. they do not overestimate their size). *Burron* et al. [20] have found that, as a group,

Table I. Diagnostic criteria for anorexia nervosa (DSM III)

A	Intense fear of becoming obese, which does not diminish as weight loss progresses
B	Disturbance of body image, e.g. claiming to 'feel fat' even when emaciated
C	Weight loss of at least 25% of original body weight or, if under 18 years of age, weight loss from original body weight plus projected weight gain expected from growth charts may be combined to make the 25%
D	Refusal to maintain body weight over a minimal normal weight for age and height
E	No known physical illness that would account for the weight loss

anorectics have no more body image disturbance than normal-weight controls yet the degree of the disturbance in body image is correlated with prognosis [21] (those with less evidence of a perceptual disturbance of body image have a better prognosis).

A third criticism of the criteria is that it lacks psychological criteria except body image disturbance. Although in our opinion this is a valid criticism, it is worth noting that the entire DSM III attempts to describe conditions rather than postulate etiology. A fourth criticism of the DSM III criteria is that the strict weight criteria (which are derived from the *Feighner* et al. [17] research criteria) may result in appropriate treatment being withheld from patients who have not yet lost 25% of their original body weight. Furthermore, since it has been noted [22] that a significant percentage of patients are underweight prior to weight loss, waiting until they meet the strict weight criteria can be particularly hazardous. A fifth criticism is that certain symptoms that occur commonly in anorexia nervosa are not even mentioned, such as shoplifting.

Diagnosis of Bulimia

The DSM III criteria for bulimia are listed in table II. The essential characteristics are episodic rapid ingestion of large quantities of food in a short period of time, termination of the episode with discomfort (often associated with self-induced vomiting), and feelings of guilt and self-contempt after the binge. Unlike patients with anorexia nervosa, there is usually awareness that the eating pattern is not normal; furthermore, although the binge-eating and purging is frequently viewed as a shameful secret, many patients present themselves for psychiatric treatment. Frequently, bulimic patients abuse barbiturates, alcohol, amphetamines or cocaine intermittently. Many normal-weight bulimics complain of 'feeling fat' and although body image

Table II. Diagnostic criteria for bulimia (DSM III)

A	Recurrent episodes of binge-eating (rapid consumption of a large amount of food in a discrete period of time, usually less than 2 h)
B	At least three of the following:
	(1) Consumption of high-caloric, easily ingested food during a binge
	(2) Inconspicuous eating during a binge
	(3) Termination of such eating episodes by abdominal pain, sleep, social interruption, or self-induced vomiting
	(4) Repeated attempts to lose weight by severely restrictive diets, self-induced vomiting, or use of cathartics or diuretics
	(5) Frequent weight fluctuations greater than 10lb (4.5 kg) due to alternating binges and fasts
C	Awareness that the eating pattern is abnormal and fear of not being able to stop eating voluntarily
D	Depressed mood and self-depreciating thoughts following eating binges
E	The bulimic episodes are not due to anorexia nervosa or any known physical disorder

disturbances have not been as rigorously studied as with anorectic patients, it is likely that perceptual and attitudinal disturbances are relatively common.

The relationship between the syndrome bulimia and anorexia nervosa and obesity is not clear. About 50% of the patients with anorexia nervosa have as a symptom episodes of binge-eating [23] and perhaps 50% of the patients with the syndrome bulimia have a past history suggestive of anorexia nervosa [24]. On the other hand, it may be that there is an important relationship between the bulimia syndrome and obesity. In 1959, *Stunkard* [25] described the 'binge-eating syndrome' as a subtype of obesity in individuals in whom stress precipitates binge-eating which is followed by remorse. In 1982, *Powers* [26] reported that about 25% of a group of 200 obese patients acknowledged binge-eating 1 time per week and said that the episode was followed by guilt; although all patients had made attempts to lose weight, it was usually not by severely restrictive diets, self-induced vomiting, use of cathartics or diuretics. In view of these findings, and recent evidence [27] that patients with bulimia and bulimic anorexia tend to be heavier before onset of the disorder than patients with restricting anorexia and have stronger family histories of obesity, it may be that bulimia is more closely related to obesity than to anorexia nervosa. In this vein, it is worth noting that some researchers believe the three conditions are on a continuum, and *Palmer* [28] postulates a 'dietary chaos syndrome'.

Subtypes

One current trend in the study of anorexia nervosa is to divide patients into restricting and bulimic subtypes. Restricting anorectics are those who unremittingly control food intake, whereas bulimic anorectics periodically engage in binge-eating. These two subtypes have been compared clinically and epidemiologically [27, 29]. Bulimic anorectics have been found to be more impulsive, more outgoing, more emotionally disturbed, more likely to be depressed and more likely to purge in various ways. Although the restricting-bulimic dualism is interesting, it is important to recognize that the studies may simply be studying patients at different points in the course of their illness: i.e. some bulimic anorectics may have developed binge-eating after having the disorder for some time. Also, as noted in chapter 13, binge-eating may begin in a response to a weight restoration program which rewards rapid weight gain with little attention to psychodynamic issues.

In terms of subtypes of bulimia, it may be useful to distinguish normal weight and obese subgroups as well as groups with or without a history of anorexia nervosa. Groups with or without purging behaviors (including vomiting, use of cathartics and diuretics) may differ epidemiologically and prognostically. The presence or absence of overexercising may be important. Exercise may have different meanings (e.g. it may be used to control appetite or it may be used to purge the food). It may have different etiological and prognostic importance, depending upon the way in which it is used.

Certain patients have been considered atypical anorectis. For example, some patients have been identified who have failed to grow in height and weight [30]. The patients may be 25% below projected weight from growth charts, yet not have the characteristic preoccupation with food and weight. This absence may reflect the fact that they have not lost weight and thus are not in a state of semistarvation, which produces characteristic cognitive defects [31]. *Yates* et al. [32] have described a group of male distance runners who do not meet the rigid weight criteria for anorexia nervosa and who tend to be older, but who have psychological profiles which are similar to those of anorectic patients. These researchers have wondered if running may be a male analogue of anorexia nervosa, especially if indulged in a ritualistic and obsessive fashion. Finally, *Ryle* [33] and more recently *Launer* [34] have described 'tardive anorexia' which occurs in middle to older age females. These women have been described as emaciated, 'sparrow-like' women, constantly obsessed with gastrointestinal functions, and living socially isolated lives. We have seen 4 elderly women who fit this description, but in 3 patients it was clear from the history that the first episode of dramatic weight loss occurred before age 25.

Differential Diagnosis

The psychiatric conditions which can mimic anorexia nervosa include schizophrenia, depression, conversion disorders and phobic neuroses. Although *Bruch* [12] proposed that the core problem in anorexia nervosa and schizophrenia is the same – i.e. both groups of patients have a deficient sense of identity – this idea has not been proven. There appear to be some anorectic patients in whom the diagnosis of schizophrenia later seems appropriate, but in a rigorous study by *Dally* [35], less than 1% or 1 out of 140 of the patients were eventually diagnosed as schizophrenic. Case 4, presented in chapter 2, is an example of a patient whose initial presentation was no different from others with anorexia nervosa but who then developed a florid psychosis.

The psychiatric differential diagnosis of bulimia is often more difficult. It is often unclear if the bulimia is a cause or a consequence of the commonly associated depressive symptoms or if the bulimia is, in and of itself, an atypical presentation of depression. Furthermore, many reports of patients with bulimia have DSM III Axis II diagnoses, especially borderline personality. These issues are addressed in chapter 4 and in chapter 16. Rarely, schizophrenia presents with binge-eating. We have seen 2 such patients, but in each, delusions about food and eating were readily identified.

Distinguishing various physical conditions from anorexia nervosa and bulimia is discussed in chapter 12. As is mentioned in several chapters (see particularly chapters 9 and 13) it is important to recognize the psychobiological effects of semistarvation which occur in anorexia nervosa and perhaps in more subtle forms in bulimia.

Epidemiology

Incidence and Prevalence

Although it is likely that recent medical and popular interest in anorexia nervosa has resulted in more frequent accurate diagnosis, there is convincing evidence that anorexia nervosa has increased in incidence (i.e. the number of new cases per year per 100,000 population has increased). *Theander* [36] in Sweden found an overall incidence of anorexia nervosa of 0.24 per 100,000 inhabitants from 1933 to 1960, but a rate of 0.45 per 100,000 inhabitants from 1951 to 1960. *Willi and Grossman* [37] have studied a defined region in Switzerland and have found that the incidence of anorexia nervosa increased significantly from 0.38 per 100,000 from 1956–1958 to 1.12 per 100,000 from 1973–1975. Both of these studies were retrospective but were carefully performed and cautiously interpreted.

Prevalence (number of cases in the population at risk at any given time) has been studied by *Nylander* [38], *Crisp* et al. [39] and *Szmukler* [40]. *Nylander* [38], in Sweden, concluded that anorexia nervosa was present in about 1 in 150 adolescent girls. *Crisp* et al. [39] compared prevalence among adolescent girls in private and state schools and found that about 1 in 200 had anorexia nervosa in the private schools and about 1 in 550 in the state schools. *Szmukler* [40] found that about 1 in 120 girls age 14–18 from upper socioeconomic classes had anorexia nervosa.

Less is known about the incidence and prevalence of the syndrome bulimia, but preliminary data indicate it may be more prevalent, at least in the USA, than anorexia nervosa. *Halmi* et al. [41] found that 13% of college coeds who completed a questionnaire met the essential criteria for a probable diagnosis of bulimia; although nearly 10% reported use of self-induced vomiting, less than 2% utilized vomiting once a week or more. *Pyle* et al. [42] found that 7.8% of female college freshmen and 1.4% of male college freshmen met slightly modified DSM III criteria for a probable diagnosis of bulimia. In a preliminary report of a prevalence study among female adolescents (age 13–19 years), it was found that binge-eating occurred weekly or more often in 16% and that 4% of the sample reported self-induced vomiting once a week or more [43].

Sex Distribution

Both disorders are more common in females. This finding has been repeatedly documented for anorexia nervosa [44, 45]; 90–95% of the patients are female. Although less well-studied, bulimia also is apparently more common in women. In our clinic, only 2 of 100 bulimic patients have been male. However, *Pyle* et al. [42] found that about 20% of the subjects who were thought to meet the criteria for bulimia by questionnaire were male.

Socioeconomic Class

Although anorexia nervosa has been reported to be more common in upper socioeconomic classes, this may be changing. Using the *Hollingshead* [46] classification scheme, *Garfinkel and Garner* [47] note that prior to 1975,

70% of their patients came from socioeconomic classes I–II, and after 1976 only about 50% came from classes I–II and the remainder from classes III–VII. They postulate that attitudes concerning body weight, achievement and control, which predispose to anorexia nervosa, are becoming more evenly distributed throughout all socioeconomic sectors.

Geographical Distribution

Anorexia nervosa is common in the Western world, including the USA, Canada, Scandinavia and Western European countries. It probably occurs less frequently in Russia [48], and in Eastern European countries, but it is known. It is uncommon in Latin American countries and virtually unknown in China. The geographical distribution of bulimia is unknown. This puzzling geographical distribution of anorexia nervosa may relate to availability of food and cultural attitudes towards size and shape.

Age at Onset

Anorexia nervosa usually begins in adolescence with a bimodal risk at ages 14 and 18 [49]. The usual age range for onset is between 12 and 25. *Garfinkel and Garner* [47, p. 103] suspect that the disorder may be starting at later ages and in 1974 *Halmi* [50] noted that the condition began after age 25 in 13% of her patients.

Although bulimia is said to occur usually in adolescence or early adult life (DSM III) very little is actually known about the age of onset. The study by *Johnson* et al., [43] documented a significant percentage of bulimics in the high school population.

Etiology and Risk Factors

As will be emphasized in subsequent chapters, anorexia nervosa and bulimia are conditions with multiple interrelated causes and consequences. The psychodynamic factors postulated to contribute to the development of these conditions are outlined in chapter 6. Similarly, the psychobiological consequences of abnormal food intake, purging and overexercising, once the condition has begun, may contribute to its maintenance. The psychosomatic model described in chapter 8 delineates the risk factors, etiological factors and factors which maintain the disorder once initiated. Similarly, the biological factors which regulate eating behavior and the biological adaptations that occur during starvation are described in chapters 9 and 13.

Cultural Factors

Our culture is preoccupied with food, dieting behavior, size and 'fitness'. A slender svelte shape, especially in women, is considered ideal. There is a prevailing belief that 'fat is bad', even among apparently psychologically normal individuals; the idea that 'no woman can be too rich or too thin' (attributed to the Duchess of Windsor) is deeply ingrained in our culture. There is an alarming tendency for concerns about size and dieting behavior to occur in increasingly young age groups; *Szmukler* [40] documented that 52% of high school girls were dieting and 14% were already chronic dieters. There is a recent advertisement promoting the use of low calorie beverages for latency age children. Recently some groups that advocate 'fitness' have extended their activities to include adolescents (e.g. Jackie Sorenson's aerobic dancing now includes a program called 'Kicks for Kids'). Aerobic exercise and maintaining a lower weight than average may improve cardiovascular functioning and may, in fact, be partly responsible for the recent decline in cardiovascular disease. However, it is the obsessive quality of the drive for fitness and thinness which ignores known facts that is here questioned. The new Metropolitan height/weight tables are a case in point (see chapter 11 for a full discussion). These tables are published by a company which earns its profits by insuring people who are long-lived. The 1983 tables which were produced are based on lowest mortality rates and present weights that are generally higher than those from the 1959 tables. The outcry which greeted these tables was only partly based on scientific criticism of the epidemiological methods used in creating the tables. It is our opinion that our culture is so immersed in the idea that 'thin is best' that information that does not agree with this idea is immediately rejected. A second example involves the studies by *Frisch* [51]. Although there is good evidence that 17% body fat is required for the maintenance of menstrual periods, which in turn depend on normal hormonal functioning, which in turn influences a wide variety of body systems, the belief that 'fat is bad' has not been relinquished. There are proponents of a 5% fat content criterion for female fitness, even on our own campus.

It is interesting to speculate on the reasons for these cultural stereotypes about weight, food intake, size and shape. *Louderback* [52] postulates that although religion is overtly less important, our culture is still driven by conscience and anxious about salvation, but these concerns have been secularized into needs for social acceptance and upward mobility. Since our society, including physicians, stigmatizes obese individuals [53], it is perhaps not surprising that these concerns have become concretized around size and shape. *Allon* [53], who was describing self-help groups of obese individuals, has noted the religious connotations of some group dieting interactions. The dieters labeled themselves as 'good' or 'bad', depending upon whether or not they had lost or gained weight; they spoke of the 'ideal of thinness' and sometimes used religious language such as sinner, saint and absolution. There are parallel findings among anorectic and bulimic patients who describe themselves as 'good' if they fast and 'bad' if they binge. This religious connotation is mirrored in a dualistic view of food as 'good' or 'bad'; many eating-disorder patients describe protein as a 'good' food and carbohydrates as a 'bad' food. This tendency to divide food into 'good' and 'bad' types is common among all groups in our culture and was noted as early as 1943 by *Mead* [54]. She said that in the USA the resistances and acceptances of food are thought of in terms of morality. She noted that people think that they ought to eat what is good for them rather than what is palatable; conversely, food that makes the body healthy is unpalatable. She notes that this attitude is so much a part of our culture that it comes as a surprise to learn that other cultures do not have this dichotomy. In many cultures, the foods believed to make people strong and healthy are the very foods that are regularly eaten and that people like to eat. She comments that in the American home, both 'right' and 'wrong' foods are placed on the table and the child is rewarded with good tasting 'wrong' food, such as candy or cake. Children are punished by having the 'wrong' food taken away from them. The repetitive message is that what is delicious is an indulgence and what is good for you is unpalatable.

Prognosis

In a 1981 report by *Schwartz and Thompson* [55], twelve studies in the last 15 years reporting outcome for a combined total of 602 patients followed at least 2 years is presented. They conclude that the mortality rate from semistarvation is about 6%, although there was wide range between the studies. It is of importance that the highest rates of 18% [50, 56] and nearly 20% [36] occurred in the two studies with the longest follow-up periods, 14.5 and 15 years, respectively. The mortality rate from suicide is about 1%. In terms of weight and disturbed eating patterns, of those alive at follow-up, 49% had completely recovered, about 31% had some improvement in weight and 18% were unchanged. The combined mortality-morbidity thus was estimated at 56% for weight and eating-related behavior. In terms of psychiatric symptoms unrelated to food and weight, half of the 402 patients for whom data was available were impaired. Although 90% of the survivors studied were successfully employed at follow-up, only 55% were married or 'keeping company'.

Several studies [29, 57–59] have identified factors which statistically may have prognostic implications, at least in terms of weight gain. Good prognosis is associated with single marital status, higher educational achievement, higher socioeconomic class, employment in skilled or professional occupations, earlier age of onset and presentation, shorter duration of illness, less weight loss during illness and at presentation, good childhood adjustment, good relationship with parents, overactivity and admission to feelings of hunger. Poor prognosis is associated with laxative abuse, vomiting, bulimia, anxiety during eating, previous hospitalizations, denial of illness, psychosocial immaturity, psychosomatic complaints, depressive symptoms and obsessive-compulsive symptoms.

Little is known about the prognosis of bulimia, although some factors have been noted to be associated with poor outcome, at least in group treatment. These factors include a previous history of anorexia nervosa even if currently at normal weight, alcohol abuse, and coexistence of a personality disorder. These issues are discussed in chapter 16. Other factors are probably also important including presence or absence of purging behavior, length of time to diagnosis, age at onset, and marital status, but these have not been rigorously studied.

Future Directions: the Need for Prevention

Introduction

In each chapter that follows, the authors have indicated numerous areas where future research and treatment efforts should be directed. However, we believe that there is a major, overriding need to attend to the issues of prevention as regards the eating disorders. The apparent dramatic increase in incidence and some beginning indications that the geographical distribution is also increasing (e.g. the incidence in South America may be rising) are of great concern. The serious morbidity and mortality of these conditions also provide impetus to consideration of preventive efforts. The social and cultural factors in the Western world (in particular the obsession with thinness and fitness at all costs) seem to be intensifying and spreading into less developed countries. Finally, the enormous costs involved in adequate evaluation and treatment of these disorders, once they are fully developed, also provide further urgency to the need to attend to prevention.

Caplan [60] has carefully outlined the levels of prevention and the types of programs that might be designed for each level. We will briefly describe each of these levels, review the successes to date for that level, and suggest what future directions might be appropriate.

Primary Prevention

Primary prevention may be defined as efforts aimed at reducing the incidence of mental disorders in a community. It is the most ambitious level of preventive efforts and there is considerable controversy as to whether such efforts are possible or feasible given current knowledge and techniques [61]. Efforts to date at this level in regards to the eating disorders have been essentially nonexistent. However, attempts to tease out the various etiologic factors that may increase the risk of eating disorders (e.g. social/cultural and familial factors) can clearly be seen as first steps toward effective preventive intervention. Future efforts should be directed to additional research along these lines as well as methods for limiting or eliminating risk factors or for minimizing the impact of these factors on susceptible individuals.

Secondary Prevention

Secondary prevention may be defined as efforts aimed at lowering the prevalence of mental disorders by shortening the duration of existing cases via early diagnosis and prompt effective treatment. This is the level of prevention where tremendous strides have been made over the last 10 years. Early diagnosis has been greatly enhanced by the tremendous attention given anorexia nervosa and bulimia in the lay media (books, newspaper and magazine articles, radio and television shows, etc.). Similarly the professional audience has been exposed to an increasing number of articles, books, continuing education programs, etc. The development of effective treatment programs is well-documented in the chapters that follow. Despite successes to date, future efforts must ensure that public and professional attentions continue to be focused on these disorders. Also, we must continue to refine our methods for patients with the poor prognostic factors mentioned above (e.g. the bulimic patient with a past history of anorexia nervosa, alcohol abuse and/or character problems).

Tertiary Prevention

Tertiary prevention may be defined as efforts aimed at reducing the impairment which may result from mental disorders via effective rehabilitation that leads to a return to productive capacity at the patient's highest potential. Some considerable progress has been made in tertiary prevention. Many patients have been returned to productive lives both occupationally and in interpersonal relationships. However, there are few long-term follow-up studies and most treatment efforts to date have, of necessity, been focused on the acute manifestations of the eating disorders. Future directions need to include increased attention to long-term follow-up and to the development of sophisticated rehabilitation and maintenance programs for patients most severely affected.

References

1 Lacey, J.: Anorexia nervosa and a bearded female saint. Br. med. J. *285:* 1816–1817 (1982).
2 McLeod, S.: The art of starvation: a story of anorexia nervosa and survival (Schocken Books, New York 1982).
3 Hobbes, T.: Letter 1668; in Gee, medical lectures and clinical aphorisms (Oxford University Press, London 1908).
4 Reynolds, J.: A discourse on prodigious abstinence (London 1669).
5 Morton, R.: Phtisiologia – or a treatise of consumption (Smith & Walford, London 1694).
6 Hoffmann, H.: Struwwelpeter (Warne, Frederick, New York 1844).
7 Gull, W.: Address in medicine delivered before annual meeting of the British Medical Association at Oxford. Lancet *ii:* 171 (1868).
8 Gull, W.: Anorexia nervosa (apepsia hysterica, anorexia hysterica). Trans. Clin. Soc. Lond. *7:* 22–31 (1874).
9 Lesègue, C.: De l'anorexia hystérique. Archs gén. Méd. *21:* 385 (1873).
10 Albutt, T.; Rolleston, H.: A system of medicine (MacMillan, London 1908).
11 Simmonds, M.: Über embolische Prozesse in der Hypophysis. Arch. Path. Anat. *217:* 226–239 (1914).
12 Bruch, H.: Eating disorders, obesity, anorexia nervosa and the person within (Basic Books, New York 1973).
13 Crisp, A.: Anorexia nervosa: let me be (Grune & Stratton, New York 1980).
14 Minuchin, S.; Rosman, B.; Baker, L.: Psychosomatic families: anorexia nervosa in context (Harvard University Press, Cambridge 1978).
15 Seneca, cited in Lowenberg, M.; Todhunter, E.; Wilson, E.; Savage, J.; Lubawski, J.: Food and man; 2nd ed., p. 45 (Wiley & Sons, New York 1974).
16 Diagnostic and statistical manual of mental disorders (DSM III); 3rd ed. (Am. Psychiatric Ass., Washington 1980).
17 Feighner, J.; Robins, E.; Guze, S.; Woodruff, R.; Winokur, G.; Munoz, R.: Diagnostic criteria for use in psychiatric research. Archs gen. Psychiat. *26:* 57–63 (1972).
18 Fries, H.: Studies on secondary amenorrhea, anorectic behavior, and body-image perception: importance for the early recognition of anorexia nervosa; in Vigersky, Anorexia nervosa, pp. 163–176 (Raven Press, New York 1977).

19 Garfinkel, P.; Moldofsky, H.; Garner, D.; Stancer, H.; Coscino, D.: Body awareness in anorexia nervosa: disturbances in body image and satiety. Psychosom. Med. *40:* 487–498 (1978).
20 Burron, E.; Fransella, F.; Slade, P.: A reappraisal of body perception disturbance in anorexia nervosa. Psychol. Med. *7:* 235–243 (1977).
21 Goldberg, S.; Halmi, K.; Casper, R.; Eckert, E.; Davis, J.: Pretreatment predictors of weight change in anorexia nervosa; in Vigersky, Anorexia nervosa, pp. 31–42 (Raven Press, New York 1977).
22 Powers, P.; Powers, H.: In-patient treatment of anorexia nervosa. Psychosomatics (in press).
23 Garfinkel, P.; Moldofsky, H.; Garner, D.: The heterogeneity of anorexia nervosa: bulimia as a distinct subgroup. Archs gen. Psychiat. *317:* 1036–1040 (1980).
24 Pyle, R.; Mitchell, J.; Eckert, E.: Bulimia: a report of 34 cases. J. clin. Psychiat. *42:* 60–64 (1980).
25 Stunkard, A.: Eating patterns and obesity. Psychiat. Q. *33:* 284–294 (1959).
26 Powers, P.: Cultural beliefs and body image disturbances. Program in Human Nutrition, Canadian Dietetic Association, Toronto 1982.
27 Garner, D.; Garfinkel, P.; O'Shaughnessy, M.: Clinical and psychometric comparison between bulimia in anorexia nervosa and bulimia in normal weight women; in Understanding anorexia nervosa and bulimia. Report of the 4th Ross Conf. on Medical Research, pp. 6–11 (Ross Laboratories, Columbus 1983).
28 Palmer, R.: The dietary chaos syndrome: a useful new term? Br. J. med. Psychol. *32:* 187–190 (1979).
29 Beumont, P.; George, G.; Smart, D.: 'Dieters' and 'vomiters and purgers' in anorexia nervosa. Psychol. Med. *6.* 617–622 (1976).
30 Root, A.; Powers, P.: Anorexia nervosa presenting as growth retardation in adolescents. J. Adol. Hlth Care *4:* 25–30 (1983).
31 Keys, A.; Brozek, J.; Henschel, A.; Michelsen, O.; Taylor, H.: The biology of human starvation (University of Minnesota Press, Minneapolis 1950).
32 Yates, A.; Leeney, K.; Shisslak, C.: Running – an analogue of anorexia. New Engl. J. Med. *308:* 251–255 (1983).
33 Ryle, J.: Anorexia nervosa. Lancet *ii:* 893–899 (1936).
34 Launer, M.: Anorexia nervosa in late life. Br. J. med. Psychol. *51:* 375–377 (1978).
35 Dally, P.: Anorexia nervosa (Grune & Stratton, New York 1969).
36 Theander, S.: Anorexia nervosa: a psychiatric investigation of 94 female patients. Acta psychiat. scand. *214:* suppl., pp. 1–194 (1970).
37 Willi, J.; Grossman, S.: Epidemiology of anorexia nervosa in a defined region of Switzerland. Am. J. Psychiat. *140:* 564–567 (1983).
38 Nylander, I.: The feeling of being fat and dieting in a school population: an epidemiologic interview investigation. Acta socio-med. scand. *3:* 17–26 (1971).
39 Crisp, A.; Palmer, R.; Kalucy, R.: How common is anorexia nervosa? A prevalence study. Br. J. Psychiat. *218:* 549–554 (1976).
40 Szmukler, G.: Weight and food preoccupation in a population of English school girls; in Understanding anorexia nervosa and bulimia. Report of the 4th Ross Conf. on Medical Research, pp. 21–27 (Ross Laboratories, Columbus 1983).
41 Halmi, K.; Falk, J.; Schwartz, E.: BInge-eating and vomiting: a survey of a college population. Psychol. Med. *11:* 697–706 (1981).

42 Pyle, R.; Mitchell, J.; Eckert, E.; et al.: The incidence of bulimia in freshman college students. Int. J. Eating Disord. *2:* 75 (1983).
43 Johnson, C.; Lewis, C.; Love, S.; Stuckey, M.; Lewis, L.: A descriptive survey of dieting and bulimic behavior in a female high school population; in Understanding anorexia nervosa and bulimia. Report of the 4th Ross Conf. on Medical Research (Ross Laboratories, Columbus 1983).
44 Jones, D.; Fox, M.; Babigan, H.; Hatton, H.: Epidemiology of anorexia nervosa in Monroe County, New York: 1960–1976. Psychosom. Med. *42:* 551–558 (1980).
45 Bemis, K.: Current approaches to the etiology and treatment of anorexia nervosa. Psychol. Bull. *85:* 593–617 (1978).
46 Hollingshead, A.: Two factor index of social position (Yale University Press, New Haven 1965).
47 Garfinkel, P.; Garner, D.: Anorexia nervosa: a multidimensional perspective, pp. 102–103 (Brunner/Mazel, New York 1982).
48 Ushakov, G.: Anorexia nervosa; in Howells, Modern perspectives in adolescent psychiatry, vol. 4, pp. 274–289 (Brunner/Mazel, New York 1971).
49 Halmi, K.; Casper, R.; Eckert, E.; Goldberg, S.; Davis, J.: Unique features associated with age of onset of anorexia nervosa. Psychiat. Res. *1:* 209–215 (1979).
50 Halmi, K.: Anorexia nervosa: demographic and clinical features in 94 cases. Psychosom. Med. *36:* 18–26 (1974).
51 Frisch, R.: Food intake, fatness, and reproductive ability; in Vigersky, Anorexia nervosa, pp. 149–161 (Raven Press, New York 1977).
52 Louderback, L.: Fat power: whatever you weigh is right, p. 39 (Hawthorn Books, New York 1970).
53 Allon, N.: The stigma of overweight in everyday life; in Obesity in perspective. Fogarty International Center Series on Preventive Medicine, vol. 2, part 2 (Natn. Institutes of Health, Bethesda, 1973).
54 Mead, M.: Dietary patterns and food habits. J. Am. diet. Ass. *19:* 1–5 (1943).
55 Schwartz, D.; Thompson, M.: Do anorectics get well? Current research and future needs. Am. J. Psychiat. *138:* 319–323 (1981).
56 Halmi, K.; Brodland, G.; Rigas, C.: A follow-up study of seventy-nine patients with anorexia nervosa: an evaluation of prognostic factors and diagnostic criteria; in Writ, Winokur, Roff, Life history research in psychopathology, vol. 4 (University of Minnesota Press, Minneapolis 1975); cited in Schwartz and Thompson [55].
57 Seidensticker, J.; Tzagorurnis, M.: Anorexia nervosa: clinical features and long-term follow-up. J. chron. Dis. *21:* 361–367 (1968).
58 Halmi, K.; Brodland, G.; Loney, J.: Prognosis in anorexia nervosa. Ann. intern. Med. *78:* 907–909 (1973).
59 Hsu, L.; Crisp, A.; Harding, B.: Outcome of anorexia nervosa. Lancet *i:* 61–65 (1979).
60 Caplan, G.: Principles of preventive psychiatry (Basic Books, New York 1964).
61 Lamb, H.; Zusman, J.: A new look at primary prevention. Hosp. Commun. Psychiat. *32:* 843–848 (1981).
62 Powers, P.S.: Obesity: the regulation of weight (Williams & Wilkins, Baltimore 1980).

2 Psychotherapy of Anorexia Nervosa

Pauline S. Powers

Introduction

This chapter summarizes the author's experience with 150 anorexia nervosa and bulimia patients over the course of 10 years. The psychotherapy of anorexia nervosa will be discussed, and will include a conceptual framework that has been found useful in formulating a treatment plan. The general principles of psychotherapy will be discussed, and common countertransference issues encountered in treating patients will be discussed. Finally, case presentations will be used to illustrate common patterns of psychopathology. Details of the treatment of bulimia are presented in chapters 4 and 6.

Diagnostic Issues

The diagnostic criteria for anorexia nervosa are presented in detail in chapter 1, but briefly the issues relevant to the discussion of psychotherapy are as follows. Initially, there is a drive to become thinner, frequently accompanied by feelings of pleasure, or even ecstasy, at achieving lower and lower weights. Often the feeling of ecstasy is associated with, and eventually completely replaced by, a fear of becoming fat. Patients are significantly underweight, at least 25% below ideal body weight (IBW). Almost invariably, there is a disturbance in body image, and females have amenorrhea. Associated symptoms include vomiting, laxative abuse, diet pill usage, and overexercising; these behaviors are designed to promote weight loss, or maintain an emaciated state. Binge-eating also occurs, and is probably in response to a normal physiological drive to eat when semistarved. Although the problem has sometimes been conceptualized as a carbohydrate phobia, it is clearly more complex: e.g. people with elevator phobias do not get euphoric in buildings without elevators. The distinction between bulimia and anorexia nervosa is not clear. The term bulimia has been used in two different ways. As a symptom, bulimia simply means an episode of overeating, and is synonymous with binge-eating. The syndrome bulimia is defined in DSM III. These issues are discussed in chapter 1. Clinically, an important distinction in the initial evaluation is that anorexia nervosa patients are 25% below IBW, and that bulimia patients are either normal weight, above normal weight, or only marginally underweight. Probably some patients with bulimia are partially recovered anorectics; i.e. initial weight loss was achieved by dieting and purging (which was associated with bingeing), and although weight has been restored, bingeing and purging have not been relinquished. Also, among this group of bulimics with a clear-cut history of anorexia nervosa are inadequately or inappropriately treated patients who may develop 'iatrogenic' bulimia.

An anorectic patient, who had lost weight by fasting, was hospitalized by her endocrinologist, placed on a 4,000-cal diet and ordered to gain 1 lb (0.5 kg) per day so that she could be discharged in a week. In order to accomplish this task, the patient learned to binge, and sneaked extra food (since 4,000 cal was insufficient to gain 1 lb in a day). She was discharged 'improved', but quickly learned to purge and began a pernicious binge-purge cycle.

This weight restoration program rewarded an uncontrolled quick weight gain (the very circumstance that usually terrifies the patient).

Obsessive-Compulsive Symptoms in Semistarvation

Historically [1], it was thought that anorexia nervosa patients, most of whom are women, frequently had obsessive-compulsive personalities. During the period of semistarvation, patients usually obsess about food, eating and weight, and behave compulsively about food (e.g. they may repetitively read cookbooks, or prepare elaborate gourmet meals which they refuse to eat) or weight (e.g. patients may weigh themselves after each morsel that is eaten). Some patients compulsively vomit after each meal, or take laxatives ritualistically; most patients say that these behaviors are designed 'to get rid of it (the food)'. The studies by *Keys* et al.[2], recently rediscovered, suggest that many of the presenting obsessive-compulsive symptoms may be due to the state of semistarvation. While it is true that a significant percentage of patients have been found to have a preexisting obsessive-compulsive personality disorder or traits [3], and this may in fact be a risk factor for the development of anorexia nervosa, many patients have been found not to have personality disorders, and many other personality factors have been noted.

Cultural Factors

Anorexia nervosa and bulimia occur in the context of a culture preoccupied with slimness, especially in women. Anorexia nervosa is unknown or uncommon in societies where slenderness is not considered a virtue. It may be that more than half the women in the USA are on diets, and it has been estimated [4] that $ 17,000 is spent per minute in the USA for various weight loss measures. *Wooley and Wooley* [5] have described the Beverly Hills diet as 'the mass-marketing of anorexia nervosa'. Advertisements for weight loss aids are ubiquitous and are directed primarily toward women. Some of these advertisements are pernicious in their reinforcement of certain distorted beliefs. For example, one recent advertisement for a diet drink promises 'now you see it, now you don't'; this could serve as a metaphor for the anorectic who binges and purges.

Another factor that may be important relates to what has been described as the feminist therapy viewpoint [6]. This theory contends that our culture views a women's source of power as her body, and notes a profound disrespect for women. Appearance, rather than any internal sense of identity, is said to be more important for women than men. This theme (the importance of appearance) certainly is a common one among anorectics, and may partially account for the preponderance of females afflicted, but it is probably only one of several predisposing factors.

Anorexia Nervosa: Conceptual Framework

The following is one model for conceptualizing the main factors that need to be considered in devising a psychotherapeutic plan (fig. 1). Any one of many existential problems may predispose and trigger the development of a biological solution (starvation) which results in a dichotomy between mind and body. This biological solution (starvation and an emaciated state) and the mind-body dichotomy is reinforced by the development of cognitive distortions and any one of several different belief systems that prevent problem-solving.

Existential Problems

Five common existential problems will be briefly reviewed, and will include grief, family conflict, lack of preparation for the tasks of adolescence, hedonistic/ascetic conflicts and borderline personality disorders. The term

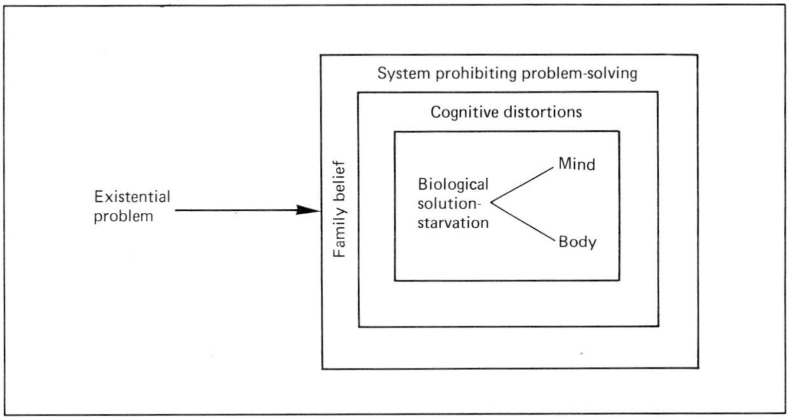

Fig. 1. Conceptual framework of major factors that facilitate and maintain anorexia nervosa.

'existential problem' is defined as any one of a variety of predisposing personality traits, psychodynamic conflicts, or situational factors.

Loss or threatened loss of a parent, sibling, or friend can precipitate the initial weight loss. In situations where the person who dies loses weight during the terminal illness, the initial weight loss by the developing anorectic may be part of the bereavement process. *Lindemann* [7] has described relatives whose inappropriate grief is characterized by assuming characteristics of the bereaved. In the patient, Carrie, described later in this chapter, anticipatory grief was particularly important. In a 53-year-old woman recently evaluated, the death of her spouse 30 years earlier precipitated her initial weight loss. The diagnosis of anorexia nervosa was not made until she had been ill more than 10 years, a factor which considerably worsened her long-term prognosis.

Covert *family conflict* is another common existential factor that has been described by several family therapists, especially *Minuchin* et al. [8] and *Selvini-Palazzoli* [9]. According to this paradigm, there may be a suspicion (often unconscious) that without a reuniting focus, something dangerous will happen to someone in the family. The emerging anorectic may be unconsciously trying to prevent parental divorce, or depression in one of the parents. *Haley* [10] has postulated that a benign concern for the family is frequently behind seemingly inexplicable behavior. Certainly the initial onset of weight loss in some anorectics does focus attention of the family to that problem, and sometimes away from other problems seemingly too difficult for the family to resolve at the time. Figure 2 is an artist's view of the transactions in one family with an anorectic member. Chapter 5 explores these issues in greater detail.

A third common existential problem is *lack of preparation for the tasks of adolescence or adulthood.* We have seen many anorectic patients whose capacity to cope independently is severely restricted. One 16-year-old girl was unable to choose her own clothes without her mother present; even in the store with her mother, she was unable to decide which clothes to try on. In other situations, the tentative steps the patient makes toward self-directed behavior are frustrated by the family.

Ms. E., age 21, could not choose a career, but thought she might become an airline stewardess. Her mother rejected this idea as 'not good enough', and described the job as 'only a waitress in the sky'. This is an isolated example in a woman whose choices had been rejected as poor throughout her life. As a consequence, she felt empty and unable to direct her own life.

It has been thought that some anorectics are attempting to avoid heterosexual development via a biological regression (inferred from the loss of secondary female sex characteristics due to starvation). A biological regression is clearly illustrated by a variety of biological systems, but particularly by the regression of the luteinizing hormone secretory patterns to prepubertal levels [11]. However, usually it is not a sexual problem per se, but rather an incapacity to cope with many tasks of adolescence, including heterosexuality, emerging independence from the family and pursuit of a vocation. The emaciated state and waif-like appearance may represent a biological regression to childhood that temporarily allows the anorectic to avoid these difficult problems, for which she is inadequately prepared. *Crisp* [12] has documented that young women who later develop anorexia nervosa statistically have an earlier menarche. The early development of a woman's body in a girl lagging behind in other areas of emotional development may be a particular risk factor.

A fourth existential problem is a *hedonistic/ascetic conflict* that is temporarily resolved by fasting and semistarvation. Adolescence is characterized by conflicting pressures toward ascetic self-denial (discipline in study, work, sports and appearance) and hedonistic drives (sexuality, eating and exercise of power). Normal adolescents resolve this conflict somewhere in the middle of the continuum between rigid self-denial and unmodulated hedonism (epitomized by 'if it feels good, do it'). Fasting and its consequence, emaciation, may come to signify to the anorectic patient that she is 'good'. The meaning attached to weight loss through fasting is achieved through the unconscious

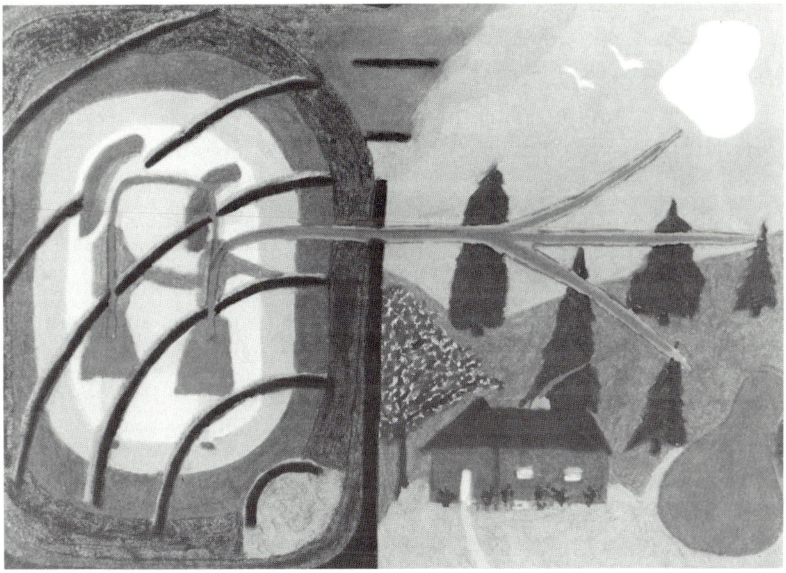

Fig. 2. An artist's interpretation of the family transactions that occur in some families containing an anorectic member. The mother and daughter are inseparably caged together. The daughter has no identity of her own. All the world can see is the daughter's illness. The lines surrounding the cage represent the derogatory remarks of the passive ineffective father (drawn by *George Maring*). Reprinted, with permission, from [27].

psychological defense mechanism of displacement; concern about how one integrates the conflicting pressures for self-denial and hedonistic pleasures are displaced to concerns about weight. The self-denial evident in fasting or very rigid dietary regimens is frequently seen in other areas of the anorectic's life (e.g. patients may hoard money, rarely spending it on any unnecessary pleasurable item). Developing anorectics often become 'better' students and employees following rigid, long and tiring schedules. Many patients who have started dating retreat from any heterosexual development. For some anorectic patients who initially resolve the ascetic/hedonistic conflict by rigid fasting and weight loss, the fear of losing control may be a real one. Some partially recovered anorectics do lapse into binge-eating, immoderate sexual activity, drinking and drug behavior. The tendency toward extremes may be more common in bulimic anorectics, and among patients who have the cognitive distortion called 'all-or-none reasoning'. This is the belief that life can be understood in terms of black or white, with no grays (the good/bad dichotomy). Thus, early in treatment, encouraging moderate weight gains and modest changes in behavior (such as spending small amounts of money, or allowing one's room to be slightly less than perfect) may help the patient avoid some of the later wide swings in attitudes and behavior.

A fifth common existential problem is best conceptualized as a *borderline personality organization. Masterson* [13, 14] has studied borderline adolescents in painstaking detail, and applied these theoretical constructs to certain patients with anorexia nervosa. According to this theory, the emerging sense of identity achieved through self-initiating behavior that begins in late infancy and toddlerhood is inhibited by the mother who withdraws affection in response to the self-directed behavior. The child fears abandonment and the ensuing depression, and learns to mold himself or herself to the mother's expectations. Over the years, a false sense of self develops, which is vigorously defended, to protect against a sense of emptiness and a lack of true identity. The false sense of self that develops is a reflection of the mother's, or family's, wish for a perfect, well-behaved, meticulous child; appearances are of paramount importance. Thus, the anorectic-to-be is postulated to have a false sense of identity heavily influenced by the need to maintain appearances, including preserving the false sense of self. The pre-anorectic with the borderline personality may start a diet innocuously (although a detailed history, that is usually not obtainable until after the patient has been in treatment for lengthy periods of time, often reveals that there has been a profoundly significant emotional precipitant). However, the weight loss resulting in emaciation may come to represent a grossly distorted symbol of the introjected false sense of self, while simultaneously and paradoxically representing the anorectic's genuine attempt to develop a truer sense of self. This dual meaning of the emaciation is one of the many factors that makes treatment of anorectics with borderline personality structures difficult.

The borderline concept of anorexia nervosa dovetails nicely with some of the theories of both *Bruch* [15] and *Minuchin* et al. [8]. *Bruch* [15] postulates that from birth onward there is behavior that originates in the infant, and behavior in the infant in response to stimuli. The family producing the disturbed child does not respond appropriately to cues coming from the infant because of their preoccupation with their own needs. Instead, the child is bombarded with expectations and demands, and learns to respond to the parents' needs, and is confused about his or her own feelings and wishes. Although *Bruch* [15] does not present this theory as a description of the development of a borderline personality, there are striking similarities. The theory of *Minuchin* et al. [8] of the family process that results in anorexia nervosa also has similarities to the borderline theory. These authors postulate that in these 'psychosomatogenic' families, enmeshment is characteristic. Enmeshment is a term used to describe the absence of personal boundaries, and the overinvolvement family members have in each other's thoughts, feelings and behavior. Thus, the emerging anorectic does not have a sense of a separate identity.

Running through these theories (the development of anorexia nervosa and borderline personality structure, *Bruch's* theory and *Minuchin's* family theory) is a common theme, namely the absence of a coherent, separate sense of identity.

Biological Solution

The biological solution of the existential conflict of the developing anorectic is semistarvation and emaciation. There are many deleterious consequences of starvation, even if the original conflict is resolved, or is no longer relevant. Not only do many physiological abnormalities develop as a consequence of starvation (see chapter 13), but many of the presenting psychological symptoms are also due to semistarvation. *Keys* et al. [2, pp. 832–833] described malnourished subjects as follows:

> 'Food and all its ramifications became the principal topic of conversation, reading and daydreams, for almost all the subjects were often caught between conflicting desires to gulp their food down ravenously and to consume it slowly so that the taste and odor of each morsel would be fully appreciated ... some of the men would dawdle for almost two hours over a meal which previously they would have consumed in a matter of minutes.'

Observations of people who were semistarved in famines, or in concentration camps, have been similar. Starving individuals are preoccupied with food.

Furthermore, irritability and angry outbursts are probably due to starvation. *Maslow* [16, p. 37] has defined hunger as an urgent need for food, and therefore a crucial physiological need. He comments that the need for food dominates a hungry man's entire existence:

> 'For the man who is extremely and dangerously hungry, no other interest exists except food ... he dreams about food, he remembers food, he emotes only about food, he perceives only food, and he wants only food.'

Maslow [16] concludes that for the hungry person, culture, politics, family and friends are irrelevant; an interest in the welfare of others is impossible if one is physiologically hungry. Many starving anorectics fit this description. Despite frequent claims to the contrary, they are often ravenously hungry. They are also profoundly egocentric at very low weights.

Although, prior to the onset of anorexia nervosa, these patients were usually highly sensitive to cultural and familial expectations, at their lowest weights they are frequently oblivious to the needs of those around them.

Mind-Body Dichotomy

The process of starvation facilitates and perpetuates an apparent split between mind and body. Cognitive and perceptual distortions are associated with starvation, and may partly be a consequence of it. The poor concentration associated with starvation may permit a ready acceptance of certain illogical beliefs without allowing the usual reality-testing efforts; or, perhaps, some of the apparent cognitive distortions are an accurate interpretation of certain unconscious or unstated family beliefs. It is hypothesized that the interaction between the physiological consequences of starvation, the dichotomization of mind and body and the incorporation of a distored family belief system produce characteristic cognitive distortions. Not only are these cognitive distortions one part of the mind-body dichotomy, but they may also become independent of the original process, and serve to perpetuate the anorexia nervosa.

These *disturbed cognitions* are discussed in greater detail in chapter 7 but, for the purpose of illustration, a few will be described. A common cognitive distortion is dichotomous, or 'all-or-none' reasoning. Events are viewed in absolute terms. The event is good or bad, right or wrong. For example, a patient may say, 'If I gain one pound, I will go on and be fat forever'. Another common example of this all-or-none reasoning is the dichotomization of foods into good and bad categories. Carbohydrates are 'bad' and protein is 'good'. These erroneous beliefs about food are frequently transformed into beliefs about the self; the anorectic who eats a candy bar (a 'bad' food) may characterize herself as 'bad'. For many anorectics, the old adage 'you are what you eat' is believed literally. With improvement in weight, and change in food beliefs, this all-or-none reasoning is frequently apparent in many other areas of the anorectic's life. One example, is, 'if I don't get straight As in school, I'll never get into college'. Another common cognitive distortion is superstitious thinking; that is, many anorectics believe in the cause-effect relationship of non-contingent events (for example, 'If I eat a sweet, it will instantly go to my stomach', or 'If I sit quietly in a chair without exercising, my hips will become huge').

Disturbances in body image are ubiquitous in the eating disorders, especially in anorexia nervosa. The earliest medical descriptions of the disorder noted the remarkable disparity between the patient's actual appearance and her perception of her appearance. The first patient evaluated by this author was in restraints on the pediatric ward, weighed 54 lb (24.5 kg) at 5 ft (152 cm) in height, was obviously and alarmingly emaciated and was exercising while complaining that she felt fat. Many patients describe themselves as initially slightly overweight, even though the great majority were normal weight or underweight [17]. A common clinical observation is that as weight loss progresses, the body image distortion worsens (i.e. even though the anorectic loses weight, she frequently feels fatter than prior to the weight loss).

Body image is a term that has been used in a variety of ways, but can be thought of as having two different components: a perceptual aspect, and an attitudinal aspect. The perceptual aspect of body image is like an inner mental blueprint of one's appearance. Although this aspect of body image is often described in visual terms (i.e., the anorectic may say 'I look fat') the major sensory components of body image are tactile and kinesthetic [18]. Since most estimates of the perceptual aspect of body image are based on the visual sensory modality, the intensity and extent of body image disturbance may be underestimated. Some patients who no longer 'see' themselves as fat may still 'feel' fat (i.e. the tactile and kinesthetic perceptual disturbance may remain even after any visual disturbance is corrected). The emotional feelings and attitudes toward one's body are the second major component of body image. Thus, patients may not only misperceive their size and shape, but may also have distorted attitudes toward their appearance; many patients describe themselves not only as fat, but ugly as well. On the other hand, some patients may take an inordinate pride in their emaciated appearance. Figure 3 is a sculpture of an anorectic woman who posed as a model for an art class; she prized her emaciated appearance, even though the art students were shocked.

One recent study [19] has shown that the incidence and extent of body image disturbances of anorectic patients are no different as a group from those of an age-matched normal population. However, several studies [19, 20] have found that the greater the identifiable degree of disturbance of body image at initial evaluation, the worse the prognosis. Although some anorectic patients do not have any indentifiable disturbance in the perceptual aspect of body image [21], this group probably represents a small minority. Another characteristic of body image is fluidity. *Crisp and Kalucy* [22] have found that estimates of size vary with the size and content of the preceding meal; after a carbohydrate-rich meal anorectics tend to overestimate size even more. A discussion of the various techniques used to assess body image and the theoretical limitations of these techniques is beyond the scope of this chapter. The interested reader is referred to *Garfinkel and Garner* [23] and *Powers* [24].

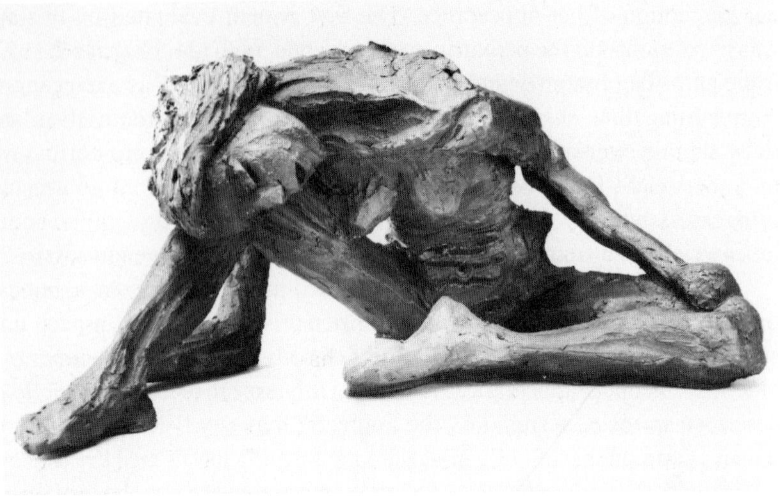

Fig. 3. This anorexia nervosa patient posed as a model for art classes. She prized her emaciated appearance and seemed oblivious to the shocked reactions of others (sculpture by *Ursula Mahlendorf*). Reprinted, with permission, from [27].

Selvini-Palazzoli's [9] work with anorectic patients is particularly relevant to the *mind-body* split that occurs, and is discussed in detail in chapter 6. She postulates that this dichotomy is frequently the result of a severe maldevelopment in object relationships. The anorectic patient may come to believe that the body has become a threatening force that must be held in check; the body becomes a symbol for all the drives experienced by the person. The anorectic believes that eating will result in an increase of the body at the expense of the mind. The anorectic equates the body with the bad incorporated object (usually the mother), which is conceptualized and felt as a negative, overpowering force. Unconsciously, and sometimes consciously, the emerging anorectic concludes it is better to oppose this force (the body), and separate it from the mind (the ego). In this situation, the body of the anorectic does not just contain the object, it is the bad object. *Selvini-Palazzoli's* [9] psychodynamic formulation seems applicable to many, but not all, anorectics.

Belief Systems Prohibiting Problem-Solving

Once the mind-body split has occurred, the problem is usually difficult to reverse, because cognitive distortions and certain belief systems prevent working directly on the original existential problem. The belief systems are usually derived from the family, and sometimes represent a distortion of the family's original meaning. For example, the anorectic patient may believe that 'one should always be independent' and, since seeking treatment from a psychiatrist entails a certain measure of dependence, the patient may try unsuccessfully for years to combat the condition alone. Since successful achievement of goals is usually important to the anorectic, repeated failure in this area may be generalized to the belief that one is a total failure at life.

Another common belief system that interferes with seeking treatment is the belief that 'parents are beyond reproach'. In this situation, the patient may correctly recognize that the parents have tried very hard, perhaps even devoted their entire lives to their children. Thus, if a major part of the positive self-evaluation of the parent is related to success as a parent, the child may understandably protect their parents from the narcissistic blow of recognizing errors. In my experience, this process is for the most part unconscious and initially rigidly defended by both patient and parents. Several other similar belief systems may prevent early effective treatment.

One family had always been viewed as a perfect family by their friends, employers and themselves. When the daughter developed anorexia nervosa, everyone was shocked and the family felt humiliated, and delayed treatment because they had not lived up to their own and others' expectations. A major curative factor was the parents' recognition that living up to perfection, and to others' expectations was not only impossible, but uncomfortable. During treatment, the mother's job was threatened and instead of behaving in a quiet, passive, 'perfect' way, she spoke out to administrators and reporters. Although her friends were surprised, her husband supported her and the daughter began to eat and gain weight.

Another common belief system is the idea that seeking help is, by definition, indicative of failure. This idea starts a round of self-criticism, and may increase the likelihood that the patient will drop out of treatment. Perhaps even more importantly, repeated visits to a care provider may be interpreted as ever-increasing proof of one's failures. Treatment itself becomes redefined as a failure.

Phases of Psychotherapy: Initial Considerations

Although certain patients may require treatment for less than a year, usually treatment is needed for 2 or more years and hospitalization is often required at some point [17]. Those patients who require less lengthy treatment usually have some or all of the following characteristics: short duration of the disorder (less than 1 year), less weight loss (less than 25% below IBW), younger age of onset, absence of bingeing and purging, presence of some sense of identity not based on rebelliousness and good candidacy for family therapy as the primary treatment modality (i.e. an intact family willing to attend regularly, and capable of relinquishing certain patterns of interaction). Although there are some patients who meet these criteria, my experience is they are a minority. However, since most centers reporting treatment of anorexia nervosa are tertiary care centers, including ours, it may be that there are a large number of patients who would respond to relatively brief (less than 1 year) interventions.

Phases of Psychotherapy: Reeducative Phase

Education about Psychotherapy

Initially, many anorectic patients need an explanation of psychotherapy, as well as guidelines for their participation. It is often helpful to start with the statement that weight loss and maintenance of an unsafe weight or abnormal eating habits are often a smokescreen for underlying conflicts. Resolving the weight or eating problem probably will not resolve these conflicts, and usually psychotherapy is needed for 1 or 2 years after weight gain. The patient is frequently concerned about her preoccupation with food, and the accompanying compulsive eating or purging behavior. Most patients are relieved to learn that these may be symptoms of starvation, and may decrease or disappear when a normal weight is reached. Education about the meaning of the other presenting symptoms is also useful. This issue is discussed in chapter 13.

Weight Restoration

In the early phase, weight restoration and psychotherapy should proceed together. It may be necessary to have one therapist provide individual psychotherapy, while another monitors the weight gain program and coordinates family interventions. Irrespective of how the responsibilities are divided, however, it is important to communicate that mind and body are not separate. Attempts to divide psychotherapy from weight gain often do not result in improvement of the patient. We have seen a number of patients who have been force-fed in a variety of ways without benefit of conjoint individual therapy, and the outcome has been poor.

For example, Erica was given insulin (to increase her appetite) by an endocrinologist who believed abnormalities in the hypothalamus cause anorexia nervosa. Not only did she lose the 10 lb (4.5 kg) she gained under this regimen in the month after discharge, but she deteriorated psychologically. Her distrust of physicians and authority figures increased, and her willingness to discuss her feelings became even more circumscribed.

On the other hand, we have also seen a number of patients who have been in individual psychotherapy, but have not been on a weight-gain program. Some patients come to understand the initial existential problem and may resolve it, but still not gain weight. Attention to the 'mind' while ignoring the 'body' models the very separation that tends to perpetuate anorexia nervosa.

Ms. L. complained repeatedly of lightheadedness to her psychiatrist. She and her psychiatrist were investigating the difficulty she had in emancipating herself from her parents, which had been correctly identified as the major precipitant for her weight loss. She went to see an internist for 'dizziness' who found she weighed 70 lb (32 kg) and had a very low serum potassium and sodium from repeated use of 50 laxatives per day. She was hospitalized and intravenous feeding started; she gained 11 lb (5 kg) in 24 h. After 3 days she was discharged and promptly lost to 68 lb (31 kg). Thus, the psychiatrist and internist, each concentrating on a limited aspect of the problem, lost the opportunity to assist the patient reintegrate her disabling mind-body dichotomy. The psychiatrist might have weighed the patient, taken her lying and standing blood pressure, measured her serum electrolytes and explained that the dizziness was due to orthostatic hypotension caused by her self-starvation and resultant dehydration. The positive relationship they had might have facilitated the patient's self-awareness of the relationship between her drive to be thin and the symptom of dizziness, thus providing a tentative link between her mind and body.

Identifying Illogical Cognitive Beliefs

During the reeducative phase, the therapist can assist the patient in identifying certain illogical cognitive beliefs. The first opportunities are usually with weight, or food-related issues. For example, Ellen, a patient recently hospitalized, said, 'If I eat when I am hungry, I will get fat', and, 'If I sit on my hips they will expand and become fat'. At a superficial level, this represented the 'all-or-none' thinking discussed earlier, but it also represented more important psychodynamic issues. Early in treatment, reeducating Ellen that hunger is an internal cue that occurs when body nutrients are depleted, and not a signal that continues once nourished, helped her cooperate with the weight restoration program. Another example of her all-or-none thinking was, 'If I rest when I am tired, I will never complete college'. When Ellen was able to discuss her experiences more openly, she recognized that she really believed that, 'If I enjoy myself, I'll get out of control'. She believed if she gained weight, there would be 'too much' of her, and if she acted on any pleasurable drives she would be in too much trouble (i.e. out of control). She condensed her fear of losing control of all her pleasurable drives (sexual, aggressive, appetitive) into a fear of obesity. Thus, a preliminary reeducative analysis of certain cognitive distortions may lead to a better understanding of major psychodynamic conflicts.

Body Image Disturbance

Body image disturbances frequently interfere with the recovery process. *Bruch* [15] believes that improvement in body image is a prerequisite for full recovery from anorexia nervosa. Most patients who perceive themselves as larger than they really are will readily acknowledge this perception, and many are aware that they are not, in fact, fat, even though they feel fat. Once a trusting relationship is established with the therapist, the patient may be able to acknowledge that others view her as emaciated. Even though parents and other relatives have usually told the anorectic repeatedly that she is emaciated, the patient may suspect their motives.

A common theme in therapy is the belief (sometimes accurate) that the parents want the patient to gain weight for the sake of appearances, so that they will not be seen as bad parents. Therefore, the therapist must not be viewed as an agent for the relatives. This may be a difficult stance for the therapist to achieve, partly because the parents may be paying for the patient's therapy. More important, however, is the fact that the therapist must maintain open lines of communication with the relatives, who may be urgently needed to help the therapist intervene in life-threatening situations. Thus, the ideal of confidentiality often cannot be strictly maintained, and may initially undermine the patient's trust in the therapist and increase the likelihood that the therapist will be viewed like a relative, with an exploitative interest in her weight gain. This problem can sometimes be avoided or minimized by outlining those situations and the manner in which the therapist will contact the relatives, and informing the patient before and after each contact with them, if it is not possible for the patient to be present. Often the patient must be in individual therapy for lengthy periods of time before various interpretations and interventions are viewed as in the patient's interest rather than in the interest of the relatives. Once this occurs, the patient may still feel fat, but be able to choose to act on the basis of logic, and ignore the misperception. Sometimes the patient may be able to substitute a statement, 'I may feel fat, but I know I am too thin, and therefore I will eat'. Sometimes anorectic patients can more easily ignore their perception of themselves as fat if they wear clothes that are not tight-fitting.

Confronting the patient with his or her inaccurate body image is difficult. Belief in one's perceptions is the cornerstone of sanity and, although most anorectics proclaim themselves mentally healthy, one common underlying fear is that they are going crazy. Thus, the therapist must help identify the misperception of size and shape as part of anorexia nervosa without undermining the patient's faith in her capacity to recognize accurately other thoughts and feelings. Usually this can be accomplished by confirming a wide variety of the patient's other accurate perceptions.

The factors that contribute to a more accurate perception of size and shape during recovery are poorly understood. Improved capacity to recognize internal body signals, including hunger and fatigue, as well as feelings of anger, sadness and happiness probably parallels improvement in body image. The preoccupation with food and the intense self-absorption that characterize anorectics at the beginning of treatment abate with weight gain and improvement in social interactions; capacity to integrate other views of the self has a beneficial effect on the patient. It is often at this stage that patients begin to compare themselves to others (usually friends or care providers, not relatives) that they consider a normal size. Some patients compare themselves to normal weight companions in the mirror. In addition to these general curative factors, there may well be specific treatment modalities that would speed improvement. Dance therapy, art therapy, or other treatment modalities based on touch and kinesthesia may be particularly useful. Physical therapy can be useful when it is not used as a means of losing weight or avoiding necessary weight gain.

Phases of Psychotherapy: Midphase Treatment of Underlying Existential Problems

Grief

In patients for whom grief has contributed significantly to the development of anorexia nervosa, individual psychotherapy is usually a major part of the management. The principles enumerated by *Lindemann* [7] for management of unresolved grief reactions are useful. Since denial is common in anorectics, a significant loss may not be acknowledged initially. Once the patient has identifed the loss, she can be assisted in recognizing the usual responses to loss including sadness, anger, guilt and sometimes relief. The anger may be particularly difficult for the patient to accept, especially if directed toward the one who died. Frequently patients are angry at physicians or nurses who cared for the loved one, and the anger may be unconsciously displaced to the therapist, especially if the therapist is a physician. Guilt about what one might have done differently, or about the quality of the relationship prior to the loss is very important. Once these feelings have been identified, the therapist can assist the patient in recognizing them as a normal and necessary part of grieving. Encouraging the patient to allow several months to elapse before expecting a decrease in the intensity or frequency of these feelings is usually helpful.

Family Conflict

The management of psychotherapy of patients in whom family dysfunction and conflict is of primary importance is discussed in chapter 5, and later in this chapter.

Lack of Preparation for Tasks of Adolescence

Anorectic patients who are unprepared for the tasks of adolescence usually require lengthy individual therapy. In this situation, family therapy may be a prerequisite to sucessful individual therapy, since a family system problem may be prohibiting natural growth and development. It is usually difficult for these patients to verbalize their concerns, and models for the psychotherapy of children can be helpful. Getting the patient to talk about almost anything may be initially difficult and require patience. Several patients have talked for months about windsurfing, electrical engineering, or needlework. Eventually the patient may allow the therapist to know how inadequate she feels in interpersonal relationships within and outside the family. The therapist often must take a more active role than in traditional psychotherapy (e.g. specific advice on coping with roommates or making friends). This author has been impressed by the extent of the passivity in some of these patients. Overtly, they appear confident, positive and self-initiating. In reality they rarely make even trivial choices, and even less often confront the major issues of their lives. This information is seldom volunteered, and much time may be required to assist the patient to acknowledge her real difficulties in coping with the usual demands of adolescence and adult life. Once certain difficulties are recognized, the patient may then require concrete assistance in certain developmental tasks. Although this group of patients may regain to a near normal weight, be successful in work, and marry, they often lead rather rigid, empty lives with frequent bouts of depression.

Ms. B., age 18, was hospitalized for 6 months at age 17 and gained to a normal weight on a behavior modification program. During her hospitalization, she was seen thrice weekly for individual psychotherapy, and once weekly in family therapy. When she achieved a normal weight, and had a positive relationship with her psychotherapist, she still was unable to make a vocational choice, had difficulty making friends and remained passive in many areas. As an outpatient, she continued in individual psychotherapy while living in a half-way house for 6 months, where she learned certain job skills and began making friends. At the end of a year of intensive treatment, she was able to hold a part-time job while living at home, maintain normal eating habits and have a few rather emotionally distant friends.

Conflict over Ascetic/Hedonistic Drives

A fourth related existential problem is a conflict over ascetic/hedonistic drives. This is usually part of a larger problem, namely inability to cope with many tasks of adolescence.

Lori, a 17-year-old girl, who was part of an enmeshed family system, had few friends and was afraid the ones she had really did not like her. She usually agreed to whatever her friends wanted to do, and genuinely enjoyed dancing and the early stages of dating. Her closest girlfriend was involved sexually with a boyfriend, and encouraged Lori to have a boyfriend and a sexual relationship. On her next date with a teenage boy she did not really like, she agreed to perform oral sex. After this experience she stopped dating, did not go out with her friends, began a stringent diet that included none of the foods she liked and induced vomiting to further her weight loss.

To this young woman, agreeing to oral sex meant the possibility of complete loss of control over her hedonistic drives and, further, that she really had no self-designed guidelines for her sexual behavior, or for herself in many other areas (i.e. she lacked a cohesive sense of identity). She responded by maintaining rigid control over all pleasurable activities. All-or-none thinking was a prominent feature in her reaction to this incident. The individual therapy of this patient was very difficult. Until her family had been successfully engaged in treatment, she was deceptive about her weight, and reluctant to talk about anything but trivial issues. It was 8 months before she spoke of the sexual incident, and many months later before she recognized the all-or-none thinking and had become confident enough to relax her guard somewhat. As her therapist, the major comments I made about the sexual incident were that it was perhaps a trifle premature for someone just beginning to date, and that it alerted her to the fact that she really did not know what she wanted for herself, sexually or otherwise.

Borderline Personality Organization

The fifth common existential problem is a borderline personality organization. It is my impression that this problem occurs more often in anorectic patients who binge and purge. The psychotherapeutic strategy used with borderline patients is a modification of *Masterson's* [13] approach to borderline adolescents, and has three phases. The first phase is to contain the acting-out behavior, namely fasting, bingeing and purging. This first phase usually requires hospitalization. The second phase is reeducative psychotherapy, in which the connection between behavior and emotions is brought to the patient's awareness.

Terri had refused to eat sufficient quantities of food to gain 1 lb (0.5 kg) in a prescribed period of time, and had been restricted to her room by the behavior therapist administering the weight restoration program. She vomited after the behavior therapist left the room. She later told her psychotherapist that she had vomited, and the therapist inquired about preceding events and her feelings about the room restriction. The patient acknowledged that she was angry. The psychotherapist commented that when the patient was angry (a feeling), she vomited (a behavior).

This reeducative phase may last several months. Initially, examples of connections between thoughts or feelings and behavior may center around food, but soon other areas of functioning come under scrutiny. In the third phase, intensive insight-oriented psychotherapy may be possible during which a genuine sense of self slowly develops.

Phases of Psychotherapy: Termination Phase

In patients for whom long-term psychotherapy has been required, termination is often neither gradual nor smooth. Although some patients may be improved physically and emotionally, they may still act on the basis of all-or-none reasoning and suddenly drop out of therapy. Other patients may continue through the termination phase, expressing only relief and not expressing sadness or anger at no longer seeing the therapist. This usually reflects the still-held belief that going to therapy is, in and of itself, proof of failure.

In the final phase, it is important to help the patient and family try to predict signs of a recurrence (including onset of another weight loss), and to have available to them sources of assistance. Usually it helps to end with an invitation for the patient to return if any signs of relapse develop. One patient, now at normal weight and married for several years, comes for an appointment every year or two when she becomes preoccupied with food. A review of the psychodynamic issues that fostered the development of anorexia in her teens, and identification of the current stressor, plus a reassurance that she is at normal weight and not fat, usually suffice.

Phases of Psychotherapy: Family Intervention

Need for Family Intervention

Family intervention is nearly always necessary, although family therapy is not always appropriate. Family intervention is often a necessary prerequisite for individual therapy to proceed. Since a family belief system (or distortion of it) often interferes with seeking or accepting treatment, this issue must usually be confronted at some point during treatment. Whenever an anorectic patient is living in the parental home, it is usually wise to include the whole family in the initial evaluation. Not only can the necessary treatment be outlined to the entire family, including the patient, but the need for family therapy can be assessed. If a family belief system is preventing treatment, and it is identified, there are several ways of assisting the family. For example, the idea that one is either completely dependent or completely independent may be believed by the entire family. The family may be assisted in identifying intermediate points on the continuum between dependence and independence. This problem is vividly illustrated by Ms. R and her family.

When Ms. R is attending college and living in a dormitory, her parents do not call or write, and she travels about by bus, bicycle and in friends' cars. When she is at home, during the summer, her mother will not allow her to drive to her appointment with her therapist. The message is that when she is at home, she is completely dependent, and when away from home, completely independent. In fact, when she is away from home, she is at a loss as to how to make friends, whom to date, is lonely and depressed and really needs continuing age-appropriate nurturance from her family. Assisting her family to recognize this need, and then act on this awareness, has been part of the focus of family intervention. However, the major modality of treatment for her has been individual psychotherapy, in which she has been encouraged to admit her dependence needs, and find suitable ways of meeting them.

Intensity of Family Intervention

During the course of treatment, the intensity of family involvement depends on the individual situation, and on the phase of therapy. Since usually more than one therapist is involved, especially if family therapy is indicated, frequent communication is needed among therapists. For some patients, especially for those who are younger, with less weight loss, without bingeing and purging, and with relatively short duration of the illness, family therapy may be the primary, or only, treatment modality. For other patients, family involvement may be minimal, either because the patient is already emancipated, or because the family is unable to participate actively in treatment. Even in this situation, however, it is usually necessary to provide some information to the family, especially if the patient is hospitalized, to assist the family in encouraging the patient to remain in treatment.

Intervention with the Spouse

Patients who are married often need marital therapy, or their spouses may also need individual therapy. The prognosis for married patients is poorer than for single patients [20]. Although the reasons for this finding are not known, the following are suggested as hypotheses. First, emotional and chronological distance from one's nuclear family (the situation in which the precursors of the disorder frequently develop) may make it difficult for the patient to reconstruct the original feelings, thoughts and belief systems that fostered the development of anorexia nervosa. Second, many married patients have had the disorder longer, another factor known to worsen prognosis. Third, patients who marry while they have anorexia nervosa may choose mates who reinforce the factors that maintain the disorder. Fourth, some spouses of anorectics are immature, and have serious psychological problems of their own.

Mrs. T was quite thin (100 lb/45 kg at 5 ft 7 inches/170 cm) when she married, but had been in treatment several years for anorexia nervosa,.and had gained 25 lb (11 kg) from her lowest weight of 75 lb (34 kg). Bingeing and purging had decreased. However, she remained very dependent on her parents. After her marriage, the couple moved away from her parental home; she developed compulsive bingeing and purging which occurred 6–10 times per day. Her husband's response was to forbid contact with her family, and to analyze repeatedly her relationship with her parents, blaming them for her problems. Despite repeated requests that he not discuss the factors resulting in the increased bingeing and purging, and the recommendation that she see her parents regularly, her husband intensified his criticism of her family and her symptoms worsened. It was learned that her husband wanted her to be dependent only on him, that he had few friends and had an antagonistic relationship with his own family. In this situation, Mrs. T's dependence problems were attracive to her husband, and thus were less available to psychotherapeutic intervention. He himself also had serious characterologic problems which intensified her conflicts.

General Principles of Psychotherapy

Problems with Neutral Stance

Certain general principles of psychotherapy require modification with anorexia nervosa patients. Often it is necessary to allow the patient to know more about the therapist than is customary. 'Transparency', a term used by *Jourard* [25] to mean that the therapist's emotions are apparent to an observer, is often helpful. The traditional psychoanalytic stance, in which the therapist is a non-disclosing blank screen onto which the patient projects feelings, is often ineffective with anorexia nervosa patients. This may be because many anorectics have a grave distrust of the therapist, project their own intense anger and then withdraw from the therapist, who is perceived as highly dangerous. In other patients, the sense of emptiness and lack of sense of self are worsened when the therapist remains distant. On the other hand, it is important not to be too open, as this may be interpreted as intrusive by the patient, who may be afraid of being consumed or overwhelmed by another person.

Need for the Therapist to Take Active Role

Early in treatment it is often necessary to explain the purpose of psychotherapy, and to take a more active role than is usually necessary. It may be useful to explain that therapy is the process of understanding one's emotions, thoughts and motivations in order to decide whether or not to change; the role of the therapist is not to be omniscient, but rather to guide the patient's own self-awareness.

Another complicating factor, especially early in treatment, is that the therapist often has to take certain actions. For example, it may be necessary to weigh the patient, order certain blood tests, or hospitalize the patient. In this early phase, individual and family psychodynamics are often poorly understood, and the impact of actions taken by the therapist may not be fully recognized until much later in treatment. Many traditionally trained therapists find it difficult to abandon the less active role appropriate for psychoanalysis, or intensive psychodynamic therapy, for the more active role appropriate for these patients. The need to incorporate these aspects of an ongoing evaluation into the therapy relationship will require considerable practice for many.

Timing and Levels of Interpretation

Another general principle of psychotherapy with anorexia nervosa patients is to avoid premature interpretations. Some patients believe 'mother knows best', and it is wise to avoid replaying this as 'therapist knows best'. Interpretations are often experienced as confrontations by these patients, and confrontation without a relationship is nearly always resented. Therefore, challenging interpretations early in therapy are countertherapeutic until an empathic, somewhat more trusting, relationship is established. When interpretations are offered, it is helpful to start with the least threatening level of interpretation, or even to limit oneself to clarification. The following example illustrates the point.

Ms. L. is a 29-year-old, 5 ft 2 inches (157 cm) tall, 75 lb (34 kg) woman, who maintained rigid control over her eating and her sexual activities. She was very fond of her father, and had been 'daddy's little girl' until she was a teenager, when she began acting out with drugs, alcohol and sex. The initial psychodynamic formulation was that she was fearful of losing control of her hedonistic impulses, and that this had developed in the context of a reawakening of the intense oedipal urges in adolescence. In her second psychotherapy session, she related a dream that she had when her weight loss began in her early twenties. She dreamt that her mother had died, and she had to go home and take care of her father. She awoke frightened and called her mother to find out if she was well. I did not comment on this dream, because she had just started therapy. In the fourth session she revealed a great deal about her life at ages 9 and 10, and told of an imaginary brother that looked much like a favored paternal uncle; she indirectly alluded to her loneliness at the time she invented this brother, and to the fact that her father had frequently been gone on business trips during this time. At the close of the session she said that she did not know how she got this way – thinking about food all the time – and asked if there was any hope for recovery. I said yes, that her ability to think in psychological terms, as she had when she recognized a connection between her loneliness and the invention of an imaginary brother, would help her unravel the reasons for needing to maintain a dangerously low weight. Alghough I thought this was a mild interpretation, she responded with surprise that she had not thought of that connection. It is important to note that I did not mention the fact that it was an imaginary brother, rather than a sister, in the dream, nor did I suggest that there might be some connection between her father's absence and the invention of the imaginary brother. I thought these might be too threatening to her; even the seemingly mild restatement of her remarks came as a surprise.

Use of Dreams and Slips of Speech

As with other psychotherapy patients, dreams can be very useful. The same principle of avoiding premature interpretations applies to dream interpretation.

Ms. C. is a 27-year-old woman, who is now near her ideal weight. In an early session she reported a dream. She dreamt that she was walking down the aisle to be married, escorted by her father, when she suddenly turned to him and said she had changed her mind. She had expected him to be angry, because there were hundreds of people at the wedding, but he was not angry. She awoke embarrassed. This dream had many levels of meaning, and has been a focal point for later stages of her treatment. At a superficial level, she spoke at length about her ambivalence about marriage, especially her fear that she will lose her own sense of identity. At another level, she recognized her fear of emancipation from her nuclear family, and at still another level of interpretation, she recognized her strong relationship with her father and his (and her) wish to remain living together. These various levels of interpretation were apparent at the time she reported the dream, but only as therapy progressed was she able to recognize and integrate all the meanings.

Freudian slips by the patient (and the therapist) can also be useful. For example, several patients have said 'emancipated' when they seem to mean 'emaciated'. These have all been intelligent, well-educated women, and thus the slip has been viewed as a statement of unconscious truth. However, in none of the patients was it helpful to inquire about the slip, and none were able to make any connection between weight loss and the sense of freedom from their families until much later in the course of treatment. Another Freudian slip was made by a woman whose 30th birthday was a few days away; she actually weighed 79 lb (36 kg) but said she weighed 29 lb (13 kg) on several occasions during one session. Inquiring about her repeated mistake in weight led to a discussion of her fear of turning 30, and her wish that she were younger.

Countertransference Issues

Treatment of anorexia nervosa is time-consuming, and arouses feelings within the therapist. Balancing the physiological hazards of starvation and bingeing and purging, against the emotional welfare of the patient and the family system difficulties requires knowledge, experience and an adequate support system for the therapist. Usually one therapist is insufficient to manage the panoply of difficulties presented by the patient and family. The treatment team will be described in detail in chapter 10, but most important is quick, frequent and easy communication among team members. Since many patients have a borderline personality disorder, splitting is a common defense mechanism, and there is a marked tendency for the treatment team to become divided and quarrel with one another. *Cohen* [26] has described an anorectic patient whose bingeing worsened when the treatment team was quarrelling internally. Resolution of the difficulty within the team was paralleled by a decrease in bingeing behavior in the patient. Since many of these patients have learned to be exquisitely sensitive to non-verbal and covert messages, such intrateam conflicts can be particularly countertherapeutic.

Another common countertransference problem is siding with either the patient or the family. The experience, training and life stage of the therapist, and the therapist's own neurotic conflicts, determine the vulnerability to this problem. Since a family system problem is often an integral part of the dilemma, and since all members of the system participate in maintaining the system's equilibrium, no one person is to blame for the problem, and siding with anyone is usually not helpful. Periodic consultation from other team members, or formal supervision, can be helpful in recognizing and avoiding this particular countertransference problem.

Case Illustrations

Case 1. Carrie is a 16-year-old girl, the second of 4 children, aged 15–21 years. She began losing weight down to 75 lb (34 kg), had amenorrhea, obsessions about food, unusual handling of food, and occasional vomiting or laxative abuse when her family forced her to eat. Initially she dieted in order to lose weight, but then lost her appetite as well. At about the same time she began to lose weight, her father, a heavy smoker, as is she, began to develop shortness of breath and lost 30 lb (13 kg). He fainted once when he was shopping with her. At the time she was evaluated, he had decided to go for an evaluation, and was hospitalized for workup for possible cancer of the lung. He was at another hospital at the time she was hospitalized for treatment of anorexia nervosa.

Carrie maintained she was not worried about her weight loss, nor was she worried about her father. A few days after she had been hospitalized, her father's workup was completed, and it was learned that he had inoperable cancer of the lung. While crying, she would say that she had no reason to be sad, but when asked about her father, she would say how fond she was of him. After a few individual therapy sessions, she was able to speak openly of her sadness about his illness, her awareness months earlier that he was ill and her wish to take his symptoms away, even if it meant dying in place of him. When he was short of breath, she became short of breath.

Her father had made several unwise financial decisions just before the cancer was diagnosed, had changed jobs and had no health insurance; although this caused severe problems in the entire family, no one complained. Family sessions revealed a close family, with everyone feeling guilty, sad and angry about the father's illness, but all had great difficulty expressing these feelings. Carrie's illness, in terms of the family's psychodynamics, allowed them a relatively safe focus on which to vent their anger. During treatment, the parents began to recognize the difficulty they had in expressing their feelings and the impact this might have on their children.

Carrie gained to 93 lb (42 kg) in the hospital, and as an outpatient she gained to 105 lb (47 kg). Her father received experimental chemotherapy, and initially did well. She still spends much time with him, but now attends school, has a job and has started going out with her friends. She cries when she thinks of her father, but now can accept his as a normal response. She voices fears that she will not be able to come to therapy if she gains to a normal weight, and is afraid of her feelings if her father does die. She is reassured by the therapist that achieving a normal weight does not mean all the problems are resolved.

Treatment was relatively straightforward. One theme was a severe anticipatory grief reaction, including taking on the mannerisms and symptoms of the ill: increased smoking, weight loss and shortness of breath. The anorexia nervosa served as a protective device for Carrie; the obsessions resulted in a decreased awareness of her father's illness. Another theme was the impact of the weight loss on the family; it 'helped' the family by providing a focus for their anger. They believed Carrie more able to 'take it' than the father, who felt guilty about both his financial errors and his failure to spend more time with his family when he was well.

Case 2. Laura is a 14-year-old girl who was referred for individual and family therapy, following approximately 2 months of inpatient treatment for anorexia nervosa. She gained 10 lb (4.5 kg) in the hospital with a behavior management program, but contended throughout that she had no problem. Her interactions with her psychiatrist were angry accusations, filled with recriminations about the weight restoration program. Family and individual therapy were suggested in the hope that some of the crucial unresolved maturational issues might be identified and mastered by the patient.

Her father was a soft-spoken, highly successful lawyer. Her mother was a guilt-ridden woman with inflexible rules for her daughters and teenage son. She bitterly resented her role as a housewife and mother. Laura had an elder sister who was said to be her mother's favorite, but actually was less favored by the mother than was Laura. The family interaction patterns commonly described in anorexia nervosa were present. There was an absence of intergenerational boundaries (e.g. the father covertly sided with the patient against the mother) and there were rigid fixed patterns of interaction (e.g. attempts to change Laura's violin practice schedule met with overt resistance from the entire family). Enmeshment was present (e.g. when a cold remedy for Laura's sister was prescribed, the father dosed both daughters 'to prevent' Laura from developing a cold) and there was a lack of conflict resolution (i.e. either emotionally charged topics were avoided or occasionally there were prolonged unresolved quarrels).

As therapy progressed, it was learned that Laura rejected her mother's homemaker life style as undesirable, and was striving to emulate her father in career aspirations. An example of the avoidance stance adopted by the family was reflected in their surprise that Laura might have difficulty integrating her career aspirations and her feminine identity (since no woman in her family had completed college or worked outside the home for longer than a few months). Laura's quarrels with her mother were overdetermined, but a major, initially unstated, reason was her mother's anger and guilt over Laura's wholesale rejection of the traditional acceptable female role. Several times Laura said she did not want to gain sufficient weight for her menstrual periods to begin. Thus, at one level of interpretation, her weight loss can be seen as a rejection of what she perceived as the only available feminine role.

Laura had been seen by her parents as 'just like her sister', and it was only with the development of anorexia nervosa that any differences were noted by her mother. These were usually viewed as negative differences. One way I worked with Laura was to focus on her ability to perceive correctly interactions in the family, in spite of both her tendency to blame others and severe obsessive-compulsive and paranoid personality traits. Like many people with strong paranoid traits, she often correctly identified in a few words the major issues. I identified with her capacity to see things as they were, e.g. that her mother frequently did take her sister's side (this was guilt and reaction formation on her mother's part). I would then comment, 'Your sister really needs your mother. After all, your sister has great difficulty verbalizing her genuine feelings, because (unlike you) she is afraid of anyone's anger'.

Another major area of difficulty was the ascetic/hedonistic conflict which Laura had resolved on the ascetic side. She did not like physical education because she was embarrassed about dressing in gym clothes. It was agreed that she would be excused from this class if she would go out with a friend once per weekend. This was an attempt to assist her in reducing her marked asceticism.

Another theme was an unresolved oedipal conflict. There was a covert alliance between Laura and her father to exclude her mother. Much of Laura's guilt was related to an unconscious wish to possess her father. In one sense, she had succeeded (via the covert alliance); this was another factor that promoted the wholesale rejection of sexuality by semistarvation. Initially, the family therapist attempted to get the father to set rules about eating. This did not really work well, because he did it in a 'kind' way, leaving the mother to become angry. Later in treatment, when Laura really was making friends, her father did genuinely become angry about her refusal to eat normally, yelled in a dramatic and decisive way and took his wife out for the evening. This resulted in improvement in Laura, with a return to more normal eating patterns. There was a gradual reuniting of the parents and the eventual development of a very sophisticated parental style.

Case 3. Ms. B. is a 20-year-old woman with premorbid obsessive-compulsive traits. Her major identification was with her father, but she had a real wish to be closer to her mother. The entire family was preoccupied with appearances, but they were also genuinely concerned with one another's welfare. Her paternal female cousin had anorexia nervosa. Overt problems began 6 months prior to evaluation, when she entered an exercise class at 5 ft 6 inches (167 cm), 120 lb (54 kg), and lost down to 95 lb (43 kg). Her mother described the group as a 'cult' that had 'brainwashed' her daughter with repetitive chants of 'think thin' during the exercises. Ms. B. was described as a 'sweet easy child' who did not know what she herself was really like. She said that she was supposed to be responsible, polite, and 'keep up appearances', but did not know what she wanted from life. At about the same time that she started to lose weight, she decided to defend a co-worker who was being fired for reasons she thought were unfair, to the surprise (and embarrassment) of her family. She organized, very capably, a large protest, and wrote letters to influential members of the community; however, her efforts did not result in the rehiring of the co-worker. She was also about to graduate from college with a major in business. She had really wanted to become a nurse, but her boyfriend thought is was not suitable. Her strivings toward a coherent self-identity were frustrated at every turn. It was postulated that weight loss became a smokescreen for this frustration.

Neither she nor her family would agree to hospitalization, but she agreed to go home to convalesce. She was able to speak openly about the feelings of incompetence she had about herself and her lack of a sense of purpose. She was seen by the same therapist for both individual and family therapy. She was seen several times with her mother, and they reflected on the mother's role in the family. The family was helped to see her as an individual, not as the quiet, sweet, uninvolved, overly polite person they always thought she was, but rather as a crusading, strong-willed woman.

Case 4. Ms. J. is a 21-year-old woman who was 64 lb (29 kg) and 5 ft (152 cm) tall at the time of her evaluation. She began gaining weight in early adolescence, and was 165 lb (75 kg) at age 14. She maintained this weight until age 20, when she decided to go on a diet, began eating less and exercising more, until she reached 64 lb (29 kg). She obsessed about food and followed a vegetarian 'pure' diet, but had no bulimic spells and did not purge. She thought she might be too thin at her admission weight, but thought she was fat at 100 lb (45 kg). The mental status examination revealed she was denying the severity of the problems, but there was no evidence of a thought disorder or perceptual distortions, other than a misperception of her actual size. She was cachectic, with a blood pressure of 86 over 50 mm Hg, had cyanotic nailbeds and cyanotic upper torso. She was hospitalized, and promptly became acutely psychotic. She chanted 'the answer is in the CAT scan', urinated on the floor, had auditory hallucinations and a marked formal thought disorder.

A computerized tomography revealed enlarged ventricles and cerebral atrophy. She was treated with antipsychotics. Gradually her auditory hallucinations abated, she was able to think clearly without delusional ideation and ate normally. However, she still had a blunted affect and related poorly to others. 6 months later she was 20 lb (9 kg) over her premorbid weight, lived at home, was not working and had few friends.

In this patient, the presenting picture was no different than that of other anorexia nervosa patients seen by this author. Closer examination of her early history revealed that she had been a schizoid child, and that her parents had been quite protective of her, perhaps recognizing her vulnerability. It is hypothesized that maintenance of a low weight was a final defense against an emerging psychosis. The possibility that the psychosis was related to her starved state was considered, but seemed unlikely, in view of the fact that she continued to have psychotic symptoms after the initial phase of fluid and electrolyte replacement.

Conclusion

The psychotherapy of anorexia nervosa is most likely to be effective in the context of a weight restoration program. A conceptual model of the development and maintenance of the disorder is presented. Existential conflict may be resolved via self-starvation which is associated with the emergence of a mind/body dichotomy and cognitive distortions. Family belief systems, in actual or distorted form, may prevent successful treatment and thus must be addressed early. In the initial phase of psychotherapy, emphasis is on educating the patient about psychotherapy, integrating psychotherapeutic efforts with weight restoration and gradually modifying illogical cognitive beliefs and body image disturbances. In the midphase of therapy the underlying existential problems are addressed. During the termination phase, the patient and family are helped to learn how to predict recurrence and seek help. The general principles of insight-oriented psychotherapy must be appropriately modified to adequately meet the needs of these patients. Countertransference problems are common and require careful attention.

References

1 Janet, P.: Les obsessions et la psychasthénie (Alcan, Paris 1919).
2 Keys, A.; Brozek, J.; Henschel, A.; Mickelsen, O.; Taylor, H.: The biology of human starvation (University of Minnesota Press, Minneapolis 1950).
3 Dally, P.: Anorexia nervosa (Heinemann, London 1969).
4 Powers, P.: Social and cultural factors in obesity; in Powers, Obesity: the regulation of weight, pp. 201–243 (Williams & Wilkins, Baltimore 1980).
5 Wooley, O.; Wooley, S.: The Beverly Hills eating disorder: the mass marketing of anorexia nervosa. Int. J. Eating Disord. *1:* 57–68 (1981).
6 Wooley, O.; Wooley, S.; Dyrenforth, S.: Obesity and women. II. A neglected feminist topic. Women's Stud. Int. Q. *2:* 81–92 (1979).
7 Lindemann, E.: Symptomatology and management of acute grief. Am. J. Psychiat. *101:* 141–148 (1944).
8 Minuchin, S.; Roseman, B.; Baker, L.: Psychosomatic families: anorexia nervosa in context (Harvard University Press, Cambridge 1978).
9 Selvini-Palazzoli, M.: Self-starvation. From the intrapsychic to the transpersonal approach to anorexia nervosa (Aronson, New York 1978).
10 Haley, J.: Leaving home: the therapy of disturbed young people (McGraw-Hill, New York 1980).
11 Boyer, R.; Katz, J.; Finkelstein, J.; Kapen, M.; Weiner, H.; Weitzman, E.; Hellman, L.: Anorexia nervosa: immaturity of the 24-hour luteinizing hormone secretory pattern. New Engl. J. Med. *291:* 861–865 (1974).
12 Crisp, A.: Anorexia nervosa: 'feeding disorder', 'nervous malnutrition' or 'weight phobia'? Wld Rev. Nutr. Diet., vol. 12, pp. 452–504 (Karger, Basel 1970).
13 Masterson, J.: Treatment of the borderline adolescent: a developmental approach (Wiley & Sons, New York 1972).
14 Masterson, J.: Primary anorexia nervosa in the borderline adolescent: an object-relations review; in Hartocollis, Borderline personality disorders (International Universities Press, New York 1977).
15 Bruch, H.: Eating disorders. Obesity, anorexia nervosa and the person within (Basic Books, New York 1973).
16 Maslow, A.: Motivation and personality (Harper & Row, New York 1970).
17 Powers, P.; Powers, H.: Inpatient treatment of anorexia nervosa. Psychosomatics (in press).
18 Gerstmann, J.: Psychological and phenomenological aspects of disorders of the body image. J. nerv. ment. Dis. *126:* 499–512 (1958).
19 Burron, E.; Franella, F.; Slade, P.: A reappraisal of body perception disturbance in anorexia nervosa. Psychol. Med. *7:* 235–243 (1977).
20 Goldberg, S.; Halmi, K.; Casper, R.; Eckert, E.; Davis, J.: Pretreatment predictors of

weight change in anorexia nervosa; in Vigersky, Anorexia nervosa, pp. 31–42 (Raven Press, New York 1977).

21 Garfinkel, P.; Moldofsky, H.; Garner, D.; Stancer, H.; Coscina, D.: Body awareness in anorexia nervosa: disturbances in body image and satiety. Psychosom. Med. *40:* 487–498 (1978).

22 Crisp, A.; Kalucy, R.: Aspects of the perceptual disorder in anorexia nervosa. Br. J. med. Psychol. *47:* 349–361 (1974).

23 Garfinkel, P.; Garner, D.: Perceptual and conceptual disturbances; in Garfinkel, Garner, Anorexia nervosa: a multidimensional perspective, pp. 123–163 (Brunner/Mazel, New York 1982).

24 Powers, P.: Psychiatric considerations in obesity; in Powers, Obesity: the regulation of weight, pp. 158–178 (Williams & Wilkins, Baltimore 1980).

25 Jourard, S.: The transparent self (Van Nostrand, New York 1971).

26 Cohen, S.: Hostile interaction in a general hospital ward leading to disturbed behavior and bulimia in anorexia nervosa: its successful management. Post-grad. med. J. *54:* 361–363 (1978).

27 Powers, P.: Obesity: the regulation of weight (Williams & Wilkins, Baltimore 1980).

3 Somatic and Behavioral Treatment of Anorexia Nervosa and Bulimia

Katherine A. Halmi

Introduction

Somatic and behavioral treatments of anorexia nervosa are closely related and intertwined. A discussion of somatic treatment in anorexia nervosa and bulimia must include the medical management as well as drug and other physiological treatments. Medical management and drug treatment are most effective when they are combined with behavioral treatment.

The immediate aim of treatment should be to restore the patient's nutritional state to normal. Mere emaciation can cause irritability, depression, preoccupation with food and sleep disturbance [1]. It is difficult to accomplish a behavioral change with psychotherapy in an emaciated patient who is suffering the psychological effects of starvation. If the anorectic patient has been ill for less than 4 months, is not bingeing or vomiting, and has parents who are willing to cooperate in family therapy, then it is likely outpatient therapy will be effective. For those more severely ill patients, the structured environment of a hospitalized treatment program is necessary for nutritional rehabilitation.

Drug Treatment: Anorexia Nervosa

Drugs can be useful adjuncts in the treatment of anorexia nervosa but there are very few randomly assigned, double-blind controlled drug studies in patients with anorexia nervosa. All open drug trials are contaminated with the concomitant use of psychotherapy and/or some type of behavioral contingency program.

Chlorpromazine

The first drug used in the treatment of anorexia nervosa was the dopamine blocker, chlorpromazine [2, 3]. Although patients receiving chlorpromazine in these studies also had other therapies such as bed rest, insulin or supportive psychotherapy, the authors thought chlorpromazine contributed significantly to weight gain in the patients. It is my clinical impression that chlorpromazine is effective in reducing the anxiety in severely obsessive-compulsive anorectic patients and hence contributes to a faster rate of weight gain by enabling the patients to take in more food with reduced anxiety. However, there is no controlled study of chlorpromazine in the treatment of anorexia nervosa.

Antidepressants

Anorexia nervosa patients have many depressive symptoms, such as sleep disturbance, irritability, admission to feeling depressed and difficulty concentrating [4]. Some anorectic patients have biological depression signs such as dexamethasone resistance, decreased 3-methoxy-4-hydroxy-phenylglycol (MHPG) secretion and an impaired growth hormone response to *L*-dopa [4]. Because of these observations anorectic patients have been treated with a variety of antidepressant medications.

Two open trials of amitriptyline in anorectics indicated that this drug may be effective for inducing weight gain [5, 6]. More recently a double-blind controlled study has shown that amitriptyline is effective in reducing depression as measured on the Hamilton Depression Rating Scale but not in producing a statistically significant weight gain in anorectic patients [7]. The maximum dose of amitriptyline used was 160 mg/day. Because of the side-effect problems of hypotension and tachycardia, it is necessary to start amitriptyline at a low dosage, as low as 40 mg/day in severely emaciated anorectics and then gradually increase the dose as the patients become more medically stable.

Another antidepressant used in Europe to treat anorectic patients is chlomiprimine. In a randomly assigned double-blind controlled study of chlomiprimine (50 mg just before sleep) in 16 anorectic patients, there was no main effect of the drug on weight gain. All patients reached their target weight in this study and there was no difference in the rate of weight gain between the clomipramine group and placebo group [8]. Although clomipramine was significantly associated with increased hunger, appetite and caloric intake (the former two items were measured by analog scales), it was not associated with increased rate of weight gain. The authors thought this might be due to increased activity in the drug patients. The study just described was on hospitalized anorectics who were also put at bed rest and given individual psychotherapy.

Cyproheptadine

In a collaborative study conducted at two hospitals [7], discussed earlier, cyproheptadine, an antihistaminic drug, was shown to significantly induce weight gain compared to placebo and to significantly reduce Hamilton Depression Score Ratings compared to both placebo and amitriptyline groups. High doses of cyproheptadine, 32 mg/day, were given. Since cyproheptadine is a relatively safe drug with no complicating side effects, such as hypotension, disturbance of cardiac rhythm and undesirable interactions with other drugs, it is an especially attractive drug to use.

Metoclopramide

Anorexia nervosa patients often complain of feeling full after they have ingested a relatively small amount of food. Some of their complaints may have a physiological basis since delayed gastric emptying is present in many anorectic patients [9]. Metoclopramide, a drug which increases lower esophageal sphincter pressure, increases gastric motility and suppresses vomiting has been shown in a double-blind crossover study to enhance gastric emptying, improve meal tolerance, reduce postprandial epigastric pain, reduce early satiety and reduce vomiting in 7 anorexia nervosa patients [10]. In this study the patients took one 10-mg tablet of metoclopramide 30 min before each meal and at bedtime. The patients received at least 1 month of treatment. This drug should be considered as an adjunct treatment for anorexia nervosa.

Miscellaneous Drugs

Other drugs used to treat anorexia nervosa have been either reported as case reports or have had equivocal or negative results. These drugs will briefly be mentioned.

Lithium was shown in a double-blind placebo trial with a small number of anorectic patients to have no overall effect on weight gain. It should be noted that this drug is particularly risky to use in anorectic patients because of the possibility of rapid toxicity from severely restricted fluid intake, self-induced vomiting and laxative or diuretic abuse [11].

In an open trial with 9 anorectic patients *L*-dopa was associated with less than 1 kg of weight gain in 4 patients. It is difficult to interpret much from this study since the maximum dosage of the drug ranged from 1 to 3 g/day and the duration of the treatment ranged from 16 to 27 days [12].

Naloxone was infused in anorexia nervosa patients to determine its effect on weight gain and lipolysis [13]. These patients were also on a behavior therapy program and some received amitriptyline. There was virtually no standardized methodology so that naloxone was administered in some patients for 1 week and in others for 11 weeks. The naloxone was also given at different periods in the hospital stay. Because this study was complicated with other treatments and had virtually no systematic methodology, no conclusions can be made on the effect of naloxone in the treatment of anorexia nervosa.

A single case report of the use of phenoxybenzamine, an alpha-adrenergic blocking agent does not provide enthusiastic evidence for using this drug in anorectic patients. The patient on 30 mg/day developed postural hypotension and nausea. It was reported that during the time the patient was on the drug, weight gain was present, and during the period of 2 days when the drug was discontinued for side effects, the patient lost weight [14].

Drug Treatment: Bulimia

Antidepressants

A number of antidepressants have also been used to treat bulimia. Imipramine was studied in a randomly assigned double-blind protocol with 11 patients receiving imipramine and 11 patients receiving a placebo. Although drug compliance is usually a difficult problem in outpatient bulimics, there was enough compliance in this study to produce a drug effect. Imipramine was associated with reduced frequency of binge-eating, decreased intensity of binges, decreased preoccupation with food, greater subjective global improvement and decreased depression as measured by the Hamilton Depression Scale [15].

Another antidepressant assessed in the treatment of bulimia is mianserin. It was thought that this tetracyclic piperazino-azepine, shown to be effective in the treatment of depression, would have an advantage over tricyclic antidepressants because of less anticholinergic effects and lack of cardiotoxicity. In a randomly assigned double-blind controlled study of 50 patients, mianserin was found to have no effect on reducing bingeing behavior, altering eating behavior or improving depression as measured from a variety of scales [16].

Because the mood disturbance of some patients with bulimia has been equated to that of patients with atypical depression, some clinicians have been treating bulimics with monoamine oxidase inhibitors (MAOIs). In an open trial study of 6 patients (5 treated with phenelzine and 1 treated with tranylcypromine), all 6 showed a significant reduction in binge-eating [17]. This initial result certainly justifies a double-blind treatment study. The effect of MAOIs on bulimia could be independent of their antidepressant activity. The use of MAOIs requires strict adherence to a tyramine-free diet. Some bulimic patients will have difficulty complying with this diet. For outpatients on MAOIs, dietary compliance should be assessed frequently and hospitalization may be necessary to assure the adherence of some patients.

Anticonvulsants

The anticonvulsant drug, phenytoin, has been studied in an open trial [18] and in a placebo double-blind crossover trial in the treatment of bulimia [19]. The latter study was a double-blind crossover study of 19 bulimic subjects comparing phenytoin with placebo. There was a significant decrease in binges among subjects who received phenytoin following placebo; but there was no difference among subjects receiving phenytoin preceding placebo, although the latter group showed a decrease in binges from pretreatment to treatment levels. In this study there was no association between EEG abnormalities and response to the medication. Phenytoin was effective in preventing binges at serum levels as low as 5 μg/ml.

Terminating Medication

There are no studies to give guidelines on when to terminate medication such as antidepressants or phenytoin in treating bulimic patients. It is probably wise to continue the medication 2–3 months after the patient is symptom-free and then gradually reduce the medication. Until more controlled treatment studies are done to serve as guidelines it will be necessary to use the 'best clinical judgment'.

Drug Treatment: Recommendations

After reviewing all these studies, the clinician is left with the decision as to how to decide what drug to use, if any, in the treatment of anorectic and bulimic patients. Taking into account the review just presented, it seems reasonable to recommend that, if an anorectic patient has a predominance of depressive symptomatology, a trial on amitriptyline or cyproheptadine is warranted. A bingeing and purging patient with anxiety and depressive symptomatology may respond to phenelzine and a bulimic patient within a normal weight range may respond to phenytoin with a reduction of bingeing episodes. Severely obsessive-compulsive and delusional anorectic patients are likely to require chlorpromazine.

Behavior Therapy: Anorexia Nervosa

Behavior therapy is especially useful in the medical management of eating disorder patients. Behavioral techniques are almost always used in the treatment of eating disorder patients but frequently the behavioral techniques are not identified as such.

Negative Reinforcement

Over 100 years ago, *Gull* [20] used a form of behavior therapy (negative reinforcement) to treat anorectic patients. He separated the patients from their families (isolated them from a noxious environment) and did not allow them access to their families until they gained weight. This is an example of negative reinforcement in which paradigm a patient works (eats) to remove an unpleasant event (isolation) from the environment. In fact, almost all treatment programs for anorexia nervosa have used this type of behavior-conditioning paradigm without recognizing it. For example, the nursing care program of *Russell* [21] and the psychotherapy program of *Crisp* [3] both require that patients be put to bed and not allowed out of bed until they have attained close to their target weight. All hospitalized treatment programs have an implicit form of negative reinforcement; i.e. in order to leave the hospital, the patients must eat.

Anorexia nervosa has been conceptualized as an eating phobia. 'They behave rather as though they suffer from an eating phobia – eating generates anxiety, and their failure to eat represents avoidance. In other words, their cessation of eating after ingesting a very small portion of a meal (or removing it from the body by self-inducing vomiting) is reinforced by anxiety reduction. From such an analysis, two treatment procedures suggest themselves: deconditioning the anxiety associated with eating and/or shaping eating behavior (and hence weight gain) by making access to powerful reinforcers contingent on eating' [22].

Systematic Desensitization

Systematic desensitization has not been effective in the treatment of anorectics. There are a few case reports of this technique used with anorectics. *Lang* [23] applied desensitization to several hierarchies of anxiety-producing social situations associated with inability to eat in a 23-year-old anorectic. Assertive training was also given to this patient. Although *Lang* [23] reported the patient gained weight, he did not report the patient's actual weight. *Hallsten* [24] paired Jacobson's relaxation technique with graded scenes of eating at home in a 12-year-old anorectic. However, *Hallsten* [24] also restricted visits by relatives and made them contingent upon weight gain in the treatment of this patient. There is only one case report of desensitization used without other treatment modalities [25]. Jacobson's relaxation technique was used to desensitize the patient to her anxiety associated with progressive weight gain and concomitant changes in appearance. The patient gained steadily throughout treatment; however, the authors did caution that the systematic desensitization alone would most likely only be effective for a subgroup of anorectic patients.

Operant Conditioning

The first explicit use of the operant conditioning paradigm in the treatment of anorexia nervosa was reported by *Bachrach* et al. [26]. Initially, social reinforcements (attention, conversation and praise) were made contingent upon eating behavior. Later, weight gain was enhanced by reinforcement deprivation in making visits and activities contingent on satisfactory eating behavior. After a while, the patient's weight stabilized at 63 lb (28 kg) and it was discovered she had been secretly vomiting. At this point reinforcements were made contingent on weight gain rather than the ingestion of food.

Very few reports on behavioral treatment of anorexia nervosa include experimental control procedures. One such report was that of *Leitenberg* et al. [27]. In 1 patient, during a 'non-reinforcement' period, an extinction technique in which complaints and comments about eating difficulties were ignored, there was no improvement in weight gain. During the 'operant' phase, ward privileges were attached to weight gain, and during this time the patient gained steadily. In a second case, the patient counted mouthfuls of food and charted her weight daily with no facilitation of weight gain. However, when she was put on a positive reinforcement regimen, she gained weight steadily. The authors state, 'The systematic desensitization strategy takes care of anxiety and lets overt behavior take care of itself, while the operant strategy takes care of behavior and lets anxiety take care of itself' [27]. In the operant conditioning strategy, the assumption is that each behavioral step forward will reduce anxiety.

Another study using an experimental design to show the efficacy of behavior therapy in inducing weight gain in anorectics was done by *Pertschuk* et al. [28]. In this study, 7 subjects were treated with an operant conditioning paradigm for a period of 13 days. Each subject received experimental behavioral treatment at a different time during hospitalization. The outcome, weight gain, was evaluated using the Rn statistic for this multiple baseline approach. For the group, the median weight gain before behavioral treatment was 0.09 kg/day, and the median weight gain over 13 behavior therapy days was 4.2 kg, or 0.32 kg/day.

In a series of 5 single case experiments, using the technique of systematic analysis, *Agras* et al. [29] were able to demonstrate the strong effect of regular feedback information of weight and calorie intake on weight gain. Without the feedback information, positive reinforcement appeared to be relatively ineffective. In this same study, the effective negative reinforcement (associating leaving the hospital with weight gain) was removed by contracting with the patient for a 12-week stay for 'research purposes' whether or not the patient gained weight. Thus, regular feedback information was shown to contribute independently to weight gain.

In a report of a series of 6 patients treated with an operant conditioning paradigm, *Blinder* et al. [30] showed that anorectic patients gained weight readily when access to activity was made contingent on a minimal daily weight gain. Since then there have been many open trial studies indicating the operant conditioning approach is effective [31–37].

In another study, *Williemier* et al. [38] compared the efficacy of an operant conditioning form of behavior therapy with a program of strict isolation, appetite-stimulating drugs and psychotherapy in 16 anorectic patients. Actually, the latter program was not free of behavioral contingencies, as it contained a strong negative reinforcer of strict isolation. In this comparison, the patients receiving the operant conditioning program had 3 times as great a rate of weight gain compared with the patients in strict isolation.

In another study, 81 anorectic patients were assigned to behavior modification or its absence [39]. In this study, which was conducted in three collaborating hospitals, there was no overall significant difference in weight gain in the two groups. Several explanations were given by the authors for lack of efficacy of behavior therapy: (1) constant reinforcers were used in all patients instead of individualized reinforcers, (2) a schedule of delayed reinforcements, given only every fifth day in this study, might not have been as effective as a schedule of more immediate daily reinforcements, and (3) the ward milieu programs and isolation, which was a form of treatment of those patients not receiving behavior therapy, may have produced a maximal possible weight gain so that behavior therapy could not be expected to do any better.

Behavior Therapy: Bulimia

During the hospital phase the bulimic patients work out a list of alternative behaviors to binge-eating. They practice these behaviors on passes from the hospital and later after they are discharged. Outpatient programs for bulimics all use some type of behavioral programs. Most of these include requiring the patient to record the food she eats and where and when it is eaten. After monitoring is established the patient contracts to eat at conventional mealtimes. Her failure to comply with this is discussed in subsequent therapy sessions. Strategies are worked out with the patient to reduce the availability of food [40].

More recently the technique of exposure and response prevention has been used in treating bulimic patients [41]. In this technique the patient is instructed to eat the amount of food that will cause her to feel a strong urge to vomit. After she does this she then stays with the therapist who encourages her to focus on her fears and discomforts until the urge to vomit vanishes. Further refinement of this last technique will undoubtedly be made in the near future.

In some outpatient programs flooding techniques are used with bulimic patients. These techniques usually require the patient to taste and handle binge items (e.g. cookies, candy bars, cakes) while the therapist describes the bulimic act and prevents the patient from vomiting. The patient may be exposed to binge foods during and after each meal or she may be requested to buy binge items in the community and refrain from bingeing [42]. In another program patients contract to maintain their present weight throughout the program and eat three prescribed meals a day [43].

Hospital Treatment: Weight-Gain Phase

Recommended Operant Conditioning Program

In an operant conditioning program, weight gain should be reinforced rather than eating behavior until the patient is able to maintain a normal weight. The reason for this is that the patients can eat a normal size meal, earn their reward and then induce vomiting and, hence, never change their weight status. Making positive reinforcements contingent only on weight gain is helpful in reducing the staff-patient arguments and stressful interactions over how and what the patient is eating, since weight is an objective measure. The use of a behavioral assessment to determine and implement individualized reinforcers and the combination of daily reinforcements with more delayed reinforcements will provide the most effective behavior therapy program.

For the patients who are hospitalized, daily weights should be measured every morning after the patient has voided and before the first feeding. Fluid intake and urine output should be measured and caloric intake should be recorded daily. Serum electrolytes must be assessed frequently in patients who are vomiting. An efficient and easy way to be certain the patients are receiving adequate amounts of vitamins, minerals, proteins, fatty acids and carbohydrates is to give all their nutrition in the form of a formula such as Sustacal. In this formula all the nutritional necessities are conveniently blended so that the patient cannot selectively discard any item. Patients are often fearful of eating certain types of foods and certainly are reluctant to eat a large quantity of food which is necessary for them to do if they are to gain weight. It is easier for most patients to take the formula which is frequently perceived as a medication than to eat an equivalent caloric amount in food. Complications such as edema, gastric distention and rarely cardiac failure may occur if the patient is refed too rapidly. To avoid this, the patient should be given a daily caloric intake to maintain her admission weight plus 50% for activity. The daily caloric intake can be increased by 50% every 5 days. If the formula is given in 6 equal feedings throughout the day, the patient will not have to ingest a large amount at any one time.

Patients who have been ill for a long time may need to take a liquid formula until they reach their target weight. Patients who are tolerating the weight gain well can be taken off the liquid formula after about 2 weeks and returned to a weight-gaining diet. After the patient has reached her target weight, it is wise to give her the amount of food to maintain that weight so she can visually conceptualize the amount of food she should be eating each day to maintain the target weight. Following 1 or 2 weeks of presenting the patient with the number of calories needed to maintain her target weight, it is important to begin to allow the patient to choose her own foods and to practice maintaining her target weight without aid from the staff. Giving the patient the autonomy to choose her own foods after she is medically normal, rather than earlier, usually results in a smoother transition to normal eating patterns.

Exposure and Response Prevention

In addition to effectively inducing weight gain, behavior therapy can be used to stop vomiting in anorectic patients. A response prevention technique is used to stop vomiting. For example, the most commonly used response prevention is to have the patients sit in a day room under staff supervision for 1 or 2 h after every meal. This constant supervision inhibits most patients from vomiting. Another technique is to have the anorectic patient exclusively use a chair commode in her room and not give her access to flush toilets. The patient is instructed that if she vomits into this commode she will have to clean it out herself. This effectively stops vomiting in most patients.

Hospital Treatment: Behavior Therapy and Medication Combined

There is only one controlled study assessing the efficacy of combining behavioral therapy with medication. This was a multicenter study of 105 anorectic patients who were randomly assigned to cyproheptadine or placebo and behavior therapy or no behavior therapy [39]. Thus, there were 4 treatment groups in this study: (1) cyproheptadine and behavior therapy, (2) cyproheptadine and no behavior therapy, (3) placebo and behavior therapy, and (4) placebo and no behavior therapy. Although a subgroup was identified that responded preferentially to cyproheptadine with increased weight gain and another subgroup was identified that responded preferentially to behavior therapy with increased weight gain, there was no subgroup of patients that responded to the combination of behavior therapy and cyproheptadine with increased weight gain. Nor did the patients assigned to the combination of the two therapies have a greater weight gain compared to the other 3 treatment groups. The fact that there was no main effect for any type of therapy in this study but only the identification of certain subgroups that responded preferentially to the cyproheptadine and behavior therapy is most likely due to the enormous heterogeneity of the patients that participated in the study. Even though they all had the diagnosis of anorexia nervosa there was considerable variation in the population group with respect to the severity of the disorder. An area for future research would be to continue to try to identify more homogeneous subgroups that will respond preferentially to a treatment.

It does make good clinical sense to combine medication with behavior therapy. For example, in the emaciated or underweight phase of anorexia nervosa, drugs will effect anorectic symptoms such as decreased gastric emptying time, hyperactivity, mood changes, obsessionality, sleep disturbance and some anorectic attitudes. Other symptoms such as 'fear of getting fat' may respond best to the exposure to the fear of weight gain by a behavioral program which requires patients to gain weight. Contrary to popular belief, exposure to weight gain is actually associated with the reduction of the fear of gaining weight and it is also associated with general psychological improvement [44].

Hospital Treatment: Weight-Maintenance Phase

If the anorectic patient has been on a weight restoration program, it is extremely unwise to discharge her as soon as she has gained to her normal weight. Although there are no controlled studies to show this, it is the clinical impression of most specialists that severely ill patients should not leave the hospital until they are actually able to eat normally and maintain a normal weight, otherwise they will relapse immediately. After anorectic patients regain to a normal weight, they must be reassessed for the need for medication. During the hospital weight-maintenance phase the combination of behavior therapy and medication may continue. For example, patients with significant residual anxiety after weight gain, or those with a more generalized anxiety, may do well to continue on antidepressants. Residual fears about food intake and weight control will continue and can be managed with continuing behavioral techniques. For example, the patients may have increased activities and privileges every day that their weight is within a normal weight range but they could be restricted to the hospital ward on the days when they are below normal weight range.

Aftercare Program

After the patient is able to eat normally and maintain her weight for a period of 2 weeks, it is time to consider discharging her to an aftercare program. There are no studies to indicate what type of aftercare program is most effective and obviously the aftercare programs have to be individualized. However, it is still possible and clinically wise to continue a combined behavioral program and, if indicated, medication in the aftercare program. Weight maintenance in the aftercare program is best managed with a behavioral contract. For a young high school student who has been physically active it is often effective to have her weighed by the school nurse every Monday and, if she is below her normal range, she cannot participate in any school sports or in gym classes for that week. Behavioral contracts for weight maintenance must be individualized and, obviously, for those patients who are not interested in physical activity, another type of contract will have to be arranged.

References

1 Keys, A.; Brozek, J.; Henschel, A.; Mickelsen, O.; Taylor, H.: The biology of human starvation (University of Minnesota Press, Minneapolis 1950).

2 Dally, P.; Sargant, W.: A new treatment of anorexia nervosa. Br. med. J. *1:* 1770–1773 (1960).

3 Crisp, A.: A treatment regimen for anorexia nervosa. Br. J. Psychiat. *112:* 505–512 (1965).

4 Halmi, K.; Sherman, B.: Prediction of treatment response in anorexia nervosa; in Obiols Ballus, Gonzalez Monclus, Developments in psychiatry, vol. 2, pp. 609–614 (Elsevier/North-Holland Biomedical Press, Amsterdam 1979).

5 Needleman, H.; Waber, D.: Use of amitriptyline in anorexia nervosa; in Vigersky, Anorexia nervosa, pp. 357–362 (Raven Press, New York 1977).

6 Mills, L.: Amitriptyline therapy in anorexia nervosa. Lancet *ii:* 687 (1976).

7 Halmi, K.; Eckert, E.; Falk, J.: Cyproheptadine, an antidepressant and weight-inducing drug for anorexia nervosa. Psychopharm. Bull. *1:* 103–105 (1983).

8 Lacey, J.; Crisp, A.: Hunger, food-intake and weight: the impact of clomiprimine on a refeeding anorexia nervosa population. Post-grad. med. J. *56:* suppl. 1, pp. 79–85 (1980).

9 Holt, S.; Ford, M.; Grant, S.; Heading, R.: Abnormal gastric emptying in primary anorexia nervosa. Br. J. Psychiat. *139:* 550–552 (1981).

10 Saleh, J.; Lebwohl, P.: Metoclopramide-induced gastric emptying in patients with anorexia-nervosa. Am. J. Gastroent., N.Y. *74:* 127–132 (1980).

11 Gross, H.; Ebert, M.; Faden, E.; Goldberg, S.; Nee, L.; Kaye, W.: A double-blind controlled trial of lithium carbonate in primary anorexia nervosa. J. clin. Psychopharmacol. *1:* 376–381 (1981).

12 Johanson, A.; Knorr, N.: *L*-Dopa as treatment of anorexia nervosa; in Vigersky, Anorexia nervosa, pp. 363–372 (Raven Press, New York 1977).

13 Moore, R.; Mills, I.; Forster, A.: Naloxone in the treatment of anorexia nervosa: effect of weight gain and lipolysis. J. R. Soc. Med. *74:* 129–131 (1981).

14 Redmond, D.; Swann, A.; Henninger, G.: Phenoxybenzamine in anorexia nervosa. Lancet *ii:* 307 (1976).

15 Pope, H.; Hudson, J.; Jonas, J.; Yurgelun-Todd, D.: Bulimia treated with imipramine: a placebo-controlled double-blind study. Am. J. Psychiat. *140:* 554–558 (1983).

16 Sabine, E.; Yonace, A.; Farrington, A.; Barratt, K.; Wakeling, A.: Bulimia nervosa: a placebo-controlled double-blind therapeutic trial of mianserin. Br. J. clin. Pharmacol. *15:* 1955–2025 (1983).

17 Walsh, T.; Steward, J.; Wright, L.; Harrison, W.; Roose, S.; Glassman, A.: Treatment of bulimia with monoamine oxidase inhibitors. Am. J. Psychiat. *139:* 1629–1630 (1982).

18 Rau, J.; Struve, F.; Green, R.: Electro-encephalographic correlates of compulsive eating. Clin. Electroenceph. *10:* 180–189 (1979).
19 Wermuth, B.; Davis, K.; Hollister, L.; Stunkard, A.: Phenytoin treatment of the binge-eating syndrome. Am. J. Psychiat. *134:* 1249–1253 (1977).
20 Gull, W.: Anorexia nervosa (apepsia histerica, anorexia histerica). Trans. Clin. Soc. Lond. *7:* 22–28 (1874).
21 Russell, G.: The management of anorexia nervosa. Symp. Anorexia nervosa and Obesity; R. Coll. Phys. Edinburgh, vol. 42, pp. 44–52 (Constable, Edinburgh 1973).
22 Brady, J.; Reiger, W.: Behavior treatment of anorexia. Proc. Int. Symp. Behav. Mod., Minneapolis 1972 (Appleton Century Crofts, New York 1972).
23 Lang, P.: Behavior therapy with a case of anorexia nervosa; in Ullman, Krosner, Case studies in behavior modification, pp. 217–223 (Holt, Rinehart & Winston, New York 1965).
24 Hallsten, E.: Adolescent anorexia nervosa treated by desensitization. Behav. Res. Therapy *3:* 87–92 (1965).
25 Schnurer, A.; Rubin, R.; Roy, A.: Systematic desensitization of anorexia nervosa seen as a weight phobia. J. Behav. Ther. exp. Psychiat. *4:* 149–153 (1973).
26 Bachrach, A.; Erwin, W.; Mohr, J.: The control of eating behavior in an anorexic by operant conditioning techniques; in Ullman, Krosner, Case studies of behavior modification, pp. 153–163 (Holt, Rinehart & Winston, New York 1965).
27 Leitenberg, H.; Agras, W.; Thomson, L.: A sequential analysis of the effect of selective positive reinforcement in modifying anorexia nervosa. Behav. Res. Therapy *6:* 211–218 (1968).
28 Pertschuk, M.-J.; Edwards, N.; Pomerleau, O.F.: A multiple baseline approach to behavioral intervention in anorexia nervosa. Behav. Res. Therapy *9:* 368–376 (1971).
29 Agras, S.; Barlow, D.; Chapin, H.; Abel, G.; Leitenberg, H.: Behavior modification of anorexia nervosa. Archs gen. Psychiat. *30:* 279–286 (1974).
30 Binder, B.; Freeman, D.; Stunkard, A.: Behavior therapy of anorexia nervosa: effectiveness of activity as a reinforcer of weight gain. Am. J. Psychiat. *126:* 1093–1098 (1970).
31 Bhanji, S.; Thompson, J.: Operant conditioning in the treatment of anorexia nervosa: a review and retrospective study of 11 cases. Br. J. Psychiat. *124:* 166–172 (1974).
32 Halmi, K.; Powers, P.; Cunningham, S.: Treatment of anorexia nervosa with behavior modification: effectiveness of formula feeding and isolation. Archs gen. Psychiat. *32:* 93–96 (1975).
33 Kehrer, H.: Behandlung der Anorexia nervosa mit Verhaltenstherapie. Med. Klin. *70:* 427–432 (1975).
34 Liebman, R.; Minuchin, S.; Baker, L.: An integrated treatment program for anorexia nervosa. Am. J. Psychiat. *131:* 432–436 (1974).
35 Rosman, B.; Minuchin, S.; Liebman, R.; Baker, L.: Input and outcome of family therapy in anorexia nervosa; in Claghorn, Successful psychotherapy, pp. 128–139 (Brunner-Mazel, New York 1976).
36 Garfinkel, P.; Moldolsky, H.; Garner, D.: The outcome of anorexia nervosa: significance of clinical features, body-image and behavior modification; in Vigersky, Anorexia nervosa, pp. 315–329 (Raven Press, New York 1977).
37 Agras, S.; Werne, J.: Behavior modification and anorexia nervosa: research foundations; in Vigersky, Anorexia nervosa, p. 291 (Raven Press, New York 1977).

38 Wulliemier, F.; Rossel, F.; Sinclair, K.: La thérapie comportemental de l'anorexie nerveuse. J. psychosom. Res. *19:* 267–272 (1975).
39 Eckert, E.; Goldberg, S.; Halmi, K.; Casper, R.; Davis, J.: Behavior therapy in anorexia nervosa. Br. J. Psychiat. *134:* 55–59 (1979).
40 Fairburn, C.: A cognitive behavioral approach to the treatment of bulimia. Psychol. Med. *11:* 707–711 (1981).
41 Rosen, J.; Leitenberg, H.: Bulimia nervosa: treatment with exposure and response prevention. Behav. Ther. *13:* 117–124 (1982).
42 Cinciripini, P.; Kornblith, S.; Turner, S.; Herson, H.: A behavioral program for the management of anorexia and bulimia. J. nerv. ment. Dis. *171:* 186–189 (1983).
43 Lacey, J.: Bulimia nervosa, binge eating and psychogenic vomiting: a controlled treatment study and long-term outcome. Br. med. J. *286:* 1609–1613 (1983).
44 Morgan, H.; Russell, G.: Value of family background in clinical features of predictors of long-term outcome in anorexia nervosa. Psychol. Med. *5:* 355–371 (1975).

4 The Treatment of Bulimia: an Overview

Joel Yager

Introduction

The clinical features of the disorder called bulimia are delineated in DSM III and described in detail in chapter 1. Bulimia is not a disease. Nor is it a simple habit. Bulimia is heterogeneous and, like pneumonia, it may result from a variety of causes. I have found it useful to conceptualize bulimia as a habit or behavioral pattern embedded in a personality, in turn embedded in a biology, and all this embedded in a culture in which bulimia seems to be developing at an increasing rate. In this regard, bulimia may be in part a culture-bound syndrome, as tied to the values and beliefs of contemporary North American and British life in the 1980s as *amok* is tied to the culture of rural Indonesia. A medical anthropologist considering causes and possible cures for the current eruption of bulimia would have a different perspective than the clinician who deals with the individual patient, or the researcher who focuses on purely biomedical aspects.

This formulation recognizes that great variation may exist at each of these levels. There are strong and weak habits, strong and weak personalities, some biologies with greater propensities for obesity than others, varying cultural pressures for preferred body shapes, and so forth. For some patients, bulimia may be the major psychiatric disorder, and the manifest problems of depression and low self-esteem may be largely secondary to the bulimic syndrome. For others, bulimia may be only the tip of the iceberg, just one among many ways in which a more central problem of drive and affect dysregulation finds expression.

Phenomenologically, bulimia shares common elements with addictions such as smoking and alcoholism, and with drive-related compulsions such as obesity. Many patients have various concurrent emotional and characterological problems, if not actual disorders: anxiety, depression, social phobias, impulsivity, emotional lability, rejection sensitivity, and problems with families and significant others. A sophisticated approach to treatment of the patient with bulimia must take these differences into account and develop individualized treatment plans, realizing that not all bulimics will respond to the same treatment. Experience has shown that many patients are not well-served by either a narrow therapeutic focus or by assembly line treatment programs.

The Treatment Literature

Professional literature on the treatment of bulimia is not extensive. At the start we would be well-advised to heed the caveat offered by *Russell* [1] regarding the results of treatment of anorexia nervosa. He cautioned that the effects of specific treatments could be assessed only when one knew something about the natural history of the 'untreated' disorder, and that all of the nonspecific effects of treatment programs had to be taken into account before specific aspects of the treatment were given credit for successful outcomes. In one of the earliest papers in this area, *Russell* [2] also contributed to an early prevailing sensibility about poor outcome for patients with bulimia, at least with regard to those with anorexia nervosa, by describing the prognosis for *bulimia nervosa* as 'ominous'. It is likely that the poor outcome in his patients reflects the fact that they required hospitalization, whereas many patients with bulimia in other series who have never been hospitalized, seem, on the whole, to be less impaired and appear, in general, to have a good prognosis with a variety of treatment approaches.

Psychodynamic Psychotherapy

The literature on the purely psychodynamic psychotherapy of bulimia is heavily anecdotal and the reported results are not spectacular [3, 4]. Behaviorally and pharmacologically oriented clinicians and researchers often comment on the fact that many of the patients they see had previously been in individual psychotherapy but were not greatly benefitted. Of course, these represent only patients who were dissatisfied with their psychotherapy, not the successes. Also, since patients with bulimia may be secretive about their eating problems, even in psychotherapy, hiding them under the guise of depression or interpersonal problems instead, some poor results with bulimic symptoms may reflect the fact that these symptoms were not adequately considered in the treatment. Furthermore, many practitioners of individual psychotherapy may not have been well-schooled in the treatment of eating disorders. Psychodynamically oriented psychotherapy, which in practice usually includes many subtle behavioral components, may not yet have received a fair trial in the treatment of bulimia. Many authorities currently agree that comprehensive treatment programs for bulimia should include, but not be limited to, components of insight-oriented psychotherapy. Our experience confirms this. Many patients resent being treated in 'purely' behavioral or 'purely' medical programs, and make their needs and desires for psychodynamic treatments known to the clinicians in no uncertain terms. The issues brought forth in psychodynamic treatment include the wide range commonly seen with predominantly late adolescent and young adult women: psychosexual development, relations with and emancipation from parents, friendships and intimacies, direction and values, femininity and role confusion, loneliness, frustrations, sense of self, trusting one's own judgment, tensions and release, gratifications, lack of assertiveness, control, lack of control and the like.

Family Therapy

In family therapies, these issues are similarly raised, and the therapy may deal with various problems regarding value conflicts, control issues, conflicting needs and expectations among family members, clarification of hidden role assignments, generational boundary confusions, distorted and misdirected concerns and ineffective communication patterns [5]. Family therapy is discussed in chapter 5.

Cognitive Psychotherapy

Cognitive behavior modification in combination with insight-oriented discussions may be more applicable to bulimic disorders. These therapies have previously been described for obese patients [6–8], for patients with anorexia nervosa [9], and more recently for patients with bulimia [10]. *Fairburn* [10] described the treatment of 11 patients, averaging 25 years of age, who had been bulimic for an average of 4 years. 5 of these patients previously had anorexia nervosa. He treated the patients individually for an average length of 7 months. He focused initially on the control of food and eating and then shifted to cognitive therapy for a broader range of problems. Treatment was divided into 2 phases. Phase 1 lasted for about 8 weeks of frequent visits, 2–3 times a week. During this time the patient was required to keep a detailed eating and behavioral diary, was educated about bulimia and was put on a rigid schedule of eating. Often the family was seen as well. In his view, once eating was regulated, vomiting took care of itself. In phase 2, patients were taught appropriate coping strategies as alternatives to their binge-eating, and a variety of cognitive psychotherapy methods were employed. Throughout treatment, the patients were given responsibility for regulating their own food intake and no outside controls were applied. By the end of the treatment, 9 of the 11 stopped bingeing and vomiting entirely, and maintained this improvement at follow-up, on the average of almost a year later. At that time, most of the patients had gained a few kilograms.

Classical Behavioral Psychotherapies

More classical behavior therapies for bulimia have been reported by several authors [11–14]. These approaches concern themselves with precise aspects of the patient's behavior. A variety of behavioral techniques have been employed including self-monitoring, targeting, graphing, stimulus control and both positive and negative reinforcements. *Long and Cordle's* [11] report is typical. They described 2 patients, 1 with bulimic anorexia nervosa and bulimia and the other with stress-related episodes of binge-eating and vomiting. These were the first 2 bulimic patients treated by these therapists, and no efforts were made to select especially suitable patients for this treatment. Therapy for the first patient involved 40 1-hour sessions over 10 months, and the second had 12 1-hour sessions over 3 months. Techniques included behavioral self-control procedures such as diary-keeping, self-monitoring, weekly self-targeting of expected behavior, display on a graph, positive reinforcement with praise, stimulus control such as relaxation training, and built-in 'time-graduated response to delay', e.g. getting the patient to not surrender to bingeing or vomiting impulses when they arose. The patients were provided with dietary education. 'Educational' sessions included many new or reformulated attributions around eating, and additional foods were introduced into the diet. Patients were also taught to identify and then alter their maladaptive thoughts. The patient with anorexia nervosa, who had binged on the average of 8 times a week, stopped binge-eating after 32 sessions. Her vomiting stopped about 1 month afterward, an observation worth noting since the two are not necessary coterminous. The second patient, who averaged 11 episodes of binge-eating and vomiting per week, stopped these behaviors completely after 7 treatment sessions. These gains were maintained in follow-ups of 9–12 months.

Whereas most behavior therapists concentrate on binge-eating and assume that improvement in vomiting will follow, *Rosen and Leitenberg* [12] took an opposite approach, suggesting that vomiting which reduced anxiety is a more appropriate focus for attention than binge-eating. They described the treatment of a 21-year-old woman, symptomatic for 6 years, who had been binge-eating about once a day but vomiting several times a day, the vomiting occurring after moderate meals as well as following large binges. Using in vivo exposure, the therapist sat with the patient while she ate large meals, junk food and snack foods either in a local restaurant or at the clinic. In sessions the patient was not permitted to vomit, but was required to eat enough to make herself slightly uncomfortable, sit through and experience the discomfort without vomiting, and express her thoughts about the discomfort until the urge to vomit passed. Each of the three types of overeating (large meals, junk foods and snack foods) was dealt with independently. The vomiting stopped after 44 days with only one breakthrough during the 10 months follow-up. These authors noted that the compulsive urges dropped off only after the subjective anxiety abated, i.e. the patient could stop the behaviors but still felt anxious about it for a while. During follow-up she gained 7 lb (3 kg), but handled it without undue difficulty.

Kenny and Solyom [13] used aversive conditioning on a patient whose treatment they described in detail. This 21-year-old woman binged and purged an average of 3 times per day for several years. In the treatment, overeating and vomiting were divided into 8 discrete steps. The patient was asked to clearly imagine doing each of these 'subroutines' in her mind, and when she had each image clearly in mind, a painful electrical shock was administered to her middle finger. 30 s elapsed between tests and the whole routine was repeated 8 times per session. Sessions were conducted daily and lasted 40–45 min. The entire 22 sessions treatment was completed over a 5-week period. She stopped vomiting entirely after the 15th session of treatment. During a 3-month follow-up she did not resume vomiting, gained no weight and developed no substitute symptoms. It is important to note that her Minnesota Multiphasic Personality Inventory (MMPI) and 16 Personality Factor Profiles were in the normal range and she was described as warm and personable. Although her work and social life were impaired due to her symptoms, she was able to work and had never been hospitalized.

To sum up, in uncontrolled trials individually administered cognitive and behavioral therapy appears to be effective in reducing and eliminating eating binges and vomiting for many patients. But it is difficult to assess what the specific therapeutic factors are. Perhaps the patients who came in for treatment were particularly ready to change and had excellent relationships with these highly involved, well-educated, active therapists. My colleagues and I have conducted a magazine-based survey that included questions about help-seeking and satisfaction among bulimic women. Only about 55% of the approximately 80 women who reported being treated with behavior modification for their eating problems were 'somewhat' or 'very satisfied' with the outcome, and indeed only a very small percentage were 'very satisfied'. This was not very different than views about dynamic psychotherapy [*Yager, Landsverk, Lee-Benner, Johnson,* unpublished]. Great variation exists in the conduct of behavior therapy, just as in individual dynamically oriented psychotherapy. Variables include the skills of the therapists in selecting and applying the right behavioral approach with a given patient, the willingness of the patients to submit to and comply with various behavior modification procedures, other clinical and motivational features of the patients and the specific patient-therapist mix. Not all behavior therapy is as elegantly or competently applied as by those who contribute to the literature, and unsuccessful treatment cases or series are rarely published.

Group Psychotherapy

Group psychotherapy, ordinarily combining psychodynamic and behavior techniques, currently enjoys increasing popularity for patients with bulimia. The empirical data base upon which this popularity rests is small but growing. A number of these earlier reports [15–18] are reviewed in chapter 16.

Johnson et al. [19] recently described the experiences of the Michael Reese Hospital group therapy project. A 12-session cognitive-behavioral group program has yielded significant reduction in binge and vomiting frequency, at least in the short run. This program includes attention to eating patterns, thoughts about body shape, femininity, interpersonal issues and related topics. Careful diaries are kept throughout. The group includes cognitive restructuring, some role-playing and relaxation-training and discussions aimed at relapse prevention.

Our own recent experiences at the University of California, Los Angeles (UCLA), confirm the value of groups, but make clear that the delineation of specific therapeutic factors may be difficult. There are currently 11 active therapy groups in our clinic with a variety of compositions and therapeutic orientations. Such elusive influences as 'group pressure' and 'expectation' (e.g. consistent and in some cases unrelenting group encouragement and demands) seem powerful. For those patients without severe personality disorders, the reduction of bingeing and vomiting behavior in cognitive-behavioral groups is often rapid and dramatic. By 2–3 months (8–12 weeks) the large majority, and in some groups all, of the patients have entirely stopped or have greatly reduced their bingeing and vomiting symptoms. That behavioral methods per se may not be necessary, over and above strong expectation, is suggested by the following observations. One group, conducted primarily along group psychodynamic lines without explicit behavioral methods, witnessed a revolt of the patients early on – they refused to fill out preliminary eating diaries and virtually sabotaged the therapists' efforts at systematic data collection from the start. Nevertheless, the group 'culture' strongly supported cessation of symptoms, and within a few months all patients stopped binge-eating and vomiting. The group met for almost a year, and in the last several months dealt exclusively with such issues as families, friendship and work relationships, sexuality, intimacy and aspirations. Bulimic symptoms per se became a thing of the past [*Thompson, Kleeman,* unpublished].

In another one of our groups that did use cognitive and behavioral methods including diaries more successfully, two thirds of the patients stopped binge-eating and vomiting within a month, and almost all the others had reduced frequency. 1 woman who was initially scheduled to join this group was out of town and missed the first month's meetings. She had been markedly bulimic for more than 10 years. When she returned and anticipated joining the group as a late starter, having heard about the progress of the other group members, she stopped binge-eating and vomiting entirely 4 days before attending her first group meeting, so as 'not to be behind the others'.

Goff has established an intensive group psychotherapy experience for bulimics at the University of Minnesota, modelled after the Alcoholics Anonymous programs. The program requires a substantial commitment of time and further demands that patients immediately stop all binge-eating and purging. For the initial 2-week phase patients are expected to attend several hours of meetings and have dinner together each week night. A less intensive group program follows for the next several months. As might be expected, there is a high drop-out rate, but for those who stay through the period of the treatment, *Goff* [unpublished] indicates that the long-term results are good.

Combined Group and Individual Treatment

We have recently described in detail a year's experience with a combined psychodynamic-behavioral group [20]. Of 19 patients who attended the group at least once, 11 remained in active treatment for a minimum of 10 months. Of these, 10 were Caucasian and 1 was black. Their average age was 23 years. At the time of initial assessment all but 1 were binge-eating and vomiting at least daily, the majority several times daily (1 binged and purged only 5 times a week). 5 were chronic laxative abusers, 5 regularly took diet pills and 4 were compulsive exercisers.

8 had previously been in outpatient psychotherapy, and 3 had psychiatric hospitalizations together with trials of various psychiatric medications. Only 1 had frank anorexia nervosa in the past, but 2 had borderline cases of

anorexia nervosa. In addition to bulimia, 6 had possible affective disorders, 3 had borderline personality disorders, 1 had an avoidant personality disorder and 1 had serious alcohol abuse. Since all but 1 were in individual therapy concurrent with group treatment and 3 were on medication, this program is best considered a multidimensional combined group and individual therapy program. At the time of follow-up, up to 18 months after this group ended, information was available on 9 of the patients. 3 had completely stopped binge-eating and vomiting, 4 had marked reduction in symptoms (3 were bingeing and vomiting no more than 3 times a week and 1 only twice per week) and 2 reported no change. Those reporting no change included 1 woman who also had a possible affective disorder, chronic post-traumatic stress disorder and ego dystonic homosexuality, and another who regularly used diet pills and laxatives. The 1 patient in the group who was not in concurrent individual therapy (and who received no medication), reduced her binges from 5/week and vomiting episodes from 10–20 per week to 3/week for each.

Techniques used in the group included education and information sharing, encouragement and support, psychodynamically based insight-oriented interpretations, strict rules regarding attendance, diaries, cognitive techniques and social skills training via role play, among others. This report discussed issues of patient selection, group composition, dropouts and many other aspects of therapy.

When we compare *Lacey's* [18] impressive results (see chapter 16) with that of the UCLA combined program, and with the medication studies to be subsequently discussed, several points merit attention. First, the level of psychopathology in *Lacey's* [18] patients seems to be far less than in the UCLA group, i.e. sicker patients were excluded. Second, his patients committed themselves (and were apparently able) to complete daily diaries, a task which many patients in a variety of settings have been reluctant to cooperate with and with which they often fail to comply. Third, the methods used were comprehensive and included attention to normal eating with carefully regulated and prescribed meals, as well as to bulimic symptoms and psychological issues.

Medications

Several types of medications have been used for the treatment of bulimia. It would appear that *some* medications offer *some* promise for *some* patients, but the picture is not at all clear. Each medication has its own advocates, but proper criteria have not been established for the selection of patients for each drug. Nor has convincing evidence been offered to show that improvement is due to specific medication effects on bulimia per se rather than to placebo effects or other less direct (e.g. antidepressant) effects.

Medications: Anticonvulsants

Diphenylhydantoin

The medication that received earliest attention for bulimia was diphenylhydantoin. *Green and Rau* [21] reported an open trial study in which 9 of 26 patients with compulsive eating disorders treated with 400 mg/day of diphenylhydantoin improved, while 17 had no response or an inadequate trial. Of the 12 patients with abnormal EEGs in this series (primarily non-specific spike and wave patterns) 6 responded, whereas only 3 of the 14 patients with normal EEGs responded. These authors further categorized a subgroup of 7 of these patients as 'true compulsive eaters': patients with irregular, unpredictable, ego-dystonic binge-eating, usually preceded by an inability to concentrate, accompanied by depersonalization and detachment, and followed by sleepiness and confusion. Using an expanded series of patients, these authors further attempted to characterize those who would best respond based on soft neurological signs and EEG findings [22]. Of 23 patients in this series who were adequately treated with diphenylhydantoin, 12 were reported improved and 11 not improved (although improvement is not further defined in this paper). No single clinical sign or EEG finding taken alone was significantly correlated with drug response. However, when the sum of all 10 soft signs plus the EEG were taken together, the resulting score was weakly but significantly correlated with improvement. The soft signs included rage attacks, headaches, dizziness, stomach aches, nausea, paresthesias, convulsions (present in only 1 of 29), perceptual disturbances, other compulsions and a family history of epilepsy (present in 2 of 28).

Moore and Rakes [23] reported the treatment of another patient who had severe episodes of binge-eating during which she ate most of her waking hours for 4–5 weeks at a time. Her EEG showed 14 and 6/s spikes in the right temporal and occipital areas while awake, and similar spikes in the left occipital area following sedation. This patient improved dramatically within 4 days after starting diphenylhydantoin 300 mg/day, and she remained symptom-free for a year. Her symptoms returned within 5 weeks of discontinuing the drug, but they disappeared entirely once again within 1 week following its resumption, and this improvement lasted for an additional 18-month period of follow-up. These authors strongly suggest that for patients with episodic ego-dystonic binge-eating an EEG should be obtained, and if abnormalities are found a trial of diphenylhydantoin should be instituted.

The most sophisticated study to date of the use of diphenylhydantoin in bulimic patients was reported by *Wermuth* et al. [24]. In this study 19 subjects completed a 12-week double-blind crossover trial using diphenylhydantoin 300 mg/day or placebo. Inclusion criteria were similar to DSM III criteria for bulimia. All subjects were women. Their average age was 26 years. Of the 19, 9 were of normal weight, 4 overweight, 5 obese, and 1 had frank anorexia nervosa. 2 had past histories of anorexia nervosa. 7 had abnormal EEGs: small sharp spikes in 4 patients, diffuse spikes in 2 patients, and bitemporal slowing (left greater than right) in 1 patient. Of the 10 patients who started with diphenylhydantoin, 7 reduced their number of binges. In 3 patients, frequency of binge episodes diminished from about 3–4 per week to about 1 per 10 days. Changes were less dramatic for the others. Of note, only 1 person reported daily binge episodes at the outset, and that patient recorded no improvement. When placebo was substituted for active drug 3 out of the 7 who had previously improved experience an increase in their binges, but none to the baseline level, and 4 experienced even further improvement. Of the 3 who did not initially improve on the drug, the switch to placebo resulted in 1 becoming worse and 2 having fewer binges. Only 2 of the 9 patients who started with placebo had slight initial improvement while the rest remained unchanged or became worse in comparison to their baseline. However, when diphenylhydantoin was substituted for placebo at the crossover, some improvement was reported by 7 of the 9 and was 'marked' for 4. To summarize, 14 of 19 patients appeared to benefit from diphenylhydantoin, although marked improvement occurred in only 6. Only 1 patient stopped binge-eating entirely whereas others typically reduced their binge frequency from about 3–4 times per week to 1 per 1–2 weeks. In this study EEG abnormalities were *not* found to be correlated with improvement. Nevertheless, the accumulated experience suggests that diphenylhydantoin can be helpful for some patients.

Carbamazepine

Recently 6 bulimic patients were treated with carbamazepine in a double-blind crossover trial [25]. Only 1 patient responded, and dramatically so. Of note, the patient had a history suggestive of bipolar disorder. She had started psychotherapy shortly before entering the project. During the initial and final 6-week period, when taking placebo, she was symptomatic. When on active drug during the study she stopped completely. This 1 case raises the interesting possibility that there may be a subgroup of bulimics with mood instability who might benefit from carbamazepine.

Medications: Antidepressants

Antidepressant medications used to treat bulimia have included monoamine oxidase inhibitors (MAOIs), tricyclic and tetracyclic drugs. Several rationales have guided these therapeutic attempts. First, a high prevalence of affective disturbance has been seen in bulimic patients, although the extent to which these features represent primary affective disorder or secondary affective disturbance is not resolved [26, 27]. The high prevalence of affective disturbance found in first-degree relatives in some, but not all, studies has contributed to the hypothesis that in some patients bulimia may represent a 'masked' affective disorder or a depressive equivalent. Second, many patients with bulimia have been described as having atypical depression, hysteroid dysphoria, or rejection sensitivity; affective and characterologic features are reported to sometimes respond to treatment with antidepressants, particularly MAOIs.

MAOIs

Walsh et al. [28] described 6 patients with bulimia and atypical depression, all of whom responded dramatically to treatment with MAOIs. These patients were women in their twenties and thirties who had been bulimic for 3–15 years. In 5 of the 6 patients bulimic episodes occurred several times per day, and in the remaining patient twice per week. 5 patients received phenelzine 60–90 mg/day, and the sixth received tranylcypromine 40 mg/day. All patients improved dramatically within several weeks, 4 having completely stopped their bulimic episodes and the other 2 having no more than 1–2 episodes per month. 1 patient remitted for 1 month only. These researchers are currently conducting a double-blind treatment study using MAOIs for bulimic patients and early results are promising.

The accumulated experience of clinicians at UCLA also indicates that MAOIs may be useful for patients who present with both atypical depression and bulimia. Many of our patients when treated with MAOIs have reported an improvement in mood and a reduction in their pressure to binge-eat. A few of our patients have been unable to tolerate the medication because they developed hypotension, and 1 patient with labile mood developed severe insomnia and became mildly hypomanic. Some patients report that the requirement to restrict certain foods from their diet while taking MAOIs has helped the treatment, since they have to be more thoughtful about what they eat during a binge. This small degree of additional awareness sometimes helps them to exert greater self-control. However, several impulsive patients have eaten 'forbidden' foods and have experienced untoward reactions to the MAOIs. 1 patient, who had prior knowledge of potential negative effects, nevertheless snorted cocaine while on phenelzine and developed hallucinosis for several days. She had used cocaine on occasion prior to taking phenelzine, but had never experienced this type of reaction. This case suggests that impulsive drug-using patients may be at particular risk and/or difficult to manage with MAOIs. Finally, before MAOIs are oversold as curative, it should be pointed out that we and others have also seen a number of patients who did not improve on MAOIs.

Tricyclic and Tetracyclic Antidepressants

Pope and Hudson [29] and *Pope* et al. [30] have reported tricyclic antidepressants to be very useful in the treatment of bulimia. They first described an uncontrolled trial in which 8 women were treated with tricyclic antidepressants alone or in combination [29]. These women were 19–49 years old and had been binge-eating from 1 to 14 times per week. In response to the drug, 3 had 'marked improvement' of greater than 90% reduction or cessation of symptoms. 1 of these patients had been binge-eating twice per day for years, another twice per day for a year, and a third once per week for 6 months. All of these patients responded only when lithium carbonate was added to the imipramine. An additional 3 of the 8 patients had 'moderate' improvement of greater than 50% reduction of symptoms. The 2 nonresponders were reported to have personality disorders, 1 borderline and 1 cyclothymic. Therapeutic blood levels were assayed for all patients.

This group then conducted a placebo-controlled double-blind study using imipramine in 22 chronically bulimic women [30]. Patients were recruited into the study by means of advertisements. All had been bulimic for at least 1 year, had binges followed by purges at least twice per week, and had no significant suicidal ideation. Of the 70 or so inquiries, about 50 individuals were not accepted into the study for not meeting study criteria. Imipramine was administered double-blind in doses of up to 200 mg/day (controlled by the patient on the basis of side effects) for 6-week periods. Of

11 patients who started on active medication, 9 completed the trial and 2 were withdrawn due to allergic reactions. Among these patients, 6 were found to have other current DSM III diagnoses including 4 with major depression or dysthymic disorder (2 of whom had personality disorders as well), 1 with simple phobia and 1 with kleptomania. Of those on active medication, 4 had marked improvement (at least 75% decrease in symptoms), 4 moderate improvement (at least 50%), and 1 no significant improvement (less than 50% decrease). In the placebo group 1 had moderate improvement, 8 had no improvement and 1 became worse. 1 additional patient was withdrawn from the study after she attempted to overdose on placebo. Follow-up 1–8 months following completion of the study revealed that 20 of the 22 patients had received a complete trial of imipramine or another antidepressant. Of these, 18 had moderate to marked reduction of binge-eating, and 7 (6 of whom had been symptomatic for 2–14 years) stopped binge-eating entirely.

These results are impressive, but several limitations of the study must be pointed out. First, the patients were specifically recruited for a medication study. One can assume that patients agreeing to participate believed that medications might be helpful, a bias not universally shared by all bulimic patients. Second, and perhaps more important, given the double-blind design, the placebo was inert rather than active (e.g. did not mimic the side effects such as dry mouth produced by imipramine). Since patients who experience side effects such as dry mouth, sedation, etc., are more likely to think they are on active drugs than those who do not, patients who believe (or who want to believe) in the efficacy of medication in the first place may be more likely to improve on active drugs for these purely psychological reasons. The same limitation applies to the diphenylhydantoin study described earlier. It is likely that those receiving active drugs were more likely to 'know' it on the basis of subjective side effects than those who were not.

This group has recently described its experiences with 65 bulimic patients treated with antidepressants, and has provided a clinical algorithm for their use. 75% of patients were at least moderately improved (although as the authors point out this may still signify a troubling level of persistent symptoms). Nevertheless, while admittedly based mostly on work with uncontrolled cases, their observations are helpful for clinicians. They discuss issues of drug refusal, compliance, side effects and their management and related clinical realities [31].

Herzog [32], in a less optimistic report, described his attempt to treat 6 of 8 adolescent bulimic patients with imipramine. Only 4 even accepted the drug, and while their affect improved initially, only 2 sustained the improvements. No mention was made of the drug effect on the bulimic symptoms. Furthermore, in a separate retrospective uncontrolled study of antidepressant treatment in 22 bulimic patients, this group reported that at 3-month follow-up, only 23% of patients maintained a response to antidepressants, defined as a 50% or greater reduction in bingeing [33].

Finally, another elegant study raises further doubts about the potential utility of related antidepressants. *Sabine* et al. [34] conducted a double-blind placebo-controlled study on 50 patients with bulimia nervosa using mianserin hydrochloride, a tetracyclic piperazino-azepine that is effective in the treatment of depression. Patients were excluded from the study if they had any other severe major psychiatric illness or weight loss of greater than 25% of original weight, or were 75% or less of ideal weight for height. At the start of the study none of the patients was in concurrent psychological treatment from any other source. In an effort to reduce the recognition of drowsiness due to mianserin all drugs were given at night. The trial lasted for 8 weeks. A dropout rate of approximately 30% was observed in both the drug and placebo groups, and those who completed the study were similar in age and clinical features. Both groups improved on measures of bulimic behaviors, eating attitudes, anxiety and depression, with no differences between the placebo and active drug group. But most notably, the number of days per week in which the subjects reported bingeing, vomiting or purging did not change throughout the trial for either group.

Here, then, are two placebo-controlled double-blind studies of antidepressants with markedly contrasting findings: imipramine seems very helpful whereas mianserin is much less helpful in reducing bulimic episodes. What can account for the differences? These two studies are not perfectly comparable on several grounds. First, imipramine and mianserin are chemically different. Mianserin, like amitryptiline, has been reported to stimulate appetite sometimes and may simply not be as useful for bulimic patients as imipramine. Second, the level of depression in the mianserin study was generally very low, whereas almost half of those in the imipramine study had a concurrent affective disorder diagnosis. This would suggest, to no one's surprise, that bulimic patients with affective disturbance may be more likely to improve on antidepressants than those without affective disturbance. Third, the nature and extent of other therapies or self-help efforts the patients might have employed once the studies began is unknown. Whereas the patients were not in other treatments at the start of the studies, neither report specified whether other forms of therapy were forbidden during the trial. And since for many of the patients the drug trials represented a major personal push toward health, some patients may have initiated other treatments as well.

It should be noted that neither of these studies are concerned with the difficult patients who have concurrent major personality disorders with features of marked emotional instability, somatic hyperreactivity and other borderline and histrionic characteristics, or with substance abusers. I would estimate that such patients represent at least 10–20% of bulimics seen in most practices, and a higher percentage of those seen in referral centers.

Other Medications

Several drugs merit brief comment, although none are of proven efficacy for bulimia. Lithium is risky at best in patients with severe purging because of the dangers related to rapid shifts of fluid and electrolytes [35]. Patients with affective instability who for other reasons require a trial of lithium should be treated only under controlled conditions – to start, preferably in a hospital.

On theoretical grounds, dopamine receptor-blocking agents might be helpful since they have been shown to block stress-induced overeating in laboratory animals [36]. But the clinically available dopamine receptor-blockers often have unpleasant subjective side effects, and their use is often accompanied by weight gain. Metoclopramide, an agent that enhances gastric emptying, has been used in occasional patients but is of questionable value [37]. There is no literature regarding the use of benzodiazepines in the treatment of bulimia. Clinical trials with alprazolam are planned.

Finally, it has been theorized that naloxone, a narcotic antagonist, might diminish the extent to which feelings of tension are reduced by binge-eating, analogous to the drug's blockade of the 'rush' following heroin administration. This possibility warrants further study.

Further Considerations in Assessment and Treatment Planning for Bulimia

The sometimes contradictory reports discussed above indicate that patients may be helped substantially by cognitive-behavioral-psychodynamic treatment individually, and/or in groups, and/or with medication.

Furthermore, for research purposes, many studies excluded those especially difficult patients whose bulimic syndrome is embedded in a more pervasive character disturbance. One tentative conclusion might be that for the less disturbed patients treated by means of the various types of therapy described above, we might borrow the felicitous phrase of *Luborsky* et al. [38], borrowed from *Lewis Carroll,* and say 'everybody has won and we all shall have prizes'. But, in fact, we really do not know that to be true. For the more disturbed patient it may be, at least thus far, that no one has won, and the prizes are all still on the shelf.

The clinician trying to devise an effective treatment plan for a given patient must, then, consider some of the more subtle issues in the treatment situation, those that are often not documented in the quantitative studies. How much do the patient and the staff believe in the efficacy of the treatment being undertaken? What other 'nonspecific' treatment methods, such as self-help groups, 'rap' sessions and other supports, are being used concurrently with the 'active' treatment? How skillful are the staff in the treatment of those conditions – how much do they know, how therapeutically optimistic are they, and how rigorous and systematic are they in applying the treatment and in 'demanding' results? The patient's willingness and ability to adhere to treatment, regardless of the type of treatment, may be a most powerful predictor of good outcome. For example, ability to adhere to all parts of a total program, such as eating regular meals, may be as powerful a determinant as all other aspects of the treatment.

Such 'ability' may actually measure how ready the patient is for treatment: the patient's motivation, willpower and ability to sustain a course of action, including improvement. For the patient who is ready, any well-devised treatment may catalyze the transformation to healthier patterns, e.g. giving up the bulimic behaviors. Is the patient really ready to change? Why now?

Can any of the current theories regarding the causes of bulimia help us select treatment? In general, the more theories that are expounded about a problem, the less we know about it. And bulimia does not lack for explanations: cultural, psychological-developmental, feminist, learning, biological theories involving adiposity and/or adolescent hormonal changes, and/or affective vulnerability and so forth. Given that bulimia is not a disease but a syndrome or disorder, quite different from one extreme to the other, each theory probably does have something meaningful to contribute, but no one theory has all the answers (and, perhaps, none of the current theories has the best answers). With such complex problems, systems-thinking and a multifaceted approach is warranted. For example, until we know more, hypertension may best be treated by combining education, diet, other aspects of self-care involving 'life-style' change, as well as medication.

Comprehensive Assessment

Treatment planning must begin with comprehensive assessment. The initial assessment should attend to the clinical features of the patient's condition as enumerated below, to the beliefs of the patient and her significant others concerning the causes and cures, and to financial and social realities. All potential therapeutic receptor sites and points of leverage must be evaluated, including biological, psychological and social. The initial assessment of bulimia must also take heed of cost-benefit implications of treatment strategies so that the disorder is not unnecessarily overmedicalized, the patient is not sent for an unnecessary series of expensive laboratory studies (but necessary tests must not be neglected) and the risks of treatment, including medication side effects, and costs in time and money are considered.

Chief Complaint

What are the patient's complaints and concerns, and why is she coming for treatment now? Given that bulimia is becoming a more socially acceptable if not downright faddish problem, the discussion of the chief complaint must ascertain the extent to which the patient's complaints about bulimia are her 'ticket of admission' to treatment, perhaps masking other problems, such as suicidality, substance abuse, affective disorder, family problems, character problems and so forth. While the bulimia is of concern, it may be presented initially as a 'smokescreen' for more pervasive and profound disorders. Ironically, just a few years ago it was often the other way around, with patients presenting as depressed, for example, but hiding their bulimia.

Since most patients with bulimia have been symptomatic for years, the reasons for the timing of their presentation are often important. Is a change in the patient's social situation pressuring her to stop the symptoms more now than a year ago? Is she first able to admit to herself the seriousness of the symptoms? Has her bulimia just been humiliatingly discovered by a family member? Is she being reluctantly coerced into treatment by someone else?

Closely associated with this aspect of the chief complaint are the patient's views about the causes of the condition (e.g. tension release, self-destructive habit, 'deep-rooted emotional problems', desire to be thin, biological, etc.) and her views about what she needs from treatment (e.g. guidance, direction, willpower or inner strength, self-awareness and insight, hypnosis, medication, threat, dietary counseling). Treatment has the highest likelihood of succeeding when it is consistent with the patient's belief systems and values. Although patients may be 'educated' in treatment into accepting new ways of understanding their problems, their initial acceptance of treatment occurs most smoothly if the treatment is consistent with their prior assumptions. Some patients may refuse to be in groups, psychodynamic therapy or behavior therapy or to take medication, for a variety of reasons, both informed and irrational. Forcing people into treatments in which they do not believe rarely works.

With the chief complaint, it is important to ascertain what the patient is willing to give up in order to rid herself of the symptoms. How strong is her motivation for change? If she has kept herself at a very low weight, is she willing to shift her desired weight upward? If stopping the bulimic behavior will require her to eat regular meals and risk gaining 5–10 lb (2.3–4.6 kg), is she willing to gain some weight?

The history of the patient's past attempts at helping herself and her experience with professional and nonprofessional help should be elicited. What did not work at all and why? What does this suggest for future treatment planning?

Eating History

The eating history should include attention to childhood development, the patient's attitudes regarding her body and weight, her detailed weight history, and the onset, frequency, severity, maintenance and course of the various primary and associated symptoms of bulimia and anorexia nervosa. It is useful to ask the patient to keep baseline diaries of these symptoms and of related behaviors, moods, thoughts and circumstances. What are the rituals and circumstances surrounding eating, fasting and purging? What is the patient's mental state and level of awareness during binges? Are medications such as diet pills, laxatives, emetics or diuretics taken? Who knows about the rituals? How are symptomatic behaviors hidden and worked into the patient's day? How costly is the binged food? How is it obtained and where does the money come from? Are there associated compulsive oral behaviors such as gum chewing, nail biting or thumbsucking? How was the onset of various symptoms related to other major milestones and life events: menarche, the development of secondary sex characteristics, early sexual interests and activities, the beginning or cessation of birth control pills, diets or smoking, the formulation or dissolution of relationships, leaving from home or returning to it, relationships with and among other family members, etc.? Does the patient ever eat normally? Does she have adequate knowledge about proper nutrition? Does she eat regular meals? Can she do this alone? Only with others? Never with others? To what extent do these symptoms interfere with family and social life, school and work?

Past Psychiatric History

Particular attention is paid to signs and symptoms of childhood and adolescent depression and to the onset of affective symptoms in relation to weight preoccupation and bulimia. Which came first is important, although this is frequently difficult to tease out. Specific therapeutic strategies are suggested when the affective disturbance is clearly felt to be primary. Characterologic issues are of equal importance: the nature, quality and durability of relationships with family and others; the modulation of thought, affect and behavior and the degree of impulsivity; sociopathic behaviors.

Associated substance abuse requires special attention: alcohol, amphetamines, cocaine, sedatives and others. Is the bulimia simply another form of substance abuse and an attempt at self-anesthesia in an impulse-ridden person? Are the other substances used in attempts to control the bulimia?

Past Medical History

What were the conditions of the mother's pregnancy? Was she taking any medication? What abnormalities occurred in delivery, neonatal and childhood periods? What were the patient's early feeding and development like? Does the patient have a physician, does the physician know about the eating disorder, and have appropriate physical and laboratory examinations been conducted? Are there dental problems, and if so, is the patient under the care of a dentist? Are the patient's menstrual periods normal? Does she have a gynecologist? Is the patient experiencing symptoms that might result from physical complications of her eating disorder?

Family History

What psychiatric and/or eating disorders are (or were) present in the patient's relatives? Whom does she resemble temperamentally and physically? Affective disturbance, alcoholism and eating/weight problems are especially relevant. What are relationships and communication like among family members and the patient? What attitudes about physical appearance, fitness, eating and individuation are held by family members? What beliefs do family members (and other significant persons) hold regarding the causes and proper treatments for the patient's problems? In what ways do they help and in what ways do they hinder help-seeking and treatment?

Social Background, Assets and Aspirations

The patient's current living situation, work/school status, networks and activities should be explored. Is she engaged in any goal-oriented activities or drifting? Is she self-reliant or dependent on others for her support? What does she expect of herself and plan for herself? Are her activities and abilities consistent with these aspirations, or is she unrealistic?

Mental Status

In addition to the usual components of the mental status examination, it is useful to try to determine the patient's basic coping styles, since these may partly determine the success or failure of certain treatment options. Patients who are information-seeking, active copers not only require education from their therapists, but also take well to professional and self-help groups. Patients with minimizing or avoidant styles may be skittish in groups. Those who are psychologically minded, or believe in psychogenesis, or have a greater sense of internal control of their destinies are more likely to profitably engage in insight-oriented therapies. Those who lack psychological mindedness or who attribute power over their lives only to outside forces may do better with directive, suggestive and behavioral therapies, where they are told what to do.

Other Components of Assessment

In addition to the clinical evaluation described above, assessment may include other components to further clarify various aspects of the patient's psychological and physical status. Although no psychological tests are definitive, we have often found the Eating Disorders Inventory, MMPI and Beck Depression Inventory to be helpful. Projective and neuropsychological testing have also been useful at times. Psychological testing is reviewed in chapter 14.

Patients with fatigue, irritability, lassitude, amenorrhea or oligomenorrhea and other specific medical complaints merit a physical examination with appropriate laboratory tests. Serum electrolytes are most useful [39, 40]. For low weight bulimics, those verging on anorexia nervosa, an EKG should be done. Although endocrine tests such as the dexamethasone suppression test and thyrotropin-releasing hormone (TRH) stimulation often yield abnormal findings [41], in practice they are of limited clinical utility and are unnecessary.

When the initial evaluation suggests that the patient's problems are sustained by forces within the family that might be amenable to change, or that the family contains resources that can potentially benefit the patient, it is useful to see the whole family, or at least those members most likely to be important for the treatment.

For the occasional patient whose clinical picture strongly suggests alterations in consciousness with episodic, totally uncontrollable bingeing rampages, an EEG should be considered, although in our experience positive findings have been rare.

Treatment Recommendations

Following the initial assessment, a series of treatment recommendations can be offered. Practically speaking, these must take into account the patient's beliefs and desires, financial means, and the available treatment resources. The patient's various problems must be given priority, and the most pressing addressed first. In developing a treatment algorithm the following decisions must be made.

Decision Regarding Hospitalization

In our experience, and in *Fairburn's* [42], hospitalization for bulimia should be recommended for any or all of the following circumstances. First, the patient has failed ordinarily high-potency, well-designed outpatient treatments and continues to demonstrate unremitting, severe bulimic behavior that jeopardizes health due to electrolyte or cardiac problems. Second, a medication trial on an antidepressant or lithium is indicated, but adequate safe monitoring or compliance is unlikely as an outpatient. Third, the patient is suicidal.

Patients' bulimic behaviors can virtually always be restrained, if not stopped, in closely monitored inpatient settings. Some patients feel that they are unable to keep themselves from bingeing and purging without such external control and find this respite useful. We have seen a number of patients consolidate the symptomatic gains made during inpatient hospitalization and remain much improved following discharge from the hospital, especially if they continue in outpatient treatment. However, we have also seen symptoms return rapidly following discharge. To date, systematic follow-up studies concerning the efficacy of hospital treatment for bulimia have not been conducted.

Decision Regarding Individual and/or Group Treatment

Several factors enter this decision, and no single answer can apply to all patients. Generally speaking, patients who do well in individual treatment can do well (sometimes more quickly) in combined treatment, and may do well in group treatment alone, particularly if they are otherwise in reasonably good psychological health. The skills of the therapists will determine the microconduct of therapy. In general, we believe that a combined dynamic-cognitive-behavioral approach, one that builds in expectations for change within a context of appropriate, meaningful and humane contingencies, has the best chance for sustained success. The addition of group therapy should always be considered for the patient in individual treatment alone who is not making progress at an acceptable rate.

In our experience patients with major characterological problems, particularly impulsivity and other borderline features, should not be immediately started in a group, and never without concurrent individual therapy. We saw many such patients attend only a few group sessions before leaving disruptively, or be unable to sustain participation in a manner that was constructive for other group members. Therefore, we have started to insist that the patients with obvious character problems start with a 'trial' of individual therapy alone before being admitted to a group, even when the patient has come to the clinic specifically seeking group treatment. After 1 or 2 months of individual treatment the individual therapist should be able to gauge the patient's commitment, staying power, tendency to distort and suitability for group therapy.

Decision Regarding Medication

When a patient initially presents with features of major depression, antidepressant medications should be offered at the start. For the patient who has been in active psychotherapeutic treatment for 2 months but is not making progress, a reassessment of the treatment plan is in order and medication should be considered. Anticonvulsants should be considered when patients present with the intermittent episodic binges described earlier.

Decision Regarding Family Intervention

Assuming the therapist is skillful in dealing with whole families, family members should be seen when they appear to be retarding improvement, or when they may offer some therapeutic leverage. Pertinent members of the patient's family of origin (parents and siblings) and/or family of insertion (spouse, children, in-laws) should be involved as needed. We have found family groups to help family members gain useful perspectives and techniques.

Decision Regarding Nutritional Counseling

For those patients who are inadequately informed about proper nutrition, counseling may be useful. Although many patients are quite knowledgeable about nutritional and caloric values of most foods, some are less informed and find sessions with a dietician to be an important adjunct to treatment.

Components of a Combined Therapy Program

To be successful, therapy must occur in a setting in which basic positive regard, honesty, genuineness, acceptance, warmth and flexibility are present. The patient's self-esteem and basic narcissistic needs must be appreciated and dealt with respectfully. In this context, the caring therapist can keep up gentle but firm expectations for improvement, always at a level which the therapist feels is realistic for the patient, yet not so great as to ensure failure. The therapist must consistently (but only genuinely) encourage the patient by constantly pointing out that she truly has the capacity for improvement at the pace that is being set. While respect and caring may be to some extent noncontingent, the regard of the therapist nevertheless has some expectations for the patient's improvement. With this background, the following components should be included.

Use of Diaries or Journals

At the start of treatment a diary or journal may help the patient to focus attention on the details of the binges and purges, together with their antecedents and consequences. Some patients take well to diaries, finding the required rigidity and structure to be reassuring. Others resent them, finding the task to be demeaning and infantile. As with other behavioral problems, some patients find that the discipline of keeping a diary may itself be therapeutic and help them to cut back on the frequency of binges and purges. However, many patients do not, and it is noteworthy that in the mianserin study previously described, daily diary-keeping (which was part of the control and active drug groups) did not result in a decrease in frequency of symptoms [34].

Nevertheless, a combination of encouragement and diary-keeping can be useful. Some patients are eager to graph a decrease in the number of binge and vomiting episodes per day or week. Others find more satisfaction in recording an increase in the number of binge- and/or purge-free days.

Normal, Planned Eating

Many bulimic patients rarely eat normal meals. We have found that as patients build normal meals into their days, a practice we strongly insist upon from the start, they find it easier to stop binge-eating. For some, binges are triggered by hunger which results from relative starvation during nonbinge periods. Dietary consultations and educational readings are used. Some patients require relatively rigid meal programs at the start, to prevent them from being overwhelmed and undone by too many choices. Introducing and insisting upon a normal meal plan is consistent with the general therapeutic principle of not stripping away certain defenses (e.g. compulsive ones such as binge-eating and purging) until they are replaced with better ones, or until the person has something else on which to rely (e.g. regular meals).

Basic Information about Bulimia

The therapist needs to provide information about the nature and treatment of bulimia and to encourage patients by telling stories about other patients who have done well, and how and why they did it. In addition to that which the therapist can provide, some recent popular books such as those by *Cauwels* [43] and by *Squire* [44] are very helpful. We also encourage patients to join national self-help groups for patients with eating disorders and to read their regularly published newsletters.

Patients' Beliefs and Attitudes

Important attitudes concerning her body, sense of worth, identity, values, goals, future, feminism, relations with parents, siblings and men need to be reviewed. The purpose is to identify distorted cognitions and self-defeating states of mind. Cognitive therapy/insight-oriented corrections of the misperceptions and faulty self-statements are appropriate. Techniques include interpretation, confrontation, distancing, externalization, thought-stopping, substitution and related strategies. Many of the faulty assumptions are similar to those described for patients with anorexia nervosa [9] and depression [45]. Realistic weight and body image goals must be set.

Appropriate Gratifications and Coping Mechanisms

Alternative gratifications and coping mechanisms to promote adaptive methods of tension reduction, direct methods of conflict resolution and problem-solving and mastery experiences need to be substituted for bulimic behaviors. The aim here is to help patients cope directly with their problems (e.g. deal with boyfriend, boss or mother) so that tension previously discharged through binge-eating may be averted. Substitute activities such as exercise may be helpful. In general, 'positive addictions' are encouraged [46], but not to the point where one all-consuming compulsion is simply substituted for another. Some patients have found the discussion by *Merzer* [47] called 'instead of eating', or '121 things to do instead of stuffing your face', helpful. For example, 1 patient came to realize that binge-eating helped her ignore the fact that she was lonely and desired affection. She bought a dog after not having had a pet for years and found that this new relationship helped mobilize her efforts to reduce her bulimic symptoms.

Environmental Contingencies

The environmental contingencies that promote symptoms must be analyzed and altered or controlled. These include space, time, setting and people. Just as behaviorally oriented weight reduction programs pay attention to where and when meals are taken, treatment programs for bulimia may benefit from a similar concern. Families, work-setting, roommates and other elements may constitute binge-evoking or binge-inhibiting salient environments [48].

Contracts

Contracts involving both positive and negative contingencies have been useful. Rewards may work if the initial incentive to improve is high and the rewards are meaningful. A negative contingency program may be considered for the recalcitrant patient, only if the therapist has an excellent relationship with the patient and believes that the patient is genuinely capable of making the planned degree of change. In my view, the proposed negative contingencies should never require the patient to perform a destructive or immoral act, but should be sufficiently powerful to assure success. The contingency must be individualized and meaningful. It is useful to have a contract written out, dated and signed. In one typical plan the negative contingency was introduced after a patient had been in treatment for several months and only 'pretended to get better'. But in my view, she had the capacity and was 'ripe' for change. The patient agreed that if she did not stop bingeing and purging within 2 weeks, I could mail to her boyfriend a letter she had written describing her bulimia. She vehemently did not want him to know about it. This plan was completely effective. She stopped her bulimic symptoms within the 2 weeks and has remained free of them for more than a year. With such a strategy it is critical that the patient's self-esteem be carefully supported throughout.

Persistent Food Preoccupations

Psychological immunization is helpful for persistent food preoccupation and periodic backsliding. Since many patients experience persistent food preoccupation at least for a while following cessation of their bingeing and purging behaviors, they need to be informed that this is common, so that when it happens they do not become utterly demoralized and completely give into their cravings. Similarly, careful analysis of situations most likely to evoke a nostalgic return of symptoms, and awareness that a small backslide need not herald an avalanche, may help prepare patients to contend with such temptations and minor transgressions [49, 50].

Mental Imagery Techniques

Finally, mental imagery techniques may enable patients to bypass ruminative, intellectualized defenses [51]. Some patients have only a limited capacity to image. But many who engage in these methods have found them to facilitate remarkably personal development and even to catalyze transformative changes, particularly in the adolescent and young adult still in the process of identity formation. For such patients, new levels of self-awareness and maturation may occur. Through imagery, I have seen several patients rapidly reconceptualize their bulimic symptoms, and see them for the first time as ineffective and defensive. In these patients, imagery appeared to help the patients more easily give up or grow beyond their bulimic symptoms.

Concluding Remarks

Bulimia is an extremely varied syndrome found in patients with a variety of character types, coping styles and associated psychiatric problems. Proper treatment of any given patient must take into account all of these differences as well as the patient's own attitudes and beliefs about treatment. The therapist must fully assess the biological, psychological, behavioral and social spheres so that unique aspects of each person's problem are understood and appreciated in the formulation of the treatment plan. A number of psychotherapeutic and medical techniques are available. Further research is necessary to pinpoint the specific therapeutic factors in these techniques, to better determine which type of patients are best treated by which treatments and to develop effective treatment methods for the significant minority of patients with severe character problems and/or anorexia nervosa whose bulimia is difficult to treat successfully with any of the currently available approaches.

References

1 Russell, G.: General management of anorexia nervosa and difficulties in assessing the efficacy of treatment; in Vigersky, Anorexia nervosa (Raven Press, New York 1977).
2 Russell, G.: Bulimia nervosa: an ominous variant of anorexia nervosa. Psychol. Med. *9:* 429–448 (1979).
3 Bruch, H.: Eating disorders: obesity, anorexia nervosa and the person within (Basic Books, New York 1973).
4 Wilson, C.: Fear of being fat: the treatment of anorexia nervosa and bulimia (Aronson, New York 1983).
5 Yager, J.: Anorexia nervosa and the family; in Lansky, Family therapy and major psychopathology (Grune & Stratton, New York 1981).
6 Stuart, R.; Davis, B.: Slim chance in a fat world (Research Press, Champaign 1972).
7 Mahoney, M.; Mahoney, K.: Permanent weight control (Norton, New York 1976).
8 Meichenbaum, D.: Cognitive-behavior modification (Plenum Press, New York 1977).
9 Garner, D.; Garfinkel, P.; Bemis, K.: A multidimensional psychotherapy for anorexia nervosa. Int. J. Eating Disord. *1:* 3–46 (1982).
10 Fairburn, C.: A cognitive behavioral approach to the treatment of bulimia. Psychol. Med. *11:* 707–711 (1981).
11 Long, C.; Cordle, C.: Psychological treatment of binge eating and self-induced vomiting. Br. J. med. Psychol. *55:* 139–145 (1982).
12 Rosen, J.; Leitenberg, H.: Bulimia nervosa: treatment with exposure and response prevention. Behav. Ther. *13:* 117–124 (1982).
13 Kenny, F.; Solyom, L.: The treatment of compulsive vomiting through faradic disruption of mental images. Can. med. Ass. J. *105:* 1071–1073 (1971).
14 Greenberg, D.; Marks, I.: Behavioral psychotherapy of uncommon referrals. Br. J. Psychiat. *141:* 148–153 (1982).
15 Boskind-Lodahl, M.; White, W.: The definition and treatment of bulimarexia in college women – a pilot study. J. Am. Coll. Hlth Ass. *27:* 84–87 (1978).
16 White, W.; Boskind-Lodahl, M.: An experiential-behavioral approach to the treatment of bulimarexia. Psychotherapy *18:* 501–507 (1981).
17 Dixon, K.; Kiecolt-Glaser, J.: An integrated group therapy approach to bulimia. Proc. 134th Am. Psychiatric Ass. Meet., New Orleans 1981.

18 Lacey, J.: Bulimia nervosa, binge-eating and psychogenic vomiting: a controlled treatment study and long-term outcome. Br. med. J. *286:* 1609–1613 (1983).
19 Johnson, C.; Connors, M.; Stuckey, M.: Short-term group treatment of bulimia. Int. J. Eating Disord. *2:* 199–208 (1983).
20 Roy-Byrne, P.; Lee-Benner, K.; Yager, J.: Group therapy for bulimia: a year's experience. Int. J. Eating Disord. *3:* 97–116 (1984).
21 Green, R.; Rau, J.: The use of diphenylhydantoin in compulsive eating disorders: further studies; in Vigersky, Anorexia nervosa (Raven Press, New York 1977).
22 Rau, J.; Green, R.: Soft neurological correlates of compulsive eaters. J. nerv. ment. Dis. *166:* 425–437 (1978).
23 Moore, S.; Rakes, S.: Binge-eating – therapeutic response to diphenylhydantoin: case report. J. clin. Psychiat. *43:* 385–386 (1982).
24 Wermuth, B.; Davis, K.; Hollister, L.; Stunkard, A.: Phenytoin treatment of the binge-eating syndrome. Am. J. Psychiat. *134:* 1249–1252 (1977).
25 Kaplan, A.; Garfinkel, P.; Darby, P.; Garner, D.: Carbamazepine in the treatment of bulimia. Am. J. Psychiat. *140:* 1225–1226 (1983).
26 Hudson, J.; Laffer, P.; Pope, H.: Bulimia related to affective disorder by family history and response to dexamethasone suppression test. Am. J. Psychiat. *139:* 685–687 (1982).
27 Walsh, B.; Poose, S.; Glassman, A.; Gladis, M.; Sadick, C.; Wright, L.: Eating disorders and depression. Proc. 136th Annu. Meet. Am. Psychiatric Ass., New York 1983.
28 Walsh, B.; Stewart, J.; Wright, L.; Harrison, W.; Roose, S.; Glassman, A.: Treatment of bulimia with monoamine oxidase inhibitors. Am. J. Psychiat. *139:* 1629–1630 (1982).
29 Pope, H., Jr.; Hudson, J.: Treatment of bulimia with antidepressants. Psychopharmacology *78:* 176–179 (1982).
30 Pope, H., Jr.; Hudson, J.; Jonas, J.; Yurgelum-Todd, D.: Bulimia treated with imipramine: a placebo-controlled, double-blind study. Am. J. Psychiat. *140:* 554–558 (1983).
31 Pope, H., Jr.; Hudson, J.; Jonas, J.: Antidepressant treatment of bulimia: preliminary experience and practical recommendations. J. clin. Psychopharm. *3:* 274–281 (1983).
32 Herzog, D.: Bulimia in the adolescent. Am. J. Dis. Child. *130:* 985–989 (1982).
33 Brotman, A.; Herzog, D.; Woods, S.: Antidepressant treatment of bulimia: the relationship between bingeing and depressive symptomatology. J. clin. Psychiat. (in press, 1983).
34 Sabine, E.; Yonace, A.; Farringon, A.; Barratt, K.; Wakeling, A.: Bulimia nervosa: a placebo-controlled, double-blind therapeutic trial of mianserin. Br. J. clin. Pharmacol. *15:* 1955–2025 (1983).
35 Barcai, A.: Lithium in anorexia nervosa: a pilot report on two patients. Acta psychiat. scand. *5:* 97–101 (1977).
36 Antelman, S.; Caggiula, A.: Tails of stress-related behavior: a neuropharmacological analysis; in Hanin, Animal models in psychiatry and neurology (Pergamon Press, Oxford 1977).
37 Saleh, J.; Lebwohl, P.: Metoclopramide-induced gastric emptying in patients with anorexia nervosa. Am. J. Gastroent., N.Y. *74:* 127–132 (1980).
38 Luborsky, L.; Singer, B.; Luborsky, L.: Comparative studies of psychotherapies: is it

true that 'everyone has won and all must have prizes'?. Archs gen. Psychiat. *32:* 995–1008 (1975).
39 Mitchell, J.; Bantle, J.: Metabolic and endocrine investigations in women of normal weight with the bulimia syndrome. Biol. Psychiat. *18:* 355–365 (1983).
40 Mitchell, J.; Pyle, R.; Eckert, E.; Hatsukami, D.; Letz, R.: Electrolyte and other physiological abnormalities in patients with bulimia. Psychol. Med. *13:* 273–278 (1983).
41 Gwirtsman, H.; Roy-Bryne, P.; Yager, J.; Gerner, R.: Neuroendocrine abnormalities in bulimia. Am. J. Psychiat. *140:* 559–563 (1983).
42 Fairburn, C.: Binge-eating and its management. Br. J. Psychiat. *141:* 631–633 (1982).
43 Cauwels, J.: Bulimia: the binge-purge compulsion (Doubleday, New York 1983).
44 Squire, S.: The slender balance: causes and cures for bulimia, anorexia and the weight loss/weight gain seesaw (Putnam, New York 1983).
45 Beck, A.: Cognitive therapy and the emotional disorders (International Universities Press, New York 1976).
46 Glasser, W.: Positive addiction (Harper & Row, New York 1976).
47 Merzer, M.: Winning the diet wars: a rescue plan for those who love to eat (Harcourt, Brace, Jovanovich, New York 1980).
48 Loro, A.; Orleans, C.: Binge-eating in obesity: preliminary findings and guidelines for behavioral analysis and treatment. Addict. Behav. *6:* 155–166 (1981).
49 Cummings, C.; Gordon, J.; Marlatt, G.: Relapse: prevention and prediction; in Miller, The addictive behaviors (Pergamon Press, New York 1980).
50 Marlatt, G.; Gordon, J.: Relapse prevention (Guilford Press, New York 1983).
51 Kosbab, P.: Imagery techniques in psychiatry. Archs gen. Psychiat. *31:* 283–290 (1974).

5 Family Therapy of the Eating Disorders

Sharon Glick Miller

Introduction

This paper will address some of the issues in the family therapy of anorexia nervosa. Although bulimia will not be directly addressed, many of the therapeutic issues raised apply to this illness as well. The treatment of anorexia nervosa by means of family therapy will be viewed within the context of current thought in systemic family therapy. Issues pertaining to the role of family therapy within the larger treatment context of anorexia nervosa will also be addressed. Finally, recommendations for utilizing family intervention in the evaluation and treatment of anorexia nervosa will be presented.

The literature contains several descriptive references to the families of patients with anorexia nervosa [1–6]. They have a limited utility to the family therapy of the eating disorders, and will not be reviewed here. One limitation arises from the fact that one can, at best, conclude that the individuals in these families exhibit a range of personality organization and dynamics. More crucial, however, is that many do not reflect a systemic view of the family. Characteristics of each family member are looked at individually or dyadically (the parts of a whole), while not addressing the complex dynamic transactions between the parts and the phenomenon of the whole. It is like assessing two parts of hydrogen and one part of oxygen while not commenting on the compound of water. Exceptions to this can be found in the work of *Minuchin* et al. [7] and *Selvini-Palazzoli* [8]. They have been the major contributors to the understanding and treatment of the families of these patients, and it is their work that is most often associated with the family therapy of anorexia nervosa. Their work will therefore be reviewed here in some detail.

The Contribution of Minuchin

Characteristics of Psychosomatic Families

With respect to the literature on anorexia nervosa, *Minuchin* et al. [7] are best known for their delineation of the structural characteristics of the families with an anorectic member. These characteristics are not seen as unique to anorexia nervosa, but as characteristic of all 'psychosomatic families'. *Minuchin* and his colleagues identified five characteristics associated with these families: enmeshment, overprotection, rigidity, lack of conflict resolution and involvement of the psychosomatic individual in the regulation of family conflict.

Enmeshment refers to a transactional style in families in which the boundaries between members are inappropriately blurred or diffuse. Dyadic transactions rarely occur, but become triadic or group transactions that confuse the issue being raised between members. Family members may be hyperresponsive to each other. There is a high degree of concern expressed for each other's welfare (i.e. overprotection), especially in relation to the symptomatic individual. The consequences of an enmeshed transactional style may be one of the important factors in symptom development. The intense sense of belonging in this system severely restricts individual autonomy. Family members have poorly differentiated perceptions of one another and of themselves. Further, enmeshment severely impairs the family's ability to respond adaptively to normal developmental crises that occur during its life cycle. This is the rigidity to which *Minuchin* et al. refer. An enmeshed system is one that is 'too richly cross-joined'. If anyone in the system attempts 'to find a new solution and to introduce the kind of random searching that is the essence of trial and error, adaptation will not be possible' [9, p. 463].

Lack of conflict resolution refers to the presence of sequences which appear to control the expression of conflict within specific dyads. It exists in families that have a low threshold for conflict and results in issues not being negotiated or resolved. Conflict between members may be denied or avoided. For example, if one member confronts, the other avoids; both chronically bicker while avoiding any real confrontation, or both may focus on a problem with a third, uniting to either protect or blame him while detouring their conflict.

Involvement of the psychosomatic individual in the regulation of family conflict is in some ways the most important characteristic and yet, ironically, is the one that is often not cited in papers making reference to this typology.

Minuchin et al. [7, p. 32] have commented that it is this characteristic, more so than the others, that highlighted the 'circularity of feedback that necessitated the move to a new order of explanation'. The importance of the fifth characteristic rests in the fact that unlike the preceding four characteristics which describe the family context of the psychosomatic individual and inadvertently infer a one-way causal link, this fifth characteristic underlies the fact that a more complex, bidirectional or multidimensional process is involved. The observation that the psychosomatic individual not only is brought in, but also brings himself in as a means of regulating the emergence of conflict perceived as threatening to the system, necessitates a move from a strictly linear to a systemic view of the symptomatology.

This typology undoubtedly has some limitations. However, it is proposed here that the problems associated with this typology arise less from its inherent limitations and more from a misunderstanding of its intent, scope, or underlying model.

The typology is limited by virtue of being a typology – i.e. it oversimplifies a complex process. Although it highlights key transactional patterns in the family, it lacks the richness and complexity found in nature. One must remember that any typology is but an artifact, in this case, one that allows us to look at certain redundancies in family interaction.

Further, although attempting to describe something that emerges from transactions over time, it is expressed in concrete terms. This, as well as the use of the term 'psychosomatic families', facilitates the misunderstanding that is a major difficulty with this typology. While anorexia nervosa is deemed only to be embedded in this structural pattern, it is easily misinterpreted as having been caused by the family structure.

Normative Model of a Well-Functioning Family

It is helpful to understand that the typology grew out of a general study of family structure in which categories of organization were established. What emerged secondarily from this study was the apparent connection between certain patterns of family organization and certain types of problems. What emerged primarily, and what was one of the most important contributions of these authors, was the development of a normative model of a family that is functioning well. According to this model, one of the key elements of a well-functioning family is a well-defined structure. The boundaries between subsystems (e.g. each individual, the marital dyad, the parental dyad, the sibling subsystem) will be clearly differentiated. Because marital issues should remain between the spouses, the boundaries of that subsystem will be closed.

The parental subsystem will have adequately demarcated boundaries between it and the children, but will still allow the access necessary for good parenting. The sibling subsystem will also have clearly demarcated boundaries, and will be organized hierarchically, so that children are treated with acknowledgement of their developmental stages. Further, in addition to providing cohesion, the structure is adequately flexible. It can adapt to both the extrafamilial stress that may infringe upon it, or to the intrafamilial stress that may arise with the birth of a child, or the increased autonomy required by the adolescent. Finally, the boundary around the nuclear family will also be respected, although the extent is dependent on cultural, social, and economic factors.

This model is extremely useful to the family therapist in that an assessment of the family's structure and its deviance from this model gives the therapist clues needed to determine in which direction to go in reversing relationship patterns in the family. However, whereas this structural analysis serves to point the therapist in the right direction, it does not offer him an adequate blueprint for therapy. For that, he must address the more idiosyncratic aspects of the family's functioning, and attempt to delineate how the circuits in the system fit together. To clarify this, it might be useful to summarize a session *Minuchin* had with the family of an anorectic child [10].

Case 1. The family was composed of Laura, age 14, who was diagnosed as having anorexia nervosa, her parents who were in their forties, and her 2 siblings – 12-year-old Jill, and 8-year-old Steven. The family was seen after Laura had been hospitalized for observation following excessive weight loss. No physical problems were detected. Laura had begun to lose weight when she started dieting at summer camp and continued losing weight. When down to 62 lb (28 kg) the family became alarmed and sought treatment.

Obviously, the fact that this was a young adolescent from an intact family who was being seen close to the onset of the behavior makes this an easier situation in which to intervene. The point in sharing it, however, is to show how, even in *Minuchin's* work, the typology assumes a prescribed role in the assessment interview, and that the real work is in exploring how the symptom and the system (particularly the structural organization of the system) may be connected.

Minuchin begins by asking the family about the presenting problem and explores some of the history. He learns that when Laura and Jill were younger, Laura was on the heavy side. Apart from that, the girls were seen as so alike they were treated as twins. It is also learned that Laura saw a psychologist at age 6 for school problems. The psychologist felt that while nothing was basically wrong with her, she was being caught between her parents, who disagreed on how to raise the children. The problem resolved after the one visit to the psychologist.

Minuchin moves on to assess the family's interaction around the symptom. Although Laura's father has asserted that family members never disagree, when *Minuchin* asks how the parents deal with Laura when she refuses to eat, disagreement emerges. While mother will ask Laura to eat only once and then stop because she sees it upsets Laura, father will go 'on and on'. From the family's description, it appears that the father-daughter relationship is a notably charged one that is expressed around the issue of eating. However, one also sees that the powerful, domineering father is undermined by his apparent 'one-down' wife as she covertly supports Laura's refusal to eat.

Next, *Minuchin* explores parent-child expression of disagreements and learns that the 12-year-old sister, Jill, angers her father when she denies his request to comb his hair. A nightly ritual is described in which the father and children cuddle together on the parents' bed. The children massage their father's legs, scratch his back or comb his hair. He in turn does these things for them; however, in the last year, he and Laura 'seem not to have done too much for each other'. *Minuchin* also learns that during this time mother is 'always busy in the house', doing laundry or puttering in the kitchen. When asked if she likes to cuddle with her husband, she laughs and says 'yes', but when asked further if she would like him to send the children out and be with her alone, she responds 'No, absolutely not!'. Their bedroom door always remains open. In fact, the doors are usually open to everyone's rooms. If the children close their doors, father will usually open them.

One begins to see the context of Laura's symptom. Laura has been close to father, in a way being a distance regulator between her parents [11]. One may hypothesize that as she approached adolescence, conflicts emerged. While the forces of nature and society compelled a move towards increased autonomy, such a move was threatening, part of the reason being that it would rupture the parents' relationship and would be an act of disloyalty in this 'bunched-in family'. Laura's anorexia nervosa provides mother with another way to oppose father through her coalition with Laura around the issue of eating. It also allows Laura to remain close to home and close to mother. While she is still accessible to father, the sexual element is removed, as many of the sexual characteristics either do not appear or disappear with her anorexia nervosa. Laura's refusal to eat may also be seen as a pathetic attempt to assert herself as an adolescent.

One can begin to see that the blueprint for therapy comes as much from the assessment of the contextual circumstances of the symptom as from the structural assessment of the family. In fact, the structural aspects cannot be separated from the other contextual aspects. It is for this reason that the extraction of the structural components from the contextual aspects, which unintentionally occurs with reference to *Minuchin's* typology, may result in distortion and misunderstanding.

Case 2. Another example of an assessment interview by *Minuchin and Fishman* [12, pp. 234–242] will illustrate this further. Martha, age 17, had anorexia nervosa for 6 years, and alternated starvation with bingeing. She was the youngest of 3 children, the oldest 2 having married and moved out of the house. The family structure quickly became evident. Spouse conflicts were detoured through Martha, and all family members acted to avoid conflict. Generally, if two began to disagree, a third would step in to keep it contained. When Mom and Dad 'felt a fight coming on', or a disagreement escalated, they would often stop talking to each other, sometimes for as long as a month. During these silences, Martha would feel guilty, feeling that she 'should be doing something... should be making them have a more pleasant life'. She says she has 'to make them talk and enjoy their life'. When asked if she was successful, she replies, 'No. So I punish myself for this and go on a binge'. When asked how long she has 'been trying to cure them' she responds, 'I never thought about it. Now that I think about it, it's about the time the anorexia nervosa started'.

The fundamental structure quickly apparent, *Minuchin* works to elucidate the contextual circumstances unique to this family. He probes the system by challenging the family's 'preferred schema', reframing Martha from the one who is ill to the family healer. By pushing the notion of Martha being responsible for her parents, *Minuchin* hopes that they will act to reject this and create distance from her. Later *Minuchin* frames Martha as responding to parental wishes that she stay involved in this way. He exaggerates this notion, expressing concern that Martha 'will never, never leave... home'. Martha responds by expressing her fear of the outside world and stating that she does not want to leave the house.

Martha's eating disorder is therefore linked to both the parents' use of Martha and Martha's use of the parents. It further supports, and is supported by, the family structure. When *Minuchin* proceeds with a challenge to the family members' use of each other in this way, he is implicitly sanctioning a family structure that will allow appropriate distance and differentiation between parent and child. As *Minuchin* has stated 'a challenge to the family worldview is simultaneously a challenge to its interactional structure, just as a challenge to its structure is a challenge to its worldview' [10, p. 243].

Again, the structural aspects of the family cannot be separated from the dynamic process of family transactions in which the symptom is embedded. In sum, *Minuchin's* approach with families with an anorectic member should therefore be viewed as more complex and comprehensive than initially conveyed by the citation of his structural description of these families.

The Contribution of Selvini-Palazzoli

Like *Minuchin, Selvini-Palazzoli* has delineated a systemic view of anorexia nervosa, in which the illness is seen as maintaining, and being maintained, in a circular sequence of transactions. Working for many years as a child analyst and treating many with anorexia nervosa, she became discouraged by her results. Impressed by the family therapy literature and her subsequent results with this approach, she moved to a systemic view and treatment of the illness. In *Self-Starvation* [8], she documents this transition. Subsequent works delineate the development of her methodology [13–16].

Although developed independently, the models of the family system of the anorectic put forth by *Minuchin* and *Selvini-Palazzoli* contain essential similarities. Like *Minuchin, Selvini-Palazzoli* [8, p. 242] observed the enmeshed quality of the system, noting that 'the collective sense of family is so pronounced that the individual is pushed into the background'. Should an individual member define herself by expressing a wish or opinion, her statement will most likely be qualified or rejected by other family members. Also like *Minuchin, Selvini-Palazzoli* [8, p. 211] observed significant marital dysfunction, with the involvement of the symptomatic child and/or family of origin in the marital process, resulting in 'secret' coalitions and 'three-way matrimony'.

Both authors have developed treatment strategies which attempt to challenge and reduce the enmeshment of these families. However, it was *Selvini-Palazzoli* and her colleagues whose fuller development of this methodology yielded incredible results, and forced the family therapy community at large to take notice. Therapists at other centers, as well as *Selvini-Palazzoli* and her associates, continue to experiment with, expand and modify the model.

Central to this approach is the understanding that in enmeshed, or too richly cross-joined families, any direct challenge to the family belief system or organizational structure may not only be ineffective, but will most likely reinforce the very thing being challenged. Aware of this phenomenon, the therapist responds not from an adversarial position, but cooperatively and enters the system in a way that appears indirect. The intervention will positively define and convey respect for the symptom-maintaining cycle.

Therapy is conducted with one therapist in the room with the family, and one or more therapists observing behind the one-way mirror. The observers are there not as consultants to the family, but to the therapist-family system. After about an hour, the therapists convene apart from the family and decide how to conclude the session. The 'conductor' rejoins the family and concludes accordingly, usually with a carefully worded statement that counsels against change. The next appointment is then established. Once the family has been engaged and adequate information gathered to formulate a systemic hypothesis, the interval between sessions is usually 1 month. Initially this interval was utilized to accommodate families traveling long distances to the center, but *Selvini-Palazzoli* [16] observed that it seemed to be more effective than briefer intervals. This may be due to the fact that the family cannot disqualify the intervention before it has had an effect on the system. It is hypothesized that in very enmeshed families, it takes much longer for the intervention to affect the system. The long interval also helps prevent the therapist from becoming caught up in the organizational pattern of the too richly cross-joined family. An illustration will provide a flavor of this approach of *Selvini-Palazzoli* and her associates.

Case 3. Interviewing a 12-year-old anorectic, his parents and his 8-year-old brother, *Selvini-Palazzoli* et al. [13, pp. 150–152] obtained most of the information from the parents, as the identified patient, Giulio, refused to participate. Giulio presented with all the usual symptoms of anorexia nervosa. In addition, it was learned that he would spend considerable time massaging his hips and legs with a slenderizing cream. The investigators described the family as follows: This family could be characterized by the social difference between father and mother. The mother was a school teacher, while the father was a blue collar worker. He, visibly intimidated by his learned wife, spent his free time playing bocce, a popular game similar to lawn bowling. Traditionally, only men participate, drinking wine and cracking jokes. He was a champion at it, and frequently won tournaments and trophies. Giulio was not permitted to follow his father in these outings, which often occurred on Sunday: 'Daddy comes back late at night, and Giulio has to get up early and be fresh for school in the morning.' Naturally, Giulio was the best student in his class. He spent Sunday afternoons with his mother and 8-year-old brother, revising his lessons and taking long walks, during which he was gently instructed in botany and mineralogy. After the team discussion, *Selvini-Palazzoli* returned to the family and read the following: 'I have to excuse myself, Giulio, to your doctor for having doubted his diagnosis. When he told me on the telephone that you had anorexia nervosa I thought: It's impossible, he must be wrong. Anorexia nervosa is a female disease! A male can't have a female disease! And instead, that's exactly what you have Giulio! But why? We have talked for more than an hour with your parents and we cannot find anything in their behavior that can explain this strange phenomenon. Our only explanation is that there has been some kind of misunderstanding. That perhaps you've got the idea that in teaching you, and expecting obedience, good manners, good work in school, respect toward your grandparents, in expecting you to keep away from foulmouthed boys, your parents wanted a Giulietta instead of Giulio (clamorous laughter on the part of the brother, followed by a progressive, moving lightening of Giulio's face, finally bursting out in uncontrollable laughter, while the parents, embarrassed, seemed to hold their breaths). But things cannot be like this (raising the tone). Daddy and Mommy can only want that you become a man, a real man (sounds of agreement from the parents). Anyway, at this point, if this is your conviction, that in order to become a man you need a woman's disease, we agree with the path that you have chosen. We respect it. Not only do we respect it, but we think you should continue to be anorectic. And to you, parents, we recommend the same things: this feminine disease should continue, because Giulio is convinced that only with a feminine disease can he become masculine.'

By the second session, Giulio had gained weight. Apparently while returning home from the first session, the family stopped in a restaurant. Giulio immediately ordered spaghetti for himself, which he devoured to the astonishment of his parents. He continued to eat at home. Other changes took place as well. He became noncompliant at school, doing only what was minimally necessary and began to participate in bocce and wrestling. The parents, apparently reacting to the 'feminine' aspects emphasized in the therapist's comment, encouraged this participation in masculine sports. The therapy continued for another four sessions and ended with 'a fit and proud Giulio, who had just won a junior cup in bocce' [13].

Importance of Positive Connotation

Central to this approach is the positive connotation. As *Selvini-Palazzoli* [8, p. 230] has clearly stated: 'Positive connotation of transactional behavior is to us the golden road for entering, and being freely admitted into, the system and changing it.' The utility of the positive connotation goes beyond that of being a strategy for change. It guards against linear thinking by adding more complexity and helps one arrive at a systemic hypothesis. The positive connotation is not any more 'true' or less linear than a negative one, but the combination of the two linear statements prompts a more circular or systemic understanding. Systems therapists see behavior as circular... she nags because he withdraws because she nags and so on. It is noncausal. Once punctuated, causality is implied: she nags because he withdraws. However, the punctuation is arbitrary. He withdraws because she nags might be another punctuation. The positive connotation of both the symptom and the behavior of the system as a whole avoids arbitrary punctuation by placing everyone in the system on one level. Another illustration of *Selvini-Palazzoli's* work [8, p. 229] will make this clearer. During a beginning family interview, the discussion turned to the anorectic's premorbid phase. It appeared that the patient managed to get the subject around to her parents' views on sexual matters, showing them to be repressive and reactionary. Avoiding the temptation to explore this further, the therapists commented positively on the 'parents' obvious fascination with their daughter's feminine charms, and on the way in which they had succeeded in driving these charms home to the patient herself. They would certainly not have acted in the way they did had they thought her anything but highly desirable. In fact, their assessment of the situation was one in which the patient must have been in full agreement. Why else had she always been so loyal to them and never used even the slightest subterfuge to defy their prohibitions.' With this, the behaviors of both child and parental dyad are put on the same level, preventing arbitrary causal punctuations: i.e. the parents impeded their daughter's sexual development with their fears, or the daughter signalled her fears around sexual development to her parents who protected her with their restrictions.

Family therapists have long relabeled negative behaviors in a positive way to avoid the mobilization of resistance. For example, in the family where father cuddled with his children and did not allow closed doors, *Minuchin* [10, p. 13] referred to him not as intrusive but as 'loving'. Family therapists have also long implied that individual symptomatic behavior had positive functional implications for the family system [17, 18]. *Boszormenyi-Nagy and Spark* [19] noted to patients how their symptoms helped them fulfill a multigenerational script. More recently, in their work with addicts and their families, *Stanton and Todd* [20] developed the technique of ascribing 'noble intention' to the identified patient, commenting on the service the symptom served for the family. The work of *Selvini-Palazzoli* and her colleagues was instrumental, however, in the more fully developed role of the positive connotation.

Within this approach, the positive connotation is much more than a simple reframing. In addition to defining the symptom as essential to the system, symptom and system are connected in a circular definition; in other words, inherent in the positive connotation is a statement of how symptom and system activate each other. Once the patterns of the system are made explicit, 'the family must take responsibility for its own actions' [21, p. 47].

Co-Evolution and Circular Questioning

The emphasis of *Selvini-Palazzoli* and her colleagues on co-evolution and their development of the technique of circular questioning have also been important contributions to family therapy. Building on *Bateson's* [22] notion of co-evolution, a repetitive behavioral sequence (including symptomatic behavior) is seen as co-evolving with a pattern of relationships. Assessment, therefore, necessitates tracing the evolution of symptomatic behavior to its present contextual fit. This is done by noting the pattern of family alignments around the presenting problem in the present and noting if the pattern differs from the past (i.e. before the onset of the symptomatic behavior) or from the future (i.e. what the effect might be if the symptom were no longer present). Questions are aimed at obtaining this organizational information in the present (e.g. who is most upset by Sue's not eating), the past (e.g. did mother fight with father more or less after Sue was hospitalized) and the future (e.g. if Sue were to get well and move out, what effect would that have on mother). Further, *Selvini-Palazzoli* et al. [14] and *Penn* [23] have refined a method of asking questions that is rich in yielding this systemic information. The method, referred to as circular questioning, has as its basis the 'triadic question'. This type of question involves asking 1 person about the relationship between 2 or more others. The therapist then cross-references the responses, circling around the group. By superimposing the multiple single impressions, the therapist begins to experience the whole.

Selvini-Palazzoli and her associates believe that circular questioning alone may bring about change. The constant evocation of different perceptions in a family about the same relationship or event, or the noting of differences in patterns over time, often leads family members as well as the therapist to a new perspective. Also, circular questioning is particularly useful with the enmeshed families in which we usually find anorexia nervosa. Asking a family member to comment on the relationship between two other members forces that person, in a sense, to separate himself from the relationship in order to comment.

Common Elements in the Work of Minuchin and Selvini-Palazzoli

In view of the work of these therapists, what remain the important considerations in working with families presenting with an anorectic member? An answer lies in a review of the common elements of their work. Although there are clear differences in their styles and in what they choose to emphasize in their theories, they share more similarities. Both attend to similar relationship dynamics and share similar therapeutic goals. The structural elements emphasized by *Minuchin* are also present in *Selvini-Palazzoli's* work. (She has even added to the repertoire of structural interventions. For example, she cleverly devised instructing parents to do something that is kept secret from the children. This unites more closely the spouse dyad and makes it more clearly separated from the offspring. The element of secrecy intensifies it, and makes less likely the chance for the offspring to block or to be used to block this.) Similarly, while *Selvini-Palazzoli* emphasizes the strategic component of her therapeutic approach, it is also part of *Minuchin's* work. Actually, it may be argued that nearly all family therapy approaches require both a structural and a strategic component whether or not acknowledged by the therapist. Further, although using them with less frequency, *Minuchin and Fishman* [12] show a common understanding of the role of indirect 'restraint from change' intervention and include a discussion of its use in his recent work on family therapy techniques. In writing about the symptom of anorexia nervosa and the relationship system in which it is embedded, *Minuchin* and *Selvini-Palazzoli* discuss the ways in which the two are connected and reinforce each other. Although generalizing about some of the qualities of the relationship system and providing global guidelines for the therapist, each presents a mode of intervention that is system-specific. Each attends to the specific system dynamics, noting the unique way in which symptom and system fit and move together. Each attends to the specific dynamics of the therapeutic (i.e. therapist-family) system, noting the need for a direct or indirect intervention. Also, each assesses multiple subsystem levels (individual, marital, family, extended family, family-referring physician, family-therapist) both to understand how a change of events in one level will impact on another, and to decide at what level the intervention should be addressed.

Both investigators continue to refine their work with increased theoretical understanding of systems and system change. It is interesting to note that the early work of both contained an element of high drama that is no longer present. Initially, they both seemed to be responding to difficulty in introducing change in the too richly cross-joined families of anorectics. *Minuchin* et al. [7, p. 95] talked of being 'radically undermined' and noted that mild interventions had little effect. They therefore felt that therapeutic maneuvers had to be of 'high intensity' to have any impact. In this vein, they developed the family lunch session, a 3-hour interview, during the latter half of which lunch was served. The patterns maintaining the symptom were enacted, intensified and dramatically dealt with. While still used by other therapists who find this particularly effective with very young anorectics, *Minuchin* no longer employs the lunch session, finding that he can achieve the same results through less dramatic means. Similarly, *Selvini-Palazzoli's* early work with these families contained hints of an adversarial relationship. Prescriptions were given with much drama and an implicit adversarial tone. With increased understanding of the dynamics of system change in the too richly cross-joined family of anorectics, the dynamics of the therapist-family system changed, and the implicit adversarial tone was no longer a function of it.

Some Issues in the Family Therapy of the Eating Disorders

The information to be gathered in the family assessment is outlined in table I. It is obtained by observing all relevant members of the family unit together over one or more sessions.

It is important to note that systemic family therapists view symptom and system as connected and moving together. They do not see the family as causing the symptom; it is an issue of co-evolution, and not of etiology. If the therapist working with the family believes otherwise, problems will emerge in the therapist-family system that will prevent an effective working alliance. The actions of the therapist toward the parents of the symptomatic individual will have the air of 'a series of careful negotiations with kidnappers for the release of a hostage' [25, p. 192]. A split in the therapeutic system will occur between the 'good' therapist and the 'bad' family. Further, whether or not reinforced by the beliefs of the therapist, the parents' feelings of culpability need to be directly addressed; if not, they are covertly reinforced. Already feeling some degree of responsibility for the child's illness, they find confirmation of culpability when asked questions about themselves, or asked to respond differently to their child's behavior. They may subsequently respond defensively by countering the therapist's moves, or by accepting the covert blame and becoming unable to respond with the appropriate limits needed by their child. With a systemic perspective, the therapist sees symptom and system on one plane. There is no victim and therefore no blame. The therapist is free to be not only nonblaming and neutral, but supportive and committed to all members of the family.

The issue of who should participate in the family therapy is less an issue than who should be included in the therapist's conception of the problem [26]. Family therapy is not defined by who is actively involved in therapy, but by an orientation in which people are seen in the context of their family emotional system. Family therapy may therefore involve only therapist and patient in a one-to-one format [27]. Similarly, individual psychotherapy may be conducted with the presence and active involvement of family members. In general, however, it is helpful to include all involved members of the family for at least the assessment phase. If the evaluation reveals a contextual basis to the symptomatology, a family system approach is indicated. The actual membership of future sessions will depend on both what the therapist sees as most effective in achieving the therapeutic goals, and who is physically available and willing to attend.

With a family system approach, the therapist will evaluate multiple levels (i.e. individual, family, therapeutic system), and may identify problems on more than one level. The order in which they are addressed will, for the most part, depend on the level in which they appear. Although usually issues in the more external levels (e.g. therapeutic system; family) take precedence over internal levels (e.g. intrapsychic), crisis situations will need to be addressed first. For example, the anorectic in physical danger needs first to be hospitalized.

University of South Florida Eating Disorders Clinic Approach to Family Intervention

The University of South Florida Eating Disorders Clinic employs a family systems approach in the evaluation of its patients. Patients living at home with their families are seen conjointly with their families for at least an evaluation. Similarly, any married patients will be seen conjointly with their spouses as part of the evaluation. For young adults living apart from their families, the individual assessment will attend to the contextual basis of their problem, and the need for subsequent conjoint family assessment and/or intervention will be determined.

The mode of intervention is one which integrates the common elements of the various schools of family therapy. While sensitive to psychodynamic issues, intervention is at the transactional level. It is both structural and strategic, and may use either direct intervention (i.e. providing interpretation, direction, suggestions) or indirect interventions (i.e. those which appear to require the family to move in one direction, with the knowledge that the family will move in the opposite direction; or those which aim for change in one part of the system, with the goal of changing another part).

The evaluation usually occurs over two sessions (although sometimes enough information can be obtained in one). Table I delineates the information that is gathered.

Information from the initial phone contact is noted, as it is not unusual for beginning themes to emerge from that point. A conjoint session is arranged, and clear directions as to who is to attend are given.

When meeting with the family, the therapist must first 'join' with the family [28]. Each family member must be engaged. The therapist's position is neutral, conveying multigenerational fairness. The approach is such that no one feels blamed, or feels that the therapist sided with one person or another. Within the engagement phase, any impediments to the establishment of a positive working alliance are addressed. For example, parents who feel that the purpose of the evaluation is to gather evidence of their failings must be effectively reassured. Similarly, the mother of one anorectic, reacting to the instruction of her daughter's previous therapist that she not be allowed to see her daughter, needed this issue addressed at the start.

Initial questions center on the presenting problem. Not only is this less threatening to the family (after all, they are there to deal with the presenting problem), but much information can be gained from this. Learning about the rapidity with which they were able to identify the problem and their attempts at solution tells one much about problem-solving resources. Details of any previous therapy are important, as knowing what was not helpful will help the therapist determine what would be helpful. It offers information about the family's style of 'cooperating' with the therapist, which will also be helpful in formulating any intervention [29]. Further, following the sequence of behaviors around the presenting problem will reveal information about family alignments, and suggest a beginning hypothesis as to the connection

Table I. University of South Florida Family Evaluation Clinic Guide to Family Assessment

- A Initial contact
  - 1 Therapy begins at the point of the initial contact
  - 2 Note referral or phone transactions
- B How the family presents itself
  - 1 Composition – who is and is not present
  - 2 Appearance – dress, demeanor
  - 3 Beginning transactions – seating, eye contact, spokesman
- C How the family functions [24]
  - 1 Problem identification and solution
  - 2 Communication – clear or masked; direct or indirect
  - 3 Range of affect
  - 4 Affective involvement – indifferent, empathic, narcissistic, symbiotic
  - 5 Mode of behavioral control
  - 6 Individuation/differentiation; autonomy; handling differences
  - 7 Family defense mechanisms
  - 8 Family belief systems – religion, culture, values, fantasies, fears, myths, loyalties
- D How the family is structured
  - 1 Boundaries
  - 2 Coalitions/alliances
  - 3 Hierarchy
  - 4 Roles – distribution, satisfaction, idiosyncratic roles
  - 5 Rules – repetitive transactional sequences
- E History
  - 1 Past as it pertains to the present
  - 2 Genogram (graphic representation of the family tree noting the history of the relationship structure of the family)
- F Therapist-family system
  - 1 Note how family responds to therapeutic interventions
- G Integration of information/hypotheses
  - 1 What are the main problems/conflicts in the family?
  - 2 How do symptom and system activate each other?
  - 3 What are the family's resources and strengths?
  - 4 What problems should be addressed in what order and by what means?

between symptom and system. For example, mother's covert alliance with daughter around not eating (mother does not push the issue of her eating, which father does) may be a way to oppose father. This initial hypothesis can be tested, modified and expanded by further questioning. The therapist may also wish to obtain information about the family relationship patterns at the time of onset. For example, the onset of a daughter's bulimia and agoraphobia coincided with the death of her grandmother, to whom her mother was exceptionally close; her illness may prevent mother from being too preoccupied with the loss, and bring a previously peripheral father back into the picture. Similarly, the therapist also asks about the effect on the relationship pattern if the problem were to no longer exist, and again can obtain information helpful for the formation of a systemic hypothesis; for example, if Sue were to leave, mother would become seriously depressed and father would die of loneliness.

With an initial hypothesis based on information around the presenting problem, the therapist asks questions that move beyond this and test the hypothesis; for example, if the anorexia nervosa were hypothesized as a way of bringing a divorced father back to the family, questions would be asked about the mother's relationship with her estranged husband. If the hypothesis proved unfounded, a second one would be formulated which would organize subsequent questions.

Throughout the evaluation, the therapist gathers information on different levels. He needs to get a sense of each individual member and each subsystem (e.g. parental, marital, sibling). He looks at the structure of the system as a whole, and notes any deviations from the model of a well-functioning family. He gathers information about the relationship between the parts of the system, and uses the triadic question (i.e. one person is asked to comment about the relationship of another two) as the basis for getting this information. The therapist circles around and obtains multiple perspectives, the superimposition of which yields a more complex understanding of the family pattern and an understanding of how symptom and system are connected. Finally, the therapist attends to information about the therapist-family transactions. The family's reaction to various moves of the therapist will yield further information, part of which will help determine how to intervene in the system. The therapist must intervene in a way that is cooperative with the dynamics of the system.

In addition to deciding how to intervene, a decision must be made on where to intervene first. The order in which problems are addressed are, for the most part, dependent on the level in which they appear. Problems that appear on the level of therapist-family interaction will need to be addressed before family or individual issues can be addressed. For example, an evaluation revealed that the father of a bulimic, himself a pediatrician, derived much satisfaction in consulting with various professionals about his daughter's condition and entering into a collaborative role with them as a colleague. This family-therapist issue needed to be addressed before any work could be done. Similarly, issues at the family level must be addressed before those at the individual level. Frequently in the families of anorectics, the therapist must first deal with the split between the parents and establish joint parental authority. Other issues may prevail. For example, a 19-year-old developed bulimia during her first year of college. The parents had a long history of marital difficulties focused on her father's alcoholism. The daughter had aligned with mother, and encouraged her to leave father. When she moved away from home to attend school, mother divorced father and went to be with her daughter. The mother-daughter transactions around the daughter's bingeing and vomiting mirrored previous wife-husband transactions around the husband's excessive drinking and subsequent vomiting. The function the bulimia served in terms of keeping father present in the system, and the complex issues of family guilt and indebtedness needed to be addressed before many of the intrapsychic issues. Attempts to prematurely engage her in individual psychotherapy would most likely have met with difficulty. The transference relationship and/or symptomatic improvement would have aroused guilt or feelings of disloyalty and family betrayal [30]. It has also been the observation of the author that when individual and family therapy of these patients is done concurrently, the individual therapist will report significantly improved motivation in the therapy process following a significant change in the family system. This observation merits formal study.

A treatment plan is made on the basis of the information gathered in the assessment, and in accordance with the other members of the Eating Disorders Clinic Team. The frequency of the sessions and the modality employed in the session will vary according to the family. One family may be seen weekly; another who cannot tolerate 'therapy' may be seen for an ongoing 'consultation', with each consultation session spaced 3–6 weeks apart. As with all therapy, assessment continues throughout treatment. Therefore, as the therapist reassesses the system each time, he may make different decisions about membership, frequency, modality and issues to be addressed.

Recommendations for Family Intervention in the Treatment of Anorexia Nervosa and Bulimia

Those principles which are fundamental to effective family intervention in the treatment of the eating disorders are listed in table II.

The first of these is the need to assume a systemic perspective which conceptualizes the eating disorder as embedded in a pattern of relationships,

Table II. Recommendations for family intervention

1	Assume a systemic perspective
2	Assess the contextual basis of the symptom
3	Develop a systemic hypothesis
4	Plan intervention in accordance with the dynamics of the system
5	Maintain clear relationships and collaboration with other involved treatment professionals
6	Assign an appropriate role for family intervention in the total treatment plan

wherein symptom and system activate each other. This allows the therapist to be neutral and nonjudgemental, which facilitates the development of a positive working alliance with the family. The second requirement is that there be a thorough evaluation which outlines the contextual basis of the symptom. A systemic hypothesis is developed to delineate how all the parts of the system are connected and move together. The positive connotation of both the symptom and the transactional behavior in the system helps one to arrive at the systemic hypothesis. Circular or triadic based questioning is utilized to gain such information about the system. Based on this understanding, the therapist plans his intervention, deciding on what level and by what means. Issues at the therapist-family level will be addressed before issues at the individual level (except when a medical crisis requires immediate attention). The intervention must be compatible with the dynamics of the family and may be by direct comment, by requesting the family to carry out a ritual, or by instructing the family to complete a task which may be direct or indirect. It is imperative to know the other treatment professionals involved and to maintain effective collaborative relationships. Both the professionals and the family must be clear about the relationships to prevent the family splitting one professional from the other, or the inadvertent undermining of the therapeutic intervention of one professional by another. Finally, it is important to assign an appropriate role to family intervention within the overall multifaceted approach (outlined in chapter 10) essential to treatment of the eating disorders. The more context dependent the symptom(s), the more essential is a family systems approach. This does not, however, preclude the importance of attending to individual dynamics. Finally, it is important to remember that family therapy is also more effective when it takes into account the larger circuits such as the therapeutic system or the referring context.

Conclusion

There is a growing and favorable body of outcome data on the effectiveness of family and couple therapy. The dramatic results reported by *Minuchin* and *Selvini-Palazzoli* are undermined by not being part of a well-controlled study. However, subsequent well-designed and controlled studies have attested to the efficacy of family therapy with a variety of illnesses [31, 32]. Even inclusion of significant others in the individual therapy process seems to increase efficacy of treatment [33, 34]. Attention to the marital or family system of patients with eating disorders is therefore indicated. The inclusion of family evaluation as part of the assessment procedure may yield much helpful information and facilitate subsequent involvement of significant others in the treatment. Anorexia nervosa has been described on each of its many levels from neuroendocrine to culture, with reference to how these different levels of phenomena influence one another [35, 36]. The treatment of the illness must take into account these multiple levels of organization. The task is systemic. There needs to be a greater awareness of how all the parts fit and move together. This requires a different way of knowing – one that is not linear or reductionistic – but circular, complex and systemic.

References

1 Bruch, H.: Eating disorders: obesity, anorexia nervosa, and the person within (Basic Books, New York 1973).

2 Crisp, A.; Harding, B.; McGuinness, B.: Anorexia nervosa. Psychoneurotic characteristics of parents: relationship to prognosis. A quantitative study. J. psychosom. Res. *18:* 167–173 (1974).

3 Hall, A.: Family structure and relationships of 50 female anorexia nervosa patients. Aust. N.Z. J. Psychiat. *12:* 163–268 (1978).

4 Kalucy, R.; Crisp, A.; Harding, B.: A study of 56 families with anorexia nervosa. Br. J. med. Psychol. *50:* 381–395 (1977).

5 Sours, J.: Starving to death in a sea of objects: the anorexia nervosa syndrome (Aronson, New York 1982).

6 Wilson, C.: The family psychological profile of anorexia nervosa patients. J. med. Soc. N. J. *77:* 341–347 (1980).

7 Minuchin, S.; Rosman, B.; Baker, L.: Psychosomatic families (Harvard University Press, Cambridge 1977).

8 Selvini-Palazzoli, M.: Self-starvation: from individual to family therapy in the treatment of anorexia nervosa (Aronson, New York 1978).

9 Hoffman, L.: Enmeshment and the too richly cross-joined system. Family Process. *14:* 457–468 (1975).

10 Aponte, H.; Hoffman, L.: The open door: a structural approach to a family with an anorectic child. Family Process. *12:* 1–44 (1973).
11 Byng-Hall, J.: Symptom bearer as marital distance regulator: clinical implications. Family Process. *19:* 355–366 (1980).
12 Minuchin, S.; Fishman, M.: Family therapy techniques (Harvard Press, Cambridge 1981).
13 Selvini-Palazzoli, M.; Boscolo, L.; Cecchin, G.; Prata, G.: Paradox and counterparadox (Aronson, New York 1978).
14 Selvini-Palazzoli, M.; Boscolo, L.; Cecchin, G.; Prata, G.: Hypothesizing – circularity – neutrality: three guidelines for the conductor of the session. Family Process. *19:* 3–12 (1980).
15 Selvini-Palazzoli, M.; Boscolo, L.; Cecchin, G.; Prata, G.: The problem of the referring person. J. Mar. Fam. Ther. *6:* 3–9 (1980).
16 Selvini-Palazzoli, M.: Why a long interval between sessions; in Andolfi, Zwerling, Dimensions of family therapy (Guilford Press, New York 1982).
17 Watzlawick, P.; Weakland J.; Fisch, R.: Change: principles of problem formulation and problem resolution (Norton, New York 1974).
18 Steinglass, P.; Davis, D.; Berenson, D.: Observations of conjointly hospitalized 'alcoholic couples' during sobriety and intoxication. Family Process. *16:* 1–16 (1977).
19 Boszormenyi-Nagy, I.; Spark, C.: Invisible loyalties (Harper & Row, New York 1973).
20 Stanton, M.; Todd, T.; and Associates: The family therapy of drug addiction (Guilford Press, New York 1981).
21 Papp, P.: The Greek chorus and other techniques of paradoxical therapy. Family Process. *19:* 45–57 (1980).
22 Bateson, G.: Mind and nature (Dutton, New York 1978).
23 Penn, P.: Circular questioning. Family Process. *21:* 267–280 (1982).
24 Chagoya, L.; Guttman, H.: A guide to assess family functioning (unpublished, 1971).
25 Terkelson, K.: Schizophrenia and the family. II. Adverse effects of family therapy. Family Process. *22:* 191–200 (1983).
26 Haley, J.: Leaving home: the therapy of disturbed young people (McGraw-Hill, New York 1980).
27 Carter, E.; Orfandis McGoldrick, O.: Family therapy with one person and the family therapist's own family; in Guerin, Family therapy: theory and practice (Gardner Press, New York 1976).
28 Minuchin, S.: Families and family therapy (Harvard University Press, Cambridge 1977).
29 DeShazer, S.: Patterns of brief family therapy: an ecosystemic approach (Guilford Press, New York 1982).
30 Boszormenyi-Nagy, I.: Loyalty implications of the transference model in psychotherapy. Archs gen. Psychiat. *27* (1972).
31 Gurman, A.; Kniskern, D.: Family therapy outcome research: knowns and unknowns; in Gurman, Kniskern, Handbook of family therapy (Brunner/Mazel, New York 1981).
32 Faloon, I.; Boyd, J.; McGill, C.; Razani, J.; Moss, H.; Gilderman, A.: Family manage-

ment in the prevention of exacerbations of schizophrenia: a controlled study. New Engl. J. Med. *306:* 1437–1440 (1982).

33 Hafner, R.; Badenoch, A.; Fisher, J.; Swift, M.: Spouse-aided individual therapy in persisting psychiatric disorders: a systemic comparison. Family Process. *22:* 385–400 (1983).

34 Anderson, C.; Hogarty, G.; Reiss, D.: Family treatment of adult schizophrenic patients: a psycho-educational approach. Schizophrenic Bull. *6:* 490–505 (1980).

35 Garfinkel, P.; Garner, D.: Anorexia nervosa: a multidimensional perspective (Brunner/Mazel, New York 1982).

36 Piazza, E.; Piazza, N.; Rollins, N.: Anorexia nervosa: controversial aspects of therapy. Compreh. Psychiat. *21:* 177–189 (1980).

6 Symptoms: Psychodynamic Meanings and Treatment Implications

Deborah Roth, Glenn G. Golloway

Introduction

As is the case with many mental disorders, the more recent history of psychiatry is mirrored in the study of the anorexia nervosa syndrome which includes both anorexia nervosa and bulimia. The symptoms of the two conditions are similar. Since *Gull* [1] and *Lasègue* [2] described anorexia nervosa as a distinct clinical entity approximately 100 years ago, it has been thought that psychological factors may play a role in the development and thus the treatment of the disorder. There was a time when anorexia nervosa was confused with Simmond's disease [3], and even now some investigators still believe that it is purely organic. This belief is based primarily on the fact that approximately one fourth of patients manifest onset of amenorrhea prior to weight loss [4]. Recent scientific literature [5, 6] has delineated the symptoms, signs and diagnostic criteria for the anorexia nervosa syndrome, and popular literature has made the disease a veritable 'cause célèbre'. This may have contributed to the seeming explosion of reports of the syndrome in colleges and communities. It appears clear, however, that somehow the evolving role of women in society and consequent changes in sociological attitudes have played a significant part in the increasing numbers of anorectics and bulimics presenting to clinics and offices.

It is now generally agreed that primary anorexia nervosa is a fairly specific syndrome different from other conditions in which anorexia (a true loss of appetite) is a primary symptom (e.g. in depression and in certain psychoses). Early on, however, anorexia nervosa was a part of a confusing spectrum of conditions which shared similar symptomatology. In the 1920s, as interest in psychoanalysis grew, so did interest in anorexia. Analysts began turning their attention to understanding the syndrome and attempted to find a unitary formulation. Review of the literature and retrospective knowledge of the field indicates that this single formulation has not been possible. Similarly, 'psychodynamics' is not a unified system. To embrace the various psychological dynamic forces at work in a case requires familiarity with and use of several conceptual systems which must be kept more or less separate from one another. Even 'cause' must be separately defined for each system of explanation; for example, endocrine abnormalities do not 'explain' phobic avoidance of food. There is an imposing array of conceptual systems at various hierarchical levels from biological through physical and psychological organizations, from the intrapersonal to the interpersonal, then family and larger social patternings. These are not at all mutually exclusive. There are some cross-correlations between systems. So in a multifaceted syndrome, the dynamic forces also are clearly multifactorial.

Ineffectiveness of Traditional Psychoanalysis and Current Implications for Treatment

Bruch's [7] and *Selvini-Palazzoli's* [8] formulations were stimulated by the observation that traditional psychoanalysis was rather ineffective in treatment of true anorexia. As early as the 1940s, *Deutsch* [9] reported that she thought that a great deal of modification of classical analysis was necessary to achieve favorable results. Others [10, 11] have doubted the capacity of insight to produce positive changes in the anorectic. *Powers and Powers* [12] discuss the lack of correlation between 'functional recovery' and achievement of insight.

In order to understand the psychological dynamics of anorexia nervosa and bulimia, one must examine the symptoms and the patient from the point of view of multiple conceptual systems. This has important implications for treatment. In order to effectively treat anorectics and bulimics, one must thus approach the patients from several different viewpoints at once.

Diagnostic Issues

Much confusion has arisen, it seems, because of differences in definition of the anorexia syndrome. *Risen* [13], an analyst, emphasizes that anorectic symptoms may exist in various personality structures with various psychiatric diagnoses, from 'neurotic' to 'borderline' to 'schizophrenic'. *Bruch* [7] utilizes primarily psychological criteria while DSM III [6] utilizes a combination, primarily leaning toward the descriptive or phenomenological. Yet most of the patients who fit either criteria seem to represent those from the more character-disordered and borderline spectrum. According to *Risen* [13] and many other current analysts, psychoanalytic psychotherapy, behavior modification techniques, group therapy and family therapy are all useful modalities provided one understands the individual and comprehends the disorder from a developmental viewpoint.

Puzzling features about anorexia nervosa include the questions regarding what sort of forces are at work to subvert so fundamental a behavior as feeding and why these patients are so difficult to treat. The same symptoms may occur in entirely different syndromes and do not usually have the same significance. What factors cause this intense focus on these symptoms?

In severe depression there is a loss of appetite with significant weight loss attributable to depression of the vegetative functions as accompaniments of the central nervous system reduction in neurotransmitters. At the psychodynamic level, feelings of guilt and unworthiness indicate to the patient that she is undeserving of the food or its nourishing or pleasurable attributes. Much of the guilt in depression is oral guilt which classifies the acts of biting, chewing and swallowing as unacceptable aggressions which, if indulged, produce more guilt. This reaction formation produces inhibition of eating as a psychological phenomenon; in order to avoid anxiety, the ego transforms the wish or the act into its opposite expression. Thus, the wish for unrestricted indulgence becomes almost total abstention. It is concomitant with and reinforces the neurotransmitter abnormalities. To what extent the starvation enhances the chemical aspects of depression or the chemical disturbance favors emphasis of guilt, one can only guess.

In psychosis the belief that food is contaminated with poison, feces or sperm (and their concomitant aggressive or libidinal features) provides the 'rationale' to the patient for repudiation of food and eating. She is attempting to protect herself from an imagined real danger and therefore to protect herself physically. It is a 'good' thing to do, even though it interferes with functioning. At the psychological level there is an effort to protect oneself from the loss of self-esteem or the narcissistic injury of being associated with such evil interests. Wishes to bite, chew or swallow are projected onto food and its utilization which become evil acts.

Both in depression and psychosis, it is food and the act of eating which are representations of the libidinal and aggressive drives, the repudiation of which becomes the source of the anorexia. We see the same sort of displacements in primary anorexia nervosa but in a more complex network of factors.

Historical Review

Early Psychodynamic Formulations

Many early psychodynamic explanations have provided valuable material which assist in the understanding and treatment of anorexia nervosa and have contributed to the more recent hypotheses. We will review the main analytic formulations which are derived from libido theory. It should be remembered that when presented in 'analytic language' these seem to be somewhat literal representations of the then current hypothesis.

In 1941, *Masserman* [14] outlined 50 years of early analytic observations of anorexia nervosa. One of the earliest references to the disorder was in a paper by *Breuer and Freud* [15] in 1892 which mentioned chronic vomiting and anorexia carried to the point of refusal of food that they thought was of psychic origin. *Freud* [16, p. 198] in 1905 traced the possible roots of oral conflicts: 'The first of these is the oral or, as it might be called, cannibalistic pregenital sexual organization. Here sexual activity has not yet been separated from ingestion of food; nor are opposite currents within the activity differentiated. The object of both activities is the same; the sexual aim consists in the incorporation of the object, the prototype of a process which, in the form of identification, is later to play such an important psychological part.' Here *Freud* was not speaking specifically of the dynamics of anorexia, but it is clear that this formulation is relevant to the understanding of the syndrome.

In 1911, *Jones* [17] hypothesized that the symptom of neurotic vomiting represented rejection of an incorporated penis, conceived as an incestuous pregnancy, which was in accordance with *Klein's* [18, p. 269] view that little girls enjoyed 'taking the penis into the body ... to make a child from it'. In 1926, *Ferenczi* [19] described the vomiting of hyperemesis gravidarum as a means of denying the genital localization of the pregnancy and vomiting in general as a reaction to coprophagic fantasies, i.e. fantasies of ingesting feces. *Masserman* [14] described the fantasied equation which was apparently first noted by *Abraham* [20] of mother = penis = feces which explains the reaction of disgust, nausea, and vomiting to oral incorporative fantasies. Because of her power and because she 'possesses' father's penis, mother comes to be represented by the penis. The penis, in that it is at times viewed as dirty and distasteful, is equated with feces.

The 'riddance principle' was described by *Rado* [21] in 1939 as a primitive psychosomatic reaction of removing dangerous substances from the body through diarrhea and vomiting. He thought that these two activities were an attempt at eliminating the source of suffering, if necessary even by the sacrifice of a part of one's own body. *Abraham* [22] referred to cannibalistic guilt and consequent food refusal in depressive states which resulted from the unconscious desire for oral incorporation of the ambivalently held lost object.

In 1934 *Alexander* et al. [23] presented a paper concerning 'gastric neurosis'. *Masserman* [14, p. 237], in his discussion of this material, described these very orally dependent patients who adopt a 'defensive facade of great personal self-sufficiency, an exaggerated attitude of helpfulness toward others and a superficial optimism that they in turn would always be provided for'. When frustrated in their strong receptive needs, they become increasingly orally aggressive and demonstrate characteristic narcissistic protests. In the same symposium in which *Alexander* et al. [23] presented this premonitory picture of the 'good compliant girl', this idea was extended to the fantasy of the orally incorporated penis, now however involving the oral dependent position with the mother. Thus, the patient would wish to take in the penis not only because of the wish for an incestuous pregnancy, but also to possess something which would please the mother and thus be able to continue to receive from her. Therefore, vomiting could signify a conciliatory gift of the penis to the mother.

In the same symposium [23], it was noted that while genital conflicts were expressed in the neuromuscular system, it seemed that pregenital conflicts were expressed primarily by disturbances in the gastrointestinal system. *Berlin* et al. [24] in 1945 discussed the oral sadistic tendencies of the anorectic. The specifically compulsive nature of the symptom complex was delineated by *Rahman* et al. [25]. Various dietary alterations including food refusal and laxative abuse were seen as compulsive solutions to various neurotic conflicts.

In the 1930s there was extensive theoretical consideration of various colonic dysfunctions including diarrhea which may be relevant to the laxative abuse which occurs in some anorectics and bulimics. The theory was that this particular symptom represented not only elimination of the incorporated penis or the incestuous pregnancy or elimination simply of the wish to be pregnant [26], but also represented the active masculine strivings of the patient. *Wilson* [23] postulated at this symposium that diarrhea represented a basic rejection of femininity; the female role was seen as parasitically orally receptive or too aggressively castrating and therefore rejected.

Hilde Bruch's Conceptualization

Bruch [7], who has devoted much of her career to research on eating disorders, has formulated a model for the anorexia syndrome which shares some of the observations of *Selvini-Palazzoli* [8], but she arrives at her conclusions from a different point of view. *Bruch* departs, as do most analysts now, from the notion that the infant is utterly helpless; instead, the infant is viewed as capable of emitting signals and cues as to unfulfilled needs to the caretaker, who then responds in various manners. This relates to work done by *Thomas* et al. [27] who delineated nine relatively stable temperamental qualities in infancy and childhood which identified different 'types' of babies (e.g. 'difficult' and 'easy'). Infants have what appear to be distinct inborn temperaments from birth onward, and there is certainly a question of how the parent-infant 'temperament match' might affect the responses given to various cues. The child's later awareness of and sensitivity to her own needs, both biological and emotional, depends on how the early needs are responded to. Consistent appropriate responses provide the basis for the developing child's body identity and also her sense of self. 'Appropriateness' seems to relate to the adult caretakers' confirmation of child-initiated cues, acknowledging the child's needs as separate and valid. A child who has not experienced such appropriate responses might have difficulty in differentiating between biologic-physiologic disturbances and interpersonal-emotional experiences and might attribute any problem in her self-body concept to external causes. One might speculate how an 'easy' baby is responded to versus a 'difficult' child, keeping in mind the different parental temperaments. Depending on parent-child match, an 'easy' baby could either become a compliant child or a rebellious individual.

Bruch thinks that, in what would seem to be an extension of this failure to provide appropriate responses to the child's needs, there is a disturbance in the separation-individuation phase in anorexia nervosa with deficient encouragement or even prohibition of independence. Autonomy is denied and the child remains tied to the parents, thus appearing obedient and compliant. Expression of feelings is also not encouraged, so the anorectic demonstrates a limited range of emotions. The patient is deficient in a sense of separateness and feels controlled by external forces, helpless under the impact of her own bodily urges; in a counterphobic effort she overcontrols them through self-starvation. Thus, she confronts and in effect seeks out what she fears most, denying the fear and loss of control all the while.

Bruch notes that there is a fixation of style of thinking and of morality in the Piagetian preoperational and concrete operational stages. This fixation may be partially the result of disturbances in separation and individuation. Accordingly to *Piaget's* theory [28], in the sensory motor stage (birth to 2 years), the first of the four stages postulated in normal intellectual development, the child's thought is dominated by her perceptions. In the second or preoperational stage (2–7 years), the child begins the development of language and has some understanding of her actions and responses in relation to things in the world. The stage of concrete operations (7–11 years) ushers in the concept of reversibility of the thought process, which *Piaget* contends is necessary before classification and seriation can occur. Thinking is bound to direct experience, however. It is only in the fourth stage, that of formal operations, that the person is freed from the necessity for direct experience and can construct theories and make logical deductions. It appears that this last stage of formal operations which provides the ability for abstract thought is not reached at all or is incomplete in anorectics. Families and other associates of patients with anorexia nervosa tend to judge these patients as having extremely high intelligence levels, in the exceptional range. This has not been demonstrated on intelligence testing. However, as noted in chapter 14, many of these studies are open to question since they were administered when the patient was still semistarved. Although many of these girls do well in school, they do not have as high an intelligence quotient as expected [29] and display marked cognitive distortions [30] which at times seem to have an almost delusional quality. The etiology of this deficit is uncertain; one might speculate that this is so because they are so discouraged from any autonomy which is necessary for the basic social interaction needed to develop higher levels of intellectual development. In addition, development of the ability for abstraction might be challenging to the family system.

Bruch presents evidence from animal experiments and human and animal observation to support her formulation. *Bruch* [7] mentions infants' attachment to and subsequent ability to separate from their mothers as related to the mothers' response to the babies' signals of need. For example, those babies who had been overfed consistently were rated at 12 months to be distressed by separation but did not seek mother out for security. She reports the study by *Miller* et al. [31] of isolate monkeys who could not send recognizable 'messages' to others and who consumed increased amounts of food. Thus, it would appear that the seemingly innate function of appetite regulation requires organizing learning experiences early in life.

Selvini-Palazzoli's Object Relations Theory

As ego psychology and object relations theory began to become part of the literature, a new outlook was directed toward the anorexia syndrome. Thus, for the past 10–20 years most dynamic formulations have not relied on libidinal drive theory.

Selvini-Palazzoli [8] interprets anorexia from an object relations point of view. Adequate personality is dependent on development of the individual's relation with her own body as whole and existing separate from the maternal object. She bases this hypothesis on the early work done primarily by *Benedek* [32–35], *Spitz* [36–43], *Jacobson* [44, 45] and *Mahler* and her associates [46–53] on the concept of separation-individuation as a normal phase of the mother-child relationship. The mother is the first 'object' in the child's awareness. From birth to approximately the third month, the infant is in the normal 'autistic' phase where she exists solely to achieve some physical and emotional hemostasis, not able to differentiate her own attempts at tension reduction from those of her mother. At the point where the infant has even dim awareness of a need-satisfying object (other than herself), she enters into the beginning of the phase of normal 'symbiosis', in which the infant 'behaves and functions as though he and his mother were an omnipotent system – a dual unity within one common boundary' [46, p. 8]. The mother serves as a buffer against inner and outer stimuli, gradually organizing them for the infant and orienting her to her inner versus the outer world in boundary formation and sensory perception – ego functions the child will later learn to perform herself [54]. It is during this phase that the child begins to form the body image. Later, the child begins to walk and thus physically separate. This begins the separation-individuation phase, during which time the child practices her new functions, checks them with mother, and masters new skills, all the while solidifying her separate sense of identity, self and body image.

Selvini-Palazzoli posits that the child who later develops anorexia nervosa never completely achieves a sense of separateness from the maternal object, never achieves a stable and correct body image and thus misinterprets the origin and cause of many experiences as arising from herself rather than from the outside world. Early on, the child would experience her body in relation with the mother as the source of pleasure, as a good object. When defective relations with the maternal object intervene and the child does not perceive herself as distinct, she may perceive her own body as a source of unpleasant sensations, as bad itself or as inhabited by a bad object. Later 'bad' experiences would then repeat the earlier pattern set during the early incorporative phase. *Selvini-Palazzoli* [8, pp. 85–86] states: 'Psychopathological body experiences are a direct expression of a libidinal and aggressive emotional relationship with negative (exciting-rejecting) aspects of the incorporated object'.

Anorexia nervosa then is regarded by *Selvini-Palazzoli* as a kind of 'intrapersonal paranoia', the main pathogenic mechanism of which is concretization. The body is endowed with negative characteristics of the primary maternal object and is perceived as an intrusive entity whose growth must be checked. The body *is* the bad object. The mother is viewed as overprotective and does not see the child as separate from her; the mother controls the child and discourages all experiences of satisfaction apart from her. Compliance is rewarded and the child feels helpless and ineffective in all aspects of her life. Further developmental tasks become difficult and a depression secondary to the sense of helplessness ensues. The body, as a negative and threatening incorporated object, leads her to take a passive role. Self-discontent is symbolically represented by the body. Later interpersonal experiences of childhood, latency and adolescence either 'compensate for or aggravate' the consequences of the defective primary object relation.

Selvini-Palazzoli also adds a sociocultural dimension to the examination of the anorexia nervosa syndrome. She sees anorectics as women who cannot, because of inadequate personal and family resources, meet the new opportunities offered by industrialized society. These women, she feels, come from traditional families with 'obsolete' values.

The Adolescent Ascetic-Hedonistic Conflict

Consideration of development through to the adolescent phase, when the anorexia syndrome most often appears, has led at least one author [55] to comment upon normal defensive attitudes characteristic of adolescence, namely intellectualization and asceticism. In the usual course of development, as the teenager struggles with burgeoning sexuality, the resurgence of drive energy and the push for independence, she often utilizes self-denial and asceticism as an adaptive resource. The anorectic is unable to tolerate the move toward real independence and naturally falls into maladaptively overutilizing these defenses in an attempt to control her own life and the lives of those around her.

Symptoms and Their Meanings

Histrionic Symptoms

Much has been said of hysterical and obsessive-compulsive patterns in some anorectic patients. The concept of hysteria has also undergone much revision. Early on, hysteria was regarded as a neurosis attributable to defensive maneuvers designed to repress the conflicts inherent in patients with significant unresolved oedipal conflicts. Repudiation of oral impregnation fantasies is a very narrow explanation. As theorists elaborated the concept of hysteria, recognition of pre-oedipal and especially oral problems received attention. Gradually borderline and narcissistic personality patterns were considered and these topics became the new bottles into which much of the old wine of 'hysterical character disorders' was placed.

Thus, observations about hysterical features in anorexia nervosa have been given increasing support as personality theory has advanced. Study of personality development and concerns over symbiosis, separation, rapprochement and individuation along with the development (or lack of it) of object constancy became the center of attention for those seeking enhanced clarification of symptoms. 'Splitting' of the good and bad parental images was viewed to be maintained until a fusion of these images occurs with the formation of relative object constancy. This coincides with successful passage through the separation-rapprochement era, also enabling more mature reality testing and, by definition, more mature object relationships. On the other hand, arrested development along these lines is viewed as resulting in borderline personality organization or narcissistic personalities with poor formation of the sense of self. Many of the defensive maneuvers representative of the borderline and narcissistic personalities are seen in anorectics. For example, 'splitting' is almost universally noted in therapy with anorectics. The almost colossal unconcern regarding their physical state which anorectics demonstrate is very much akin to 'la belle indifférence' noted in classic conversion-hysterics.

Obsessive-Compulsive Symptoms

Similarly, pregenital factors in obsessive-compulsive symptoms and personalities were delineated early in the history of anorexia nervosa and these are classically attributed to disturbances in the anal stage of development. Literal oral and anal expulsive behavior are prominent in the anorexia syndrome. Both are consciously induced with the purpose of riddance of 'bad food' which will result in fat. These are counterphobic maneuvers aimed at control over the forbidden food. Later these maneuvers become part of the power struggle entered into with the family and the therapist. Thus, although one usually thinks of food from an 'oral' point of view, the issue of control and the power struggles that ensue forces one to recognize the anality involved in symptom formation.

It has been observed that among starving persons there is considerable emergence of obsessional rumination about food and compulsive rituals about food; this is clearly true in anorectics. Anorectic and bulimic patients ruminate about food almost constantly. Rituals regarding the size of the bite of food or what foods are acceptable or prohibited are prevalent. Hiding and hoarding of foods, especially sweets, become compulsions. Often magical thinking or special symbolic significances give rise to the rituals. Obsessive-compulsive behavior is usually thought of as a derivative of the anal stage of personality development and is related to power and control issues. What is not clear is how much of the obsessive-compulsive patterning represents what should be considered a normal shift to those patterns secondary to starvation and how much of it represents obsessive-compulsive proneness on the part of the individual prior to the onset of the starvation.

Phobic Symptoms

The issue of phobias similarly clouds the descriptive diagnostic picture. One has a hard time determining the phobic object in anorexia, i.e. what the very first link is in the chain of elaboration of symptoms. The phobic object should be symbolic of what is feared. Is it food? Is it too much food? Is it certain kinds of food? Is it fat? Is it mother's body? Is it instinctual wishes? Or is it hunger that symbolizes unacceptable urges and appetites of both a sexual and an aggressive nature? If one does not press the definitions too tightly all of the above can be, generally speaking, phobic in character. Phobias about fat or food refer to objects and are typical of hysterical phobias. Those phobias concerning weight, being like mother, etc., more likely represent displacements to ideas, and thus may be classified more clearly as obsessions. Clearly these phobias and obsessions are multidetermined and symbolic of many issues in both intrapsychic and interpersonal life. At times these beliefs border on delusions. They are certainly held to with a tenacity similar to that with which a delusion is held.

From this general point of view about phobias, much of the typical behavior of forced dieting and riddance behaviors, i.e. diuretic ingestion, laxative abuse and vomiting, are properly viewed more as avoidance behavior rather than true counterphobic behavior indulged in to prove one is not phobicly fearful. *Crisp* [56] sees the syndrome as a 'weight phobia' into which the anorectic flees as a means to gain control of adolescence itself with its phase-specific conflicts, primarily sexuality.

An Integrated Libidinal Object Relations Theory

It is essential that one understand the anorexia nervosa and bulimia syndrome and its symptoms and characteristics from both a classical libidinal-drive point of view and from the classic object relations point of view in order to fully understand and assess the patient. In this integrated theory, the libidinal symptoms are seen from an object relations point of view without denying their libidinal origins.

A common mistake is to consider anorexia a disorder which appears out of the blue and without apparent cause. The patient has usually been seen as a model child, living in a happy family without apparent conflict. This, however, is not actually the case.

Parents tend to be a little older than the norm [57–61] with the patients being born into what is usually an established, moderately successful, stable and usually fairly 'happy' family [58, 61, 62]. There is a tendency for the parents to be overachievers and to impart these values to their children. The father, though often quite successful, is said to often suffer from feelings of inadequacy. Parents tend to take credit for the accomplishments of their children, implying that this is due to their good parenting, rather than the children's abilities or effort. There is considerable emphasis on conformity on the part of the children and a tendency to disregard signals from the children about their own needs, wishes, and accomplishments.

Apparently the most crucial period in the developmental history of patients who later develop anorexia nervosa is the rapprochement subphase of individuation. The child, having succeeded in separating sufficiently from the symbiotic ties to the mother to explore the world at some length, returns to mother and attempts to get a new view of her, using some of the newly found maturity and independence gained from the accomplishments of separation. It is of great importance in the development of individuation at this stage that the child receive appropriate validation for her successes and accomplishments as well as to be treated as an individual with her own needs and wishes, etc. It is as this stage in anorectics that the pattern of family living produces insufficient validation for the child to develop an appropriate sense of individuality.

The child thus lacks the necessary reflections from the parents that would indicate that she is an autonomous individual deserving of respect and capable of independent thought and action. Any existing aspects of individuality tend to be ignored or suppressed by the family. One is supposed to do certain things whether one wants to do or not. External demands take priority over internal demands. The child at this stage finds continuing to accommodate to the parents as the only pathway open to her for a relationship with them. The child in this overaccommodating mode does not have the ability to evaluate others or their performance and therefore does not have angry rebellion at her beck and call to aid in the individuation. She can only go along, trying as best as possible to stay aloof from her own motivations.

This particular adaptation to a bad situation has some dire consequences for cognition. Development of object constancy and a stable and real opinion about herself is impaired. As a result, reality testing, which depends on successful formation of object constancy, becomes impaired. Reality testing requires the ability to recognize differences and the ability to formulate and hold an oppositional posture. The tendency is for the child to 'go along' and not to form opinions of her own. This results in the child's remaining in the preoperational and concrete stages of thinking. By early adolescence, when abstract reasoning and the ability to make evaluations and form opinions independently are ordinarily present, the potential anorectic patient finds herself behind. However, the patient's greatest deficiency in comparison with other more normal children is the serious defect in her sense of self.

It is important to note here that serious pathology is developing early on, but that it does not ordinarily show itself because of the absence of clashes between the child and the parent. The child is overcompliant and few parents would complain about a good and obedient child. The child attempts to do well in all areas and adopts a highly arbitrary value system in keeping with the parents. They work extra hard at school and generally make good grades. At school or in other social situations, real friendships are few and they tend to be followers. The child appears to everyone as having an identity, but it is in fact a sort of pseudo-identity in that so much of her own strivings and reactions to the world are suppressed or repressed in the service of accommodating to the parents. Thus, what develops in the child is more a carbon copy of the parents' identity or an 'as if' self which she believes to be more acceptable to them than her own.

When a person's adaptational patterns prove to be unsuccessful in meeting the problems of everyday living or the stresses which may occur, a period of emotional chaos known as an identity crisis occurs. Following a period of identity diffusion, realignment of the defensive patterns of the ego occurs. The person does not start fresh to develop a whole new personality. The solution to an identity crisis includes handling some of the old problems in a new way, but in keeping with the previous personality structure and the earlier lessons of personality development. The shift in anorexia nervosa is from an anal solution of passive dependency in childhood to an anal pattern of passive aggression as a means to effect a solution to daily life stresses. In a sense, this does represent an improved adaptation at a slightly higher level of functioning. This is a somewhat positive resolution of the passive dependent conflict because the anorectic patient does, in fact, take much more control of what happens to her and how the world treats her. It is our contention that the primary characteristic of anorexia is an anal battle for control where the 'enemy' is the anorectic's own instincts and her relationships with significant others. It is the frustration and failure of her former passive, dependent, accommodating behavior patterns to meet the demands of adolescence in terms of social relationships and to meet the burgeoning demands of her sexual development that brings about the crisis.

There are several reasons why the battle for control comes to be fought over food. Very often in the families of anorectics, food, eating and weight have been reasonably prominent issues. Many anorectics have had periods of bulimia or overweight to contend with where remarks were made often by the parents in terms of the need for weight loss. There are, of course, enormous cultural pressures at every turn on the young woman to retain a slim and attractive figure. In addition, the idea of being tiny, hence weak, helps insulate against the fears of growing up and taking on more adult responsibilities. In some cases, the specific wish is to get rid of fat and initial success at dieting to lose weight provides a great satisfaction. Then any sign of fattiness on her own body signals failure in her battle to control her instinctual energies. Fat is the signal of the failure. In addition, if the mother is overweight, the child may compare her body with that of her mother and desire to be different in order to assert her own independence. She attempts to rid herself of the dreaded fat which is like mother and this increases dieting and weight loss. Fatness or overweight may additionally at an unconscious level represent pregnancy in the secondary oedipal stages. Denial of this oedipal wish is played out in efforts to be thin or skinny. Being slight of weight is such a powerful goal, initially rewarded by some ecstasy from feelings of self-control, that the patient becomes obsessed with her weight and anything having to do with food. This soon changes to serious fears about being overweight; it is these fears that may be related to the tendency of these patients to overestimate their size even when seriously undernourished. The patient is preoccupied with a feared condition and thus tends to feel that her defenses against it have been inadequate. Therefore, such patients will see themselves as overweight. It is probable that some cognitive disturbances both on the basis of developmental defects and on the basis of starvation enter into this body image disturbance.

It should be observed that vomiting, taking of laxatives or diuretics and excessive exercise to a certain extent become libidinized and can become secret substitutes for other erotic practices which tempt the patient because of the onset of puberty. Many anorectics who suffer amenorrhea due to starvation and its secondary hormonal consequences are very reluctant to gain weight if this means their menses will return and remind them of their sexual longings. The patient's solution to her dilemma of an inadequate sense of self and an inadequate sense of autonomy at a time of burgeoning biological urges is to develop an ascetic denial of those urges with the hope of keeping them under control and hence not a threat. Occasional bulimic episodes represent failure of that ascetic control. It is easy for someone who is hungry for love to become hungry for food, and it is characteristic that most anorectics stay hungry most of the time. Sometimes they do finally overcome the hunger. But this is usually as a consequence of the limited diet, often primarily protein with a minimum or no carbohydrate, leading to the development of an acidotic state. The purposeful frustration of the continually experienced oral drives can also be viewed as somewhat masochistic. Here at least is a predictable and constant enemy over which control is continuously attempted. Such an ongoing masochistic battle provides an opportunity for sensations of control which provide a greater sense of ego boundaries than was the case under an approach based on continued compliance to others.

When finally the patient's peculiar dietary habits and loss of weight come to the attention of the parents, a new epoch in the dynamics of the syndrome begins. The formerly compliant girl who was no trouble has now changed into an oppositional, somewhat aggressive person, asserting her own strong 'moral' standard of thinness in opposition to the exhortations of the parents and later the treating physician to eat and gain weight. Another virtue of the choice of food as a stage on which to act out the stubborn drama of passive-aggressive rebellion is that, in a social interaction, stubbornness about eating is nearly impossible for the antagonist to overcome. The anorectic then finds herself in a peculiarly powerful position in her social interactions because stubbornness is so powerful and is, after all, ego-syntonic. Being big or fat equates with dangerous aggression and being thin equates with control of aggressions as well as control of libidinal urges. The masochistic portions of the self-imposed plan represent to some extent a masochistic self-punishment for any unacceptable urges felt or acted upon. The fantasy is to be in control of the body and therefore opposite of the compliance of the earlier stages. In the service of this self-control, which is felt by the patient to be so valuable, is the belief that almost any means, fair or foul, is appropriate when confronted by the opposition of the family. Many patients anticipate this and make elaborate excuses to justify their eating habits. Others will lie, conceal food, take it to their room and secretly dispose of it and engage in a variety of other deceits, all aimed at maintaining their chosen pathway.

One needs to keep in mind that any behavior is in some way an effort by that person to help herself. Indeed, if ordinary control of hunger for food were kept at a reasonable level, this might prove to be an appropriate solution to at least part of the difficult interpersonal problems of the adolescent anorectic both in the family and at a social level. However, what leads to the development of the syndrome is the overuse of this solution to a pathologic degree; in its severest form it becomes life-threatening. Yet, any effort to dissuade the patient about the wisdom of such stringent dieting is met with the most extreme opposition. From her point of view, someone is trying to talk her out of what she views as a successful means of helping herself. It is agreed that a variety of cognitive disturbances permits them to deny the grave threat of the illness as well as to deny the actual body size and the significance of that low weight. These cognitive difficulties enable the patient to perceive reality more as she wishes it to be rather than as it in fact is. Even when the patient becomes sufficiently ill to require hospitalization, the denial continues and the enemy shifts from the patient (her body, her drives) to the physician. Many failures of the usual form of psychotherapy have been reported by many authors. The severe negative preformed transference against the therapist, who is perceived in a parental role, justifies to the patient the same sort of deceitful, pseudoagreement and pseudocompliance that was played out against the parents. This arrangement makes it extremely difficult to establish a genuine, positive therapeutic alliance with these patients because of the tendency for them to form a pseudoalliance with a negative, hidden agenda. Game playing, maneuvers, and manipulations are standard operating procedures when anorectic patients are hospitalized and an attempt is made to strictly control their diet and to keep accurate intake and output records. Here, over and over, it is observed that the actions of patients speak louder than their words. They tend to be full of reassurance and optimism, attesting to their wishes to gain weight and to their total cooperativeness while surreptitiously disposing of food they are to eat and continuing to carry on the rebellious battle displaced onto the physician from the battle at home. To the patient, it is simple: she knows more accurately than the physician what is wrong and her way of treating herself is more desirable than the means of the physician.

What can the psychotherapist do when pitted against such an ego-syntonic solution reinforced by cognitive deficits and positive satisfactions from the adaptation that the patient has chosen? Success will depend on several things being attended to simultaneously. Hospitalization is regularly indicated in order to bring the weight under control. Behavior modification contracts have tended to work fairly well for this specific goal. It is highly desirable to split the role responsibilities between two treating physicians, one of whom handles the behavior program while the other attempts to establish genuine contact with the patient and foster the development of a positive therapeutic alliance. The psychotherapist must be aware of the tendency of the patient to sabotage such an alliance due to the negative transference. The therapist must recognize that this passive-aggressive, often openly aggressive, rebellious and stubborn stance that the patient has chosen is an effort to foster her own separation and individuation and her sense of autonomy. Therefore, in a manner of speaking, asking her to agree to eat more and give up her favored method of adaptation is equivalent to asking her to once again surrender to a state of compliance and forego what she sees as a wholesome search for autonomy and individuality.

In a sense, because of the intensity of the interaction between the patient and her parents, the patient's disorder is something that the whole family has or at least is involved in. Sessions with the whole family, with the parents separately, and with the patient individually, are all needed from time to time, trying gradually to demonstrate to the patient first that her views do represent a distortion and that she may in fact be endangering her life. One also gradually attempts to have the patient see that her difficulties are potentially solvable in a more healthy manner. Only after the patient is able to improve her sense of self and identity will the cognitive disturbances diminish and more ordinary psychotherapy become possible. In this regard, the severity of the consequences of the starvation must not be overlooked and considerable improvement in the capacity of the patient to cooperate in a genuine fashion can be expected only when the starvation is truly brought under control. The psychotherapy of anorexia nervosa is extensively discussed in chapter 2.

References

1 Gull, W.: Anorexia nervosa; in Kaufman, Herman, Evolution of psychosomatic concepts, pp. 128–138 (International University Press, New York 1964).
2 Lasègue, E.: On hysterical anorexia; in Kaufman, Herman, Evolution of psychosomatic concepts, pp. 141–155 (International University Press, New York 1964).
3 Sheldon, J.: Anorexia nervosa. Proc. R. Soc. Med. *32:* 738–741 (1939).
4 Fries, H.: Studies on secondary amenorrhea, anorectic behavior and body image per-

ception: importance for early recognition of anorexia nervosa; in Vigersky, Anorexia nervosa, pp. 163–176 (Raven Press, New York 1977).
5 Feighner, J.; Robins, E.; Guze, S.; Woodruff, R.; Winokur, G.; Munoz, R.: Diagnostic criteria for use in psychiatric research. Archs gen Psychiat. *26:* 57–73 (1972).
6 Diagnostic and statistical manual of mental disorders (DSM III); 3rd ed. (Am. Psychiatric Ass., Washington 1980).
7 Bruch, H.: Anorexia nervosa: therapy and theory. Am. J. Psychiat. *139:* 1531–1538 (1982).
8 Selvini-Palazzoli, M.: Self-starvation: from individual to family therapy in the treatment of anorexia nervosa (Aronson, New York 1978).
9 Deutsch, H.: Anorexia nervosa (with introduction by Roazen, P.). Bull. Menniger Clin. *45:* 499–511 (1981).
10 Eissler, K.: Some psychiatric aspects of anorexia nervosa, demonstrated by a case report. Psychoanal. Rev. *30:* 121–145 (1943).
11 Meyer, B.; Weinroth, L.: Observations on psychological aspects of anorexia nervosa. Psychosom. Med. *19:* 389–398 (1957).
12 Powers, P.; Powers, H.: Inpatient treatment of anorexia nervosa. Psychosomatics (in press).
13 Risen, S.: The psychoanalytic treatment of an adolescent with anorexia nervosa. Psychoanal. Stud. Child *37:* 433–459 (1982).
14 Masserman, J.: Psychodynamisms in anorexia nervosa. Psychoanal. Q. *10:* 211–241 (1941).
15 Breuer, J.; Freud, S.: On the psychical mechanism of hysterical phenomena; in Strachey, The complete psychological works of Sigmund Freud, vol. 2 (Hogarth Press, London 1953).
16 Freud, S.: Three contributions to the theory of sexuality; in Strachey, The complete psychological works of Sigmund Freud, vol. 7 (Hogarth Press, London 1953).
17 Jones, E.: The phallic phase. Papers in psychoanalysis (Wood, Baltimore 1938).
18 Klein, M.: The psychoanalysis of children (Hogarth Press, London 1932).
19 Ferenczi, S.: Theory and technique of psychoanalysis (Hogarth Press, London 1926).
20 Abraham, K.: The influence of oral eroticism on character formation; in Selected papers, vol. 1, pp. 393–406 (Hogarth Press, London 1927).
21 Rado, S.: Developments in the psychoanalytic conception and treatment of the nervosas. Psychoanal. Q. *8:* 427–437 (1939).
22 Abraham, K.: A short study of the development of the libido; in Selected papers, vol. 1, pp. 418–502 (Hogarth Press, London 1927).
23 Alexander, F.; Bacon, L.; Wilson, G.; Levey, H.; Levine, M.: The influence of psychologic factors upon gastrointestinal disturbances: a symposium. Psychoanal. Q. *3:* 501–588 (1934).
24 Berlin, I.; Boatman, M.; Sheimo, S.; Szurek, S.: Adolescent alternation of anorexia and obesity. Am. J. Orthopsychiat. *21:* 387–419 (1945).
25 Rahman, L.; Richardson, H.; Ripley, H.: Anorexia nervosa with psychiatric observations. Psychosom. Med. *1:* 335–365 (1939).
26 Waller, J.; Kaufman, M.; Deutsch, F.: Anorexia nervosa. Psychosom. Med. *2:* 3–16 (1940).
27 Thomas, A.; Chess, S.; Birch, H.: Temperament and behavior disorders in children (New York University Press, New York 1968).

28 Powers, P.; Stavens, C.; Andreasen, N.: The ontogenesis of intelligence: evaluating the Piaget theory. Compreh. Psychiat. *16:* 149–154 (1975).
29 Smart, D.; Beaumont, P.; George, G.: Some personality characteristics of patients with anorexia nervosa. Br. J. Psychiat. *128:* 57–60 (1976).
30 Garfinkel, P.; Garner, D.: Anorexia nervosa: a multidimensional perspective, pp. 123–163 (Brunner/Mazel, New York 1982).
31 Miller, R.; Mirsky, V.; Caul, W.; Sakata, T.: Hyperphagia and polydypsia in socially isolated rhesus monkeys. Science *165:* 1027–1028 (1969).
32 Benedek, T.: Adaptation of reality of early infancy. Psychoanal. Q. *7:* 200–215 (1938).
33 Benedek, T.: The psychosomatic implications of the primary unit: mother-child. Am. J. Orthopsychiat. *19:* 642–654 (1949).
34 Benedek, T.: Psychobiological aspects of mothering. Am. J. Orthopsychiat. *26:* 272–278 (1956).
35 Benedek, T.: Parenthood as a developmental phase. J. Am. psychoanal. Ass. *7:* 389–417 (1959).
36 Spitz, R.: Anaclitic depression. Psychoanal. Stud. Child *2:* 313–341 (1946).
37 Spitz, R.: The first year of life (a psychoanalytic study of normal and deviant development of object relations) (International University Press, New York 1965).
38 Spitz, R.: The smiling response: a contribution to the ontogenesis of social relations. Genet. Psychol. Monogr. *34:* 57–125 (1946).
39 Spitz, R.: No and yes: on the genesis of human communication (International University Press, New York 1957).
40 Spitz, R.: The evolution of dialogue; in Schur, Drives, affects, behavior; 2nd ed., pp. 170–190 (International University Press, New York 1965).
41 Spitz, R.: Relevancy of direct infant observations. Psychoanal. Stud. Child *5:* 66–75 (1950).
42 Spitz, R.: Hospitalism: an inquiry into the genesis of psychiatric conditions of early childhood. Psychoanal. Stud. Child *1:* 53–74 (1945).
43 Spitz, R.: Hospitalism: a follow-up report. Psychoanal. Stud. Child *2:* 313–342 (1946).
44 Jacobson, E.: Denial and repression. J. Am. Psychoanal. Ass. *5:* 61–92 (1957).
45 Jacobson, E.: The self and the object world (International University Press, New York 1964).
46 Mahler, M.: On human symbiosis and the vicissitudes of individuation (International University Press, New York 1968).
47 Mahler, M.: Thoughts about development and individuation. Psychoanal. Stud. Child *18:* 307–324 (1963).
48 Mahler, M.: Autism and symbiosis – two extreme disturbances of identity. Int. J. Psychoanal. *39:* 77–83 (1958).
49 Mahler, M.: On the significance of the normal separation-individuation phase; in Schur, Drives, affects and behavior; 2nd ed., pp. 161–169 (International University Press, New York 1965).
50 Mahler, M.; Furer, M.: Certain aspects of the separation-individuation phase. Psychoanal. Q. *32:* 1–14 (1963).
51 Mahler, M.; LaPerriere, R.: Mother-child interactions during separation-individuation. Psychoanal. Q. *34:* 483–489 (1965).

52 Mahler, M.; McDevitt, J.: Observations on adaptation and defense in statu nascendi. Psychoanal. Q. *37:* 1–21 (1968).
53 Mahler, M.; Pine, F.; Bergman, A.: The mother's reaction to her toddler's drive for individuation; in Anthony, Benedek, Parenthood (Little, Brown, Boston 1970).
54 Masterson, J.: From borderline adolescent to functioning adult: the test of time, pp. 5–39 (Brunner/Mazel, New York 1980).
55 Mogul, S.: Asceticism in adolescence and anorexia nervosa. Psychoanal. Stud. Child *35:* 155–175 (1980).
56 Crisp, A.: Anorexia: 'feeding disorder', 'nervous malnutrition', or 'weight phobia'. Wld Rev. Nutr. Diet., vol. 12, pp. 452–504 (Karger, Basel 1970).
57 Bruch, H.: Eating disorders: obesity, anorexia and the person within (Basic Books, New York 1973).
58 Dally, P.: Anorexia nervosa (Grune & Stratton, New York 1969).
59 Hall, A.: Family structure and relationships of 50 female anorexia nervosa patients. Aust. N.Z. J. Psychiat. *12:* 263–268 (1978).
60 Jensen, L.: Anorexia nervosa. Acta psychiat. scand. *203:* suppl., pp. 113–115 (1968).
61 Theander, S.: Anorexia nervosa: a psychiatric investigation of 94 female cases. Acta psychiat. scand. *214:* suppl., pp. 1–194 (1970).
62 Kendall, R.; Hall, A.; Harley, A.; Babigian, H.: The epidemiology of anorexia nervosa. Psychol. Med. *3:* 200–203 (1973).

7 Disturbances in Cognition: Implications for Treatment

Robert C. Fernandez

Introduction

In this chapter the principle disturbances in cognition that have been noted in patients with anorexia nervosa and bulimia will be reviewed. A thorough understanding and awareness of these disturbances is needed to maximize therapeutic outcome. These include the way these disturbances help to 'lock in' the condition, their contributions to the considerable countertransference problems encountered in working with these patients, the tendency to mistakenly assess the severity and the generalized nature of the disturbances and ways in which some of these disturbances are shared by the families of these patients. We will not review the perceptual disturbances. For a discussion of these and their implications for treatment see chapter 2, and for a review on the research and clinical findings see *Garfinkel and Garner* [1].

Disturbances in Cognition

Bruch [2–5] has repeatedly pointed to the conceptual disturbances in patients with anorexia nervosa. More recently several authors have begun to discuss these disturbances in greater detail and some specific approaches to their treatment [6–8]. In considering the cognitive disturbances in anorexia nervosa and bulimia, three main streams of thought will be addressed. These include *Arieti* [9], *Piaget* [10, 11] and *Bruch's* [12] elaboration of *Piaget's* theory of the ontogenesis of intelligence and *Beck's* [13] theory of cognitive disturbances in depression which have been modified by *Garner and Bemis* [14] for eating disorder patients.

Table I. Common categories of cognitive disturbances [modified and used with permission from ref. 14]

Cognitive disturbance	Examples in regard to food, weight, eating behavior, etc.	Examples from other areas
Selective abstraction, or basing a conclusion on isolated details while ignoring contradictory and more salient evidence	'I just can't control myself. Last night when I had dinner in a restaurant, I ate everything I was served although I had decided ahead of time that I was going to be very careful. I am so weak.'	'I was unfaithful once. It's no surprise my marriage is in trouble since I'm a promiscuous, awful person.'
Overgeneralization, or extracting a rule on the basis of one event and applying it to the other dissimilar situations	'When I used to eat carbohydrates, I was fat; therefore, I must avoid them now so I won't become obese.'	'I once tried to explain to my husband about something that made me sad and he didn't understand. I can't discuss anything that upsets me with him.'
Magnification, or overestimation of the significance of undesirable consequent events. Stimuli are embellished with surplus meaning not supported by an objective analysis	'Gaining five pounds would push me over the brink.' 'I've gained two pounds, so I can't wear shorts anymore.'	'I got a B on an English test. I won't get accepted to college.'
Dichotomous or all-or-none reasoning, or thinking in extreme and absolute terms. Events can be only black or white, right or wrong, good or bad	'If I'm not in complete control, I lose all control. If I can't master this area of my life, I'll lose everything.' 'If I gain one pound, I'll go on and gain a hundred pounds.'	'If I don't establish a daily routine, everything will be chaotic and I won't accomplish anything.'
Personalization and self-reference, or egocentric interpretations of impersonal events or overinterpretation of events relating to the self	'Two people laughed and whispered something to each other when I walked by. They were probably saying that I looked unattractive. I have gained three pounds.'	'I can't enjoy anything because it will be taken away.'
Superstitious thinking, or believing in the cause-effect relationship of noncontingent events	'If I eat a sweet it will be converted instantly into stomach fat.'	'My boyfriend looked very upset when he got home from work today. It must have been something I did earlier.'

Beck's Theory and Eating Disorders

Beck [13, p. 3] has studied cognitive disturbances in depression and anxiety disorders. He postulates that: 'The individual's problems are largely derived from certain distortions of reality based on erroneous premises and assumptions. These incorrect conceptions originated in defective learning during the person's cognitive development.' When significant events in the patient's life occur, they are interpreted and responded to on the basis of these faulty concepts. Therapy is focused on helping patients unravel these distortions and learn new, more realistic, ways to understand their experiences. Utilizing the categories developed by *Beck* [13], *Garner and Bemis* [14] have summarized the cognitive distortions that are common in eating disorder patients: selective abstraction, overgeneralization, magnification, all-or-none reasoning, personalization or self-reference and superstitious reasoning. Table I is a modification of their summary; examples are categorized into those that are related to food, eating behaviors, weight, etc. and those related to other areas. We have also added additional examples from our experience. *Powers* has provided a number of case examples that demonstrate these distortions in chapter 2.

Arieti's Theory and Implications for Eating Disorders

From the outset, it should be emphasized that the author does not consider the prominent cognitive disturbances in anorexia nervosa and bulimia to be the same as the formal thought disorder in schizophrenia. Certainly the accessory symptoms of schizophrenia are rarely found in anorexia nervosa patients. It has been noted that less than 1% of patients with anorexia nervosa develop the characteristic signs and symptoms of schizophrenia as specified in the DSM III (see chapter 1) and 1% is comparable to the rate of schizophrenia in the general population.

Nonetheless, it is postulated that certain of the principles enunciated by *Arieti* [9] are relevant, in modified form, to some anorexia nervosa and bulimic patients. He postulated that in schizophrenia, and some other psychopathological conditions, there are three characteristic cognitive abnormalities: the process of active concretization, teleological regression and paleological thinking which reflects the *Von Domarus* [15] principle. By the process of *concretization Arieti* means that the psyche is still capable of conceiving the abstract, but not of sustaining it, because the abstract concept is too anxiety-provoking. He posits that *teleological regression* may occur if the person is in a situation of severe anxiety and functioning at a certain level of psychological integration cannot take place or does not bring about the desired results; then there is a tendency toward functioning at lower levels of integration in order to effect those results. A third common characteristic is *paleological thought.* Unlike Aristotelian logic in which the normal person accepts identity only on the basis of identity of subjects, the person using paleological thought accepts identity on the basis of identical predicates. An example which he gives is as follows. A person is given the following information: John Doe is a person who was born in the United States; the President of the United States is a person who was born in the United States; the individual utilizing paleological thinking concludes that John Doe is the President of the United States: i.e. the identity of the predicates results in the individual assuming an identity of the subjects. This principle was first articulated by *Von Domarus* [15].

In patients with anorexia nervosa and bulimia, certain cognitions are similar, but not identical, to the *Von Domarus* principle of paleological thought. The following case example illustrates the point. Each step in the illogical thought process is identified in terms of *Garner and Bemis's* [14] paradigm and the conclusions based on the illogical sequence are then studied to determine if there is a similarity to the paleological thought processes described by *Arieti* [9].

Ms. Y. who had anorexia nervosa for many years lived next door to her parents in a duplex and shared the same telephone line. She had a hostile dependent relationship with her mother who was depressed, socially isolated, obese and unhappily married. Ms. Y. was herself depressed, socially isolated and had been unhappily married. A recurrent theme in her psychotherapy sessions was her fear that if she ate and gained weight she would become fat and be identical to her mother.

In terms of the *Garner and Bemis* [14] paradigm, her cognitive sequence might be summarized as follows:

– 'If I eat, I will gain weight' (selective abstraction – omits contradictory evidence that she will only gain weight if she eats more than needed to maintain current weight).

– 'My mother eats and is fat' (selective abstraction and magnification; her analysis leaves out salient detail – namely that mother eats or has eaten too much – and magnifies the process of eating – that eating per se is 'too much').

– 'If I gain weight, I will be fat' (selective abstraction – omits fact that she is currently too thin and needs to gain weight to be in the normal range).

– 'If I am fat, I will be just like my mother' (selective abstraction, leaves out fact that mother is depressed, unhappily married and socially isolated).

In terms of the theory proposed by *Arieti* [9], her cognitive sequence might be *reinterpreted* as follows:

– My mother (subject) is fat (predicate).
– I (subject) will be like my mother if I get fat (predicate).
– My mother and I will be the same if I get fat (illogical, partial paleological conclusion based on potential identity of the subjects).

In comparing the thinking process in this particular patient to that described by *Arieti* [9], it is important to notice that the conclusion is an 'as if' one, i.e. in the future conditional tense. The patient's plan for action was to not eat in order to avoid the identity of the subjects. The main psychodynamic factor that facilitated this illogical thought sequence was the need to deny the fact that she was in fact much like her mother – unemployed, depressed and socially isolated. In her therapy sessions, confrontation with the fact that she was very much like her mother in that she was depressed and socially isolated was not helpful. In *Arieti's* [9] terms, because she was unable to attain a certain level of psychological integration which would have allowed her to relate in an age-appropriate manner, and because this was injurious to her self-image and experienced as an inner danger, she regressed to an earlier stage of functioning (i.e. teleological regression occurred). She also experienced a phenomenon similar to what *Arieti* called active concretization in that occasionally (in situations in which she perceived herself as different from her mother – i.e. the situation was not threatening to her self-image) she could realize that she was in fact too thin; when she returned to her home her capacity to maintain this abstract concept disintegrated and she concretized her concerns about life and her capacity to cope into a fear of becoming fat.

Piaget's Theory and the Eating Disorders

Piaget's [10, 11] theory of the ontogenesis of intelligence posits that there are four stages in normal intellectual development: sensorimotor (birth to 2 years), preoperational (2–7 years), concrete operational (7–11 years) and formal operations (over 11 years). In the sensorimotor stage, the child's thoughts are dominated by his perceptions. In the preoperational stage he begins the development of language and recalls his repertoire of actions and responds to objects he encounters but his thought processes are not yet reversible – i.e. he cannot see that events are ordered. During concrete operations, reversiblity of the thought process relating to the manipulation of an object is present, but the child's thinking is still bound to direct experience. In the formal operational stage, the person can construct theories and make logical deductions without the necessity for direct experience.

Just as *Goldstein and Scheerer* [16] have postulated that the capacity for abstract thought depends on the capacity to hold two viewpoints simultaneously so *Piaget* has postulated that the ability to classify and order events depends on the ability to hold two viewpoints simultaneously and that this ability derives from social interaction and communication. He contends that the child is born egocentric – i.e. the child considers his own point of view the only one possible and is incapable of putting himself in someone else's shoes because he is unaware that the other person has a point of view. As the child begins to interact socially, this egocentricity decreases.

Bruch [12] has postulated that patients with anorexia nervosa do not progress to the stage of formal operations – i.e. that they do not reach the stage where they can make logical deductions without the necessity for direct experience. One important consideration that needs to be kept in mind for all the paradigms thus far described for the cognitive disturbances in anorexia nervosa and possibly in bulimia is that the state of starvation may be partly responsible for the cognitive distortion. *Arieti's* [9] idea that regression occurs to serve a purpose (teleological regression) may be apt in terms of Piagetian development. Regressing to a preoperational or concrete operational stage may assist the patient in denying her own incapacity to form meaningful relationships with peers yet at the same time reinforce the likelihood that the condition will continue.

Some patients with anorexia nervosa seem dominated by their perceptions. For example, after eating a moderate sized meal, they may feel bloated and fat. This intense self-awareness of various physical changes may become a serious therapeutic impediment when interpreted via a cognitive distortion – i.e. that the full feeling is evidence of impending obesity (according to *Garner and Bemis* [14] this would be an example of magnification). Most of the examples of cognitive distortions listed by *Garner and Bemis* [14] are in fact examples of preoperational and concrete operational Piagetian logic.

Implications for Psychotherapy

These disturbances play a large role in the difficulties that have been encountered in attempting psychotherapeutic interventions with these patients in particular as regards insight-oriented or uncovering psychotherapies. They seem to help 'lock in' the condition by facilitating defenses and resistances to traditional psychotherapy efforts. *Bruch* [5] has indicated that her own discouragement with results from traditional psychoanalytic approaches led her to develop what she describes as a 'fact-finding' approach in which 'therapy will attempt to repair the underlying sense of incompetence, conceptual defects and distortions, isolations and dissatisfaction' [5, p. 235]. She goes on to state that a critical aspect of the process of psychotherapy with these patients, especially the early phases, involves the gradual, deliberate and honest labeling of 'misconceptions and errors in the patient's thinking' [5, p. 239]. The importance of attending to the disturbances in cognition has also been reflected in the inclusion of extensive cognitive-educative components in virtually every multidimensional treatment approach to the eating disorders. Examples of such components and their utility are provided by *Powers* in chapter 2, *Yager* in chapter 4 and *Fernandez* in chapter 16.

Countertransference Problems

We have become aware of the great resistance to learning about and working with patients with eating disorders. These resistances and some of the steps to address them are presented in chapter 8. Therapists working with these difficult patients also encounter numerous countertransference difficulties. The cognitive disturbances can contribute significantly to these difficulties especially if the therapist does not pay careful attention to identifying and addressing them. For example, a therapist may misidentify the results of the patient's use of all-or-none thinking as a lack of motivation on the patient's part or as an attempted manipulation of the therapist. This is similar to the common experience of less-experienced therapists in working with patients with hysterical neuroses or personality disorders. When such patients describe an incident (which to the therapist clearly contains seductive messages) and their shock at the sexual advances that result, it is virtually impossible for the therapist to imagine that the patient cannot see or understand how their seductive behavior may have contributed to the sexual advances. Their unwillingness to accept, or their righteous anger directed at the therapist in response to any interpretations or clarifications often produces strong negative countertransference problems. Similarly when the patient with bulimia 'stubbornly' insists that there is no correlation between the marked dysphoria that routinely precedes her binges and the subsequent eating symptoms, it is not unusual for the therapist to experience strong feelings of anger and annoyance. Once the therapist becomes familiar with the various cognitive disturbances and with cognitive-educative techniques to address them, there is a marked reduction in these sorts of countertransference problems.

Need for Accurate Assessment

Another difficulty is that the cognitive disturbances may be noted but incorrectly assessed. For example, a common error is to accurately note the presence of the disturbances but to inaccurately believe they are limited only to ideas about food and eating behaviors. In these situations the therapist fails to note, for example, that the use of all-or-none thinking is not limited to 'good' or 'bad' foods but extends to the way the patient responds to all interpersonal situations including to the therapeutic one. For example, a patient views any small evidence of improvement as a complete recovery and she discontinues therapy. Then with the return of any symptom (e.g. a binge), the patient becomes extremely despondent and feels she is a complete failure. Another error is to fail to note how the widespread use of selective abstraction and overgeneralization severely limits the capacity of the patient to correctly abstract. This can easily reach proportions where the patient is working, in *Piaget's* terms, at the preoperational or the concrete operational stage. This, of course, further hampers the patient's development and severely impedes her ability ot learn and benefit from experience including early psychotherapy experiences.

Another error in assessment is to encounter a cognitive disturbance (e.g. an overvalued idea about food) that is held with great intensity and to incorrectly label it a delusion and therefore to incorrectly treat the patient as if she were psychotic.

Involvement of the Family

We have also noted that at times the families and/or spouses of patients with eating disorders appear to share and thereby reinforce some of the cognitive disturbances present in the patients. In many instances the patient appears to have 'learned' an incorrectly held idea or value from one or both parents, e.g. 'carbohydrates are bad food'. This may be the case although the patient may, in fact, have been taught by the parents that 'too many carbohydrates are bad for you' and distorted the teaching to 'carbohydrates are bad food'. However, in other cases the cognitive disturbances are in fact shared by both the parents or spouse and the patient, although they are usually in a more severe form in the patient. For example, the mother of a patient complained that her daughter was doing 'much worse' because she had vomited again. This assessment was made in spite of the fact that the mother was

Table II. Recommendations for addressing cognitive disturbances

Working familarity with cognitive disturbances and their various presentations
Skill at utilizing cognitive-reeducative techniques and incorporating these into various therapies
Must be addressed early in therapeutic efforts
Exacerbations at times of stress are common
Family and/or spouse intervention if disturbances shared or reinforced
Countertransference difficulties may arise

aware that the patient was controlling the frequency of her vomiting, was starting to date and make friends, and felt much happier about herself. In such cases attempts to intervene and correct the cognitive disturbances in the patient may be partially or totally hampered until an appropriate family intervention occurs.

Recommendations

For any therapist who is going to work with patients with eating disorders, careful attention to the following principles is recommended (table II). First, the therapist must develop a working familiarity with the cognitive disturbances and their various presentations. Second, the therapist should familiarize himself with the cognitive-educative methods that are available to attempt to modify these disturbances. For some therapists this will take considerable practice, especially the modification of more traditional individual therapy techniques that is required. Third, it is crucial that these disturbances be addressed early in the therapeutic efforts. The possibility of successfully reaching other therapeutic goals in the presence of significant cognitive disturbance is very limited, if not impossible. Fourth, the therapist must learn to expect relapses and to promptly respond to exacerbations of the cognitive disturbances. This is particularly common at times of increased stress including transition points in the patient's therapy (e.g. termination), or in her living situation (e.g. loss of a loved one). Fifth, the therapist must be prepared to evaluate the family and/or spouse for the presence of any shared cognitive disturbances or reinforcement of a cognitive disturbance in the patient. If such difficulties are noted a prompt intervention should be undertaken. Finally, the therapist should carefully examine any negative countertransference feelings to determine if unidentified or incorrectly assessed cognitive disturbances are causing or magnifying such feelings. Appropriate supervision or consultation may be necessary to appropriately deal with such problems.

References

1 Garfinkel, P.; Garner, D.: Anorexia nervosa, a multidimensional perspective (Brunner/Mazel, New York 1982).

2 Bruch, H.: Hunger and instinct. J. nerv. ment. Dis. *149:* 91–114 (1969).

3 Bruch, H.: Perceptual and conceptual disturbances in anorexia nervosa. Psychosom. Med. *24:* 187–194 (1962).

4 Bruch, H.: Conceptual confusion in eating disorders. J. nerv. ment. Dis. *133:* 46–54 (1961).

5 Bruch, H.: Eating disorders: obesity, anorexia nervosa, and the person within (Basic Books, New York 1973).

6 Ben-Tovim, D.; Hunter, M.; Crisp, A.: Discrimination and evaluation of shape and size in anorexia nervosa: an exploratory study. Res. Commun. Psychol. Psychiat. Behav. *2:* 241–257 (1977).

7 Ben-Tovim, D.; Whitehead, J.; Crisp, A.: A controlled study of the perception of body width in anorexia nervosa. J. psychosom. Res. *23:* 267–272 (1979).

8 Crisp, A.; Fransella, F.: Conceptual changes during recovery from anorexia nervosa. Br. J. med. Psychol. *45:* 395–405 (1972).

9 Arieti, S.: Interpretation of schizophrenia; 2nd ed. (Basic Books, New York 1974).

10 Piaget, J.: The origins of intelligence in children (International University Press, New York 1952).

11 Piaget, J.: The construction of reality in the child (Basic Books, New York 1954).

12 Bruch, H.: Preconditions for the development of anorexia nervosa. Am. J. Psychoanal. *40:* 169–172 (1980).

13 Beck, A.: Cognitive therapy and the emotional disorders (International University Press, New York 1976).

14 Garner, D.; Bemis, K.: A cognitive-behavioral approach to anorexia nervosa. Cognitive Ther. Res. *6:* 123–150 (1982).

15 Von Domarus, E.: The specific laws of logic in schizophrenia; in Kasanin, Language and thought in schizophrenia: collected papers, pp. 104–114 (University of California Press, Berkeley 1944).

16 Goldstein, K.; Scheerer, M.: Abstract and concrete behavior, an experimental study with special tests. Psychol. Monogr. *53* (1949).

8 Eating Disorders as Models for Psychosomatic Illness

Kailie Shaw, B. Ashok Raj

Introduction

West [1] writes: 'The future of psychiatric education is inextricably linked with the future of medical education in general. Advances in psychiatry will occur as new knowledge is produced by basic and applied research in the medical and behavioral sciences and from ongoing investigation in various disciplines, including our own.'

In this chapter we propose to look at the course charted for psychiatry and its implications for psychiatric education in the 1980s and 1990s. At the University of South Florida College of Medicine, the development of an Eating Disorders Program has allowed us to experiment with an educational model geared to meet the expanded training needs of future psychiatric practitioners. We will review our experience with this evolving educational model and our future plans. The chapter will conclude with a summary of our recommendations for the use of the eating disorders in psychiatric education.

Directions for Psychiatry

West [1] sees the psychiatrist of tomorrow as being more thoroughly grounded in the areas of neurobiology, endocrinology and the behavioral sciences. He envisions the psychiatrist as having increased awareness of psychosocial issues and research. The challenge is the integration of these newer areas into psychiatric education without compromising the body of knowledge accumulated by psychodynamic psychiatry.

Brodie [2], in his presidential address to the American Psychiatric Association, examined the field of psychiatry in terms of its locus, its boundaries and its future. It is his opinion that over the next decade psychiatrists will find it necessary to interface their own field of expertise with three distinct boundary areas. He views psychiatry as a discipline with three interfaces; a triangular locus bounded by: (1) the non-medical mental health disciplines; (2) the biologic front, and (3) the practice of family medicine, behavioral medicine and behavioral pediatrics. We have illustrated this concept in figure 1.

The psychiatric trainee will need the knowledge base and the skills to interact with, receive input from, and continue to educate his colleagues in the primary care specialities and in the non-medical mental health disciplines. At the same time, he will be required to have competence in and be actively involved with ongoing research along the cutting edge of epidemiology, pharmacology, experimental psychology, neurobiology and endocrinology as applied to psychiatric illness. All of this will have to be accomplished simultaneously; the integration of new fields with the established base of psychiatric theory and therapeutic expertise.

The eating disorders are splendid examples of conditions which require the psychiatrist to have a specific knowledge base, diagnostic and psychotherapeutic expertise, as well as the ability to interface effectively with non-medical mental health professionals and primary care specialists. For example, the anorectic patient may be referred by a primary care physician who may need to encourage the patient and family to seek psychiatric treatment, and it may be the primary care physician who monitors the recovered patient for relapse. During active treatment, a social worker or psychologist may provide family therapy. To effectively coordinate treatment, the psychiatrist must understand the underlying principles of family therapy, determine when and if family therapy is appropriate, and effectively collaborate with the family therapist. The psychiatrist must understand the biology of starvation so that cognitive symptoms due to starvation (e.g. poor concentration, obsessions, compulsive handling of food) are correctly identified as such, rather than as necessarily indicative of an obsessive-compulsive disorder. Rapid changes in psychiatric epidemiology (e.g. increased incidence of bulimia in the last 10 years) needs to be part of the knowledge base of a psychiatrist. Recent advances in psychopharmacologic approaches (e.g. use of monoamine oxidase inhibitors for the treatment of bulimia) are another example of the continual changes that must be integrated into the psychiatrist's knowledge base.

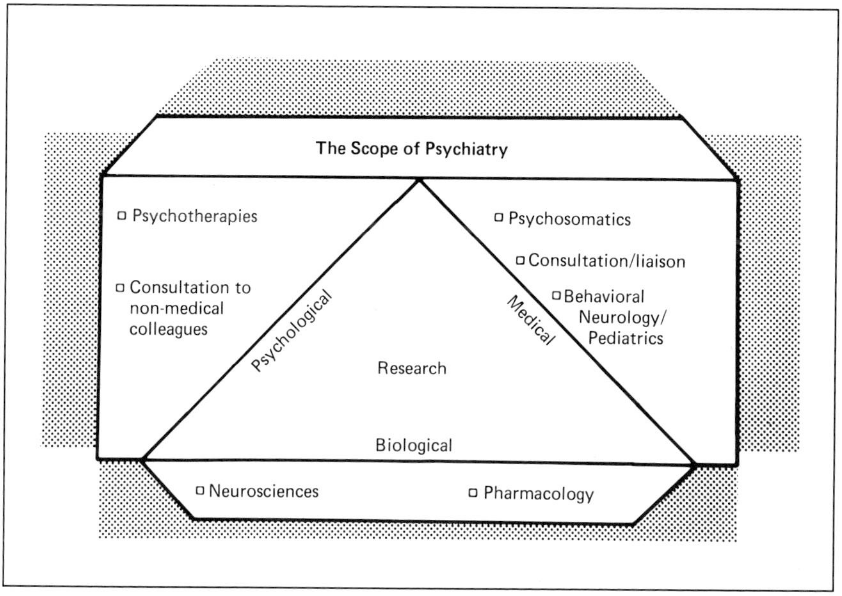

Fig. 1. The scope of psychiatry.

Priorities in Psychiatric Residency Training

Bowden et al. [3], in a pilot survey of 22 psychiatric educators, tried to determine the basic skills and knowledge considered essential to psychiatric education. Their findings showed that the highest emphasis was given to practical clinical objectives: the ability to describe the clinical manifestations and the course of psychiatric illnesses, to perform a thorough psychiatric evaluation, to establish differential diagnoses and to develop and implement an appropriate treatment plan for the major psychiatric disorders. Knowledge of normal and abnormal development was considered important, as were phase-specific conflicts of childhood, adolescence and old age. In the area of treatment skills, individual psychotherapy and psychopharmacology were considered essential; while in the area of theory, psychodynamic objectives were emphasized to a greater degree than learning theory and behavioral objectives.

We feel that these priorities may be too narrow. The need for training that will allow flexible, continued, professional development is illustrated by the eating disorders. For example, although in this study 22 psychiatric educators placed less emphasis on learning theory and behavior modification than on psychodynamic theory and psychotherapy, some of the major advances in the treatment of eating disorders have utilized behavioral and cognitive strategies, both of which have evolved, at least in part, from learning theory. Thus, what is needed is a training program that will prepare the psychiatric practitioner to incorporate new knowledge and skills into an integrated multidimensional model.

Training Sites

It is estimated that by 1990, 90% of the psychiatric beds in this country will be in general hospitals [4]. If this is the case, psychiatric training will be changed by the increased use of general hospitals for psychiatric education. Where better to foster integration with the rest of medicine? In a 1976 survey, it was estimated that only 10% of residency training time was spent in consultation/liaison psychiatry [5]. The shift towards general hospital-based psychiatry will lead to an increased need for training in psychosomatic medicine and consultation/liaison psychiatry.

There is general agreement that many patients with anorexia nervosa will require inpatient treatment at some point (see chapter 10). This is particularly true for those seen in tertiary care centers where most residents are trained. For this reason psychiatric training programs based in general hospitals are likely to include experience with patients with eating disorders.

Conceptual Models

The solutions to many multivariate problems in medicine require appropriate conceptual models for problem analysis. With problems of ever-increasing complexity, the conceptual models will of necessity be derived from interdisciplinary contributions.

A Historical Perspective

Kaplan [6] has reviewed the history of psychosomatic medicine. *Heinroth* in 1818 used the term 'psychosomatic' in relation to insomnia. Since then, the list of psychosomatic disorders was expanded to include ulcerative colitis, peptic ulcer, migraine, bronchial asthma and rheumatoid arthritis. In 1952, the term 'psychophysiological autonomic and visceral disorders' displaced the then commonly used term 'psychosomatic disorders' in the first edition of the *American Psychiatric Association's Diagnostic and Statistical Manual of Mental Disorders.* While acknowledging mind-body interaction, DSM I went a step further in recognizing that physical disease could be mediated by emotional tension. *Alexander* pointed out that conflict was a stress and that suppression of conflict could be expressed through either the voluntary nervous system or the autonomic nervous system. Prolonged alertness and tension could produce physiological disorders and eventual pathology. 'Psychophysiological disorders', the DSM II classification, did not encourage collaboration between psychiatrists and other medical specialists. The theoretical basis for this category perpetuated a simplistic unicausational concept of disease etiology. The DSM III classification attempts to address these shortcomings through the use of the multiaxial system and classifies these disorders in the category 'psychological factors affecting physical conditions'.

Henker [7] has shown that the understanding of the term psychosomatic varies widely among patients, students, general physicians and psychiatrists. Four main recurring themes are: (1) a physical disorder that is imagined; (2) a disturbance of the function of an organ mediated by emotional tensions; (3) an actual physical structural disturbance mediated by emotional tensions, and (4) an approach to any state of the body that considers both physical factors in psychic conditions and psychic factors in physical conditions.

Hidden Conceptual Models of Lazare

Lazare [8] proposes that the application of conceptual models is an implicit part of the psychiatric evaluation and treatment plan of any patient. He has sought to make explicit the four conceptual models used most commonly in clinical psychiatry: the medical, psychological, behavioral and social.

The medical model (which might be more appropriately termed the 'biological' model) views each psychiatric syndrome as a disease for which a specific cause will eventually be found related to the functional anatomy of the brain. The focus is on etiology, pathogenesis, signs and symptoms, differential diagnosis, treatment and prognosis. This model has provided the conceptual foundations for major advances in psychopharmacology, genetic and metabolic studies of psychiatric illness. In terms of eating disorders, the dopamine theory of anorexia nervosa [9] (i.e. disturbances in certain neurotransmitter tracts that pass through the hypothalamus cause characteristic signs and symptoms of the illness) is one example of a medical (or 'biological') model.

According to the psychological model, normal personality development is impaired by a variety of distortions and/or deprivations in early childhood relationships. These experiences leave the patient vulnerable to certain stresses and locked into a pattern of repeating the past in the present. Its derivative, psychotherapy, has become an accepted mainstay of the psychiatrist's therapeutic armamentarium. *Bruch's* [10] theory that anorectics-to-be are bombarded with expectations by their parents and are taught to respond to these, rather than to their own internal needs and feelings, is an example of a psychological model of anorexia nervosa.

According to the behavioral model, both neurosis and psychosis are examples of abnormal behavior that have been learned as a result of aversive events, and are maintained because they lead to positive effects, or because they avoid deleterious ones. Its derivative is behavior therapy. The many aspects of behavioral methods used in the treatment of eating disorders are outlined in chapters 2, 3, 4, and 16. A specific example is the work on relapse prevention by *Marlatt and Gorden* [11].

The social model of psychiatric illness regards symptoms as an index of social disorder. The rapid increase in the incidence of eating disorders has been conceptualized by some [12] as the consequence of the national obsession with slimness. This social model of the etiology of anorexia nervosa may explain certain puzzling epidemiological findings (e.g. the fact that 90% of anorectics are female), that women are the targets of advertisements for dieting aids and that the increase in the incidence of eating disorders has paralleled the national interest in staying 'slim and fit'.

Psychiatrists generally use one or more of these conceptual models when making clinical decisions. In practice, the choice is determined by a number of variables: the ideology of the therapist, the diagnosis, the effectiveness of available treatments, the attributes of the patient and the availability of services. In terms of anorexia nervosa and bulimia, it is clear that none of these models taken alone accounts for the disorders and that some integration is needed to understand and effectively treat afflicted patients. Although each model has some validity, there is considerable artificial separation which leads to impaired communication between professionals and unnecessary limitations in the use of treatment options.

Biopsychosocial Model

Engel [13] introduced his biopsychosocial model in 1977 to provide a greater understanding of disease and illness than the then prevalent biomedical or psychosomatic models. His model is rooted in general systems theory which holds that all levels of an organization are linked to each other in such a fashion that a change in one level necessitates a change in other levels [14]. In human terms, the organizational levels may range from atoms, molecules, cells, organs, and organ systems to the individual and his experiences, the dyad, family group, society, etc. [15]. The lower levels of this system's hierarchy are subordinate to the higher levels. There are interconnections and feedback arrangements, so that a disturbance or affliction at any level may affect any other systems level. The importance of this model becomes apparent in situations in which a strict biomedical approach is applied. Insistence on compliance with orders and treatment plans prescribed by the physician, while neglecting the psychosocical factors, frequently triggers iatrogenic psychiatric disorders. This may then generate an urgent request for psychiatric consultation. Thus, in addition to helping in evaluation the biopsychosocial approach helps to determine at which system(s) level intervention will be most effective.

A Proposed Model for Eating Disorders

At the University of South Florida, in addition to the biopsychosocial theory of disease, we have incorporated many aspects of the writings of *Kubie* [16] and *Weiner* [17]. Much attention is given to the following in our model for working with patients who have eating disorders: multiple and varied predisposing factors, individual constitutional vulnerability, initiating factors, range of intensity in the expression of the illness and sustaining factors. This model is illustrated in figure 2 and can be used equally well for any psychosomatic disorder.

Predisposing Factors

As with other conditions, the eating disorders do not occur at random. In individuals with anorexia nervosa for example, there are known individual, familial and cultural predisposing factors. Individual predisposing factors include female gender, early menarche [18] and poor self-identity [10]. Predisposing familial factors include twinning [19], older age of parents [10] and the 'psychosomatogenic' family system described by *Minuchin* et al. [20].

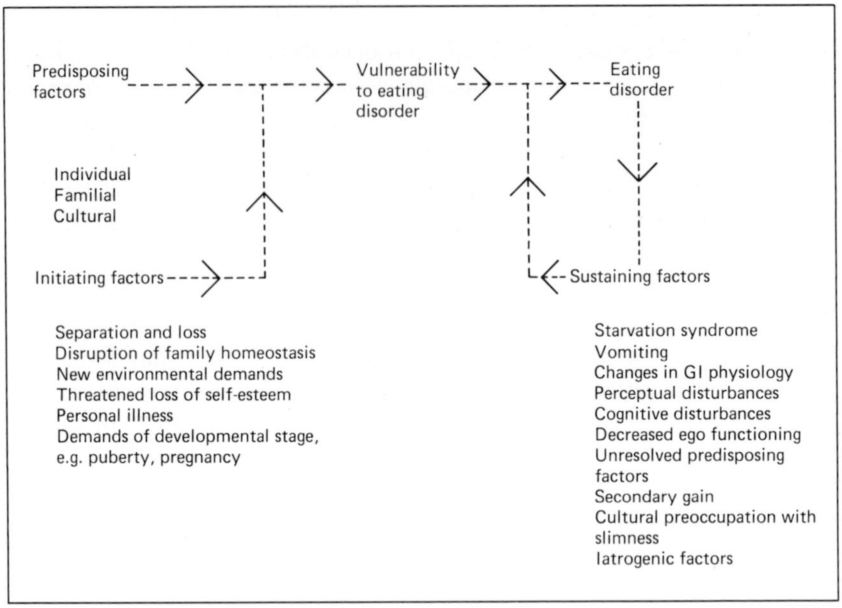

Fig. 2. Eating disorders model.

Cultural predisposing factors include upper socioeconomic class of the parents [21], living in industrialized Western society [10] and preoccupation with slenderness [12].

Initiating Factors

The onset of the disorder coincides with events in the individual's life which, according to this model, are termed initiating factors. The initiating stress must be greater than that to which the person is able to adapt. Examples of this stress may include the demands of adolescence, separation and loss, and disruption of family homeostasis. As the symptoms develop, there is variability in the intensity with which they manifest. This will influence the patient as well as the family.

Sustaining Factors

As the symptoms evolve, the individual's attempts to deal with them may produce changes that further sustain or perpetuate the disorder. For example, in anorexia nervosa, the loss of weight may alleviate anxiety and set up a reinforcement for further weight loss. The state of starvation may result in an increase in β-endorphins [22] and results (at least initially) in euphoria, thus sustaining the drive toward ever-increasing thinness. Vomiting may begin during an ill-conceived treatment plan which encourages too rapid weight gain. The vomiting may become one of the major factors that sustains the illness. Use of laxatives to increase weight loss may result in permanent damage to the gastrointestinal tract and thus make relinquishing laxatives difficult.

An Educational Model for the Eating Disorders

The eating disorders have proved valuable as a link between the biological and psychological aspects of illness and in the introduction of trainees to many of the concepts enumerated in the model above. The blatant physical manifestations of the eating disorders are useful in encouraging medical students, non-psychiatric residents and beginning psychiatric residents to look at the close association between mind and body. The trainee is then encouraged to move from this into a consideration of the biopsychosocial model and then on to the model illustrated above for understanding and treating the illness.

Medical Student Education

Our contact with the medical students begins with the Introduction to Behavioral Medicine Course at the beginning of their second year. In this course we utilize a developmental model for learning about human behavior including psychodynamic, behavioral, biological and cultural perspectives and the biopsychosocial model is introduced. Eating behaviors, and in particular the cultural aspects, are examined. In the Introduction to Psychiatry Course, later in the second year, further didactic instruction in the evaluation and treatment of the eating disorders is provided and students are offered mini-elective experiences in the Eating Disorders Clinic. Students are encouraged to seek a greater understanding of the multiplicity of the predisposing etiological risk factors, initiating stressors and the sustaining factors operative in each individual case. In the fourth year, students are offered more extensive electives that enable them to acquire some experience and beginning skills in the comprehensive multidisciplinary evaluation and treatment of patients with eating disorders.

Psychiatric Residency Training

We have developed a comprehensive plan for integrating the Eating Disorders Program throughout the 4 years of psychiatric residency training. This plan is designed to increasingly challenge the residents with additional educational opportunities. In the first year, the residents begin with rotations in Internal Medicine or Pediatrics. The eating disorders serve as a natural bridge between these rotations and the beginning of psychiatric training. Here, in a rather concrete way, the identity issues of the psychiatric resident as a physician and a psychiatrist surface. The challenge of integrating the biomedical aspects with the psychosocial ones and their relevance for understanding etiology, presentation of the illness and treatment planning is particularly valuable at this stage of training. To accomplish this, our first year trainees are assigned a half day a week for 3 months to the Eating Disorders Clinic with the educational goal of acquiring a sound theoretical base and improving their evaluation skills.

The second year of psychiatric residency is essentially an inpatient year with the educational goal of learning basic skills in inpatient evaluation and management while functioning within a multidisciplinary team. Patients with eating disorders offer the residents opportunities to learn and apply the basics of medical nutritional management, behavioral techniques, and family intervention. The residents are taught to recognize the powerful dynamics set in motion, which affect them and other members of the treatment team, and to separate patient management issues from individual psychotherapy issues. Collaboration with non-psychiatric physicians and non-medical colleagues allows for discussion and exchange of ideas, thereby promoting good patient care along with an appreciation of specialized areas of expertise. The residents may, at this time, begin to crystallize their own areas of interest and seek to be involved in ongoing research.

The third year of residency is designed to provide outpatient experience and the acquisition of increasing skills in individual, family and group psychotherapy. Patients evaluated in the Eating Disorders Program are referred to residents for psychotherapy. The chronicity of the eating disorders, the frequent presence of significant character pathology and the recurrence of stressors repeatedly challenge the residents to sharpen their therapeutic skills in individual psychotherapy and in family therapy. Group therapy for selected patients with anorexia nervosa and bulimia enables the residents to participate as co-therapists with senior faculty.

In the fourth year, the senior residents are assigned for a 6-month consultation/liaison experience at an affiliated general hospital. The residents are called to evaluate patients with eating behavior problems on a medical or pediatric service. Their familiarity with the multifactorial nature of the eating disorders, the precipitating stressors and the sustaining factors enable the residents to provide effective consultation to their medical colleagues. Liaison activities generally include assignments running staff groups on specialty units, including those dealing with eating disorders patients, consultation to self-help groups and in giving talks to community organizations. Research interests are encouraged and the residents are given opportunities to learn research design, to become familiar with current research and to participate in ongoing research projects.

A 6-month elective opportunity completes the senior year of training. Residents are required to develop and submit a proposal tailored to their individual needs and/or interests for further experience in research or clinical areas. This elective period offers an opportunity for residents to develop subspeciality-level skills in the management of the eating disorders.

Other Trainees

Residents in Pediatrics, Internal Medicine, and Family Practice are provided exposure and training in the eating disorders via the activities of the Psychiatry Consultation/Liaison Service. These residents as well as trainees from the non-medical mental health disciplines, e.g. psychology interns, are offered electives in the Eating Disorders Program.

Continuing Education

An extensive program of continuing education has been developed. This includes conferences, study groups and seminars to provide a venue for full-time residents and clinical faculty as well as other practitioners to learn more about the eating disorders. A growing awareness and interest on the part of our faculty in the eating disorders model for psychosomatic illness has resulted in its application to other areas of their teaching.

Results

The response to these educational efforts, in particular from the medical students and psychiatric residents, has been most favorable. We have been able to fully implement this plan with the exception of the training for second year psychiatry residents. At the present time, an eating disorders inpatient program is not available at the sites used for inpatient training. Instead, a limited exposure to working with inpatients with eating disorders is offered as a part of the consultation/liaison experience in the fourth year. However, we will implement our plan for second-year residents in July of 1985 when our new psychiatric facility, which will include an Eating Disorder Inpatient Program, is scheduled to open.

Dispelling the Myths

We have found that, despite our successes in our educational efforts, we encounter a continued resistance to the recognition of the seriousness and potentially lethal nature of the eating disorders on the part of many medical students, non-psychiatric physicians, psychiatrists, non-medical care personnel and the general public.

Myth: These Patients Are Not 'Really Ill'

There is a persistent belief that these patients are willful and 'not really ill'. The eating behavior symptoms mask the illness and distract from the underlying psychopathology. This myth is reinforced by the denial that results from the fact that the socioeconomic group at greatest risk for eating disorders parallels that from which the care providers are drawn. Also our current cultural bias towards thinness is so strong that it further contributes to the denial that is characteristic of this illness and to the collusion between physician and patient that may ensue.

Myth: Only an Expert Can Work with These Patients

A second persistent belief is that all eating disorder patients are so seriously disturbed that all aspects of their management require a level of skill and expertise found only in the 'expert'. Avoidance of eating disorder patients is a phenomenon seen frequently among experienced as well as novice clinicians. For example, some of our supervisors have taken the position that all eating disorder patients are too disturbed to be assigned to residents for intensive psychotherapy.

Patients with eating disorders may have major psychopathology and their management may be complicated by their enmeshment in extremely difficult families. The thought of working with such patients may certainly lead to discouragement and a sense of therapeutic nihilism. However, the question is: 'Do they pose any greater difficulties than those posed by many of the difficult patients with whom psychiatrists spend much of their time?' (e.g. patients with early onset schizophrenia, labile bipolar affective disorder, severe neuroses, or personality disorders). We think not. In fact, working with complex and difficult patients and acquiring specialized knowledge and skill, including the knowledge of when to consult with or refer to the subspecialist, is an integral part of becoming a psychiatrist.

Recommendations for an Eating Disorders Educational Program

In instituting an educational program in the eating disorders for psychiatric residents, attention to the following principles (table I) is recommended.

First, an integrated approach to the eating disorders throughout all 4 years of resident training that keeps pace with the residents' developing psychiatric skills and professional identity is most useful. Acknowledgment of the very real difficulties inherent in working with one of psychiatry's most demanding, difficult and seriously ill clinical populations is required. Close supervision which focuses on the process of the illness and is ever alert to countertransference issues is necessary. The provision of appropriate role models via the residents having an opportunity to be part of a well-functioning multidisciplinary team is the best way to encourage the development of interdisciplinary work skills. The risk of 'burnout' is reduced by ensuring that there is adequate support among team members and also that the team does not become overloaded. Sufficient psychiatric coverage is needed to make it possible for physicians to step back from a particular situation as needed. Attention should also be paid to residents' case loads to ensure that they are varied both as to types of patients and to spacing of appointments on a particular day. The range of treatment modalities used in psychotherapeutic interventions must be comprehensive and the residents will need to be helped with the difficult adjustments in their therapeutic role. The ways in

Table I. Recommendations for educational programs for psychiatry residents

1	Integrate into all four years of training
2	Attend to considerable difficulties in working with these patients
3	Supervise with careful attention to transference and countertransference issues
4	Develop interdisciplinary work skills
5	Include experience in wide range of treatment modalities
6	Provide research training and opportunities

which the considerable and predictable technical effects of these adjustments will be reflected in the transference and countertransference must be addressed. Supervisors must carefully look for and attend to the countertransference issues which surface repeatedly. Finally, active encouragement of residents to participate in ongoing research is a useful and effective way of helping them keep an appropriate perspective. Regularly scheduled time for research activity should be included in the residents' schedule.

Conclusion

The eating disorders offer an opportunity to utilize a model which goes beyond the biopsychosocial model and is applicable to all psychosomatic illness. They also offer an opportunity to develop educational programs that can evolve in the same direction as that envisioned for the field of psychiatry in the future. They require that the psychiatrist be a physician who is knowledgeable about the many advances in medicine, who seeks to appreciate the complexity and multiplicity of factors operative for the individual patient and who is able to formulate and implement a comprehensive treatment plan, drawing on the expertise of colleagues from other disciplines. As psychiatrists ask the questions required to do the above, they are inevitably led to seeking answers. If they are provided the encouragement and basic tools for competency in the area of research, they will respond in a way to further the development of psychiatry.

References

1 West, L.: The future of psychiatric education. Am. J. Psychiat. *130:* 521–528 (1973).
2 Brodie, H.K.H.: Presidential address: psychiatry – its locus and its future. Am. J. Psychiat. *140:* 965–968 (1983).
3 Bowden, C.; Humphrey, F.; Thompson, G.: Priorities in residency training. Am. J. Psychiat. *137:* 1234–1246 (1980).
4 Brooklodge Conference on Consultation Liaison Psychiatry, Kalamazoo 1982.
5 Schubert, D.; McKegney, F.: Psychiatric consultation education. Archs gen. Psychiat. *33:* 1271–1273 (1976).
6 Kaplan, H.: History of psychophysiological medicine; in Freedman, Kaplan, Sadock, Comprehensive textbook of psychiatry, vol. II, pp. 1624–1637 (Williams & Wilkins, Baltimore 1975).
7 Henker, F.: Conflicting definitions of the term psychosomatic. Psychosomatics *23:* 8–11 (1982).

8 Lazare, A.: Hidden conceptual models in clinical psychiatry. New Engl. J. Med. *288:* 345–350 (1973).
9 Barry, V.; Klawans, H.: On the role of dopamine in the pathophysiology of anorexia nervosa. J. neural Transm. *38:* 107–122 (1976).
10 Bruch, H.: Eating disorders: obesity, anorexia nervosa, and the person within (Basic Books, New York 1973).
11 Marlatt, G.; Gorden, J.: Relapse prevention (Guilford Press, New York 1983).
12 Wooley, O.; Wooley, S.: The Beverly Hills eating disorder: the mass marketing of anorexia nervosa. Int. J. Eating Disord. *1:* 57–69 (1982).
13 Engel, G.: The need for a new medical model: a challenge for biomedicine. Science *196:* 129–136 (1977).
14 Bertalanffy, L. von: General system theory. Foundations, development, applications (Braziller, New York 1968).
15 Mohl, P.: A systems approach to liaison psychiatry. Psychosomatics *21:* 457–461 (1980).
16 Kubie, L.: Multiple fallacies in the concept of schizophrenia. J. nerv. ment. Dis. *153:* 331–342 (1971).
17 Weiner, H.: Psychobiology and human disease (Elsevier/North-Holland, New York 1977).
18 Crisp, A.: Premorbid factors in adult disorders of weight with particular reference to primary anorexia nervosa: a literature review. J. psychosom. Res. *14:* 1–22 (1970).
19 Garfinkel, P.; Garner, D.: Anorexia nervosa; a multidimensional perspective, p. 170 (Brunner/Mazel, New York 1982).
20 Minuchin, S.; Rosman, B.; Baker, L.: Psychosomatic families: anorexia nervosa in context (Harvard University Press, Cambridge 1978).
21 Crisp, A.; Palmer, R.; Kalucy, R.: How common is anorexia nervosa? A prevalence study. Br. J. Psychol. *128:* 549–554 (1976).
22 Kaye, W.; Pickar, D.; Naber, D.; Ebert, M.: Cerebrospinal fluid opioid activity in anorexia nervosa. Am. J. Psychiat. *139:* 643–645 (1982).

9 Biological Aspects of Eating Behaviors

Allen W. Root

Introduction

It is extremely useful for anyone working with patients with eating disorders to be knowledgeable as to the neurobiologic aspects of these conditions. This chapter will begin with a review of the processes involved in the regulation of appetite. The metabolic consequences and endocrinologic response to malnutrition will then be considered. The chapter will conclude with a review of the immunologic effects of malnutrition.

Regulation of Appetite

The appetite is regulated through the interaction of ventromedial and lateral hypothalamic nuclei, which integrate the many neural inputs which describe the nutritional status of the individual. Basic experiments and clinical observations suggest that the 'satiety' center is located within the ventromedial hypothalamus; electrical stimulation of this area results in decreased food intake, while its destruction leads to hyperphagia and obesity [1]. The 'feeding' center is located within the lateral hypothalamus; electrical stimulation of this area leads to excessive food intake, while its destruction inhibits feeding. The regulation of feeding is indeed more complex than the concept of two controlling centers suggests. Also involved in feeding behavior are neural tracts and many neurotransmitters. Serotonin agonists, beta-adrenergic agonists, several peptides, glucose, fatty acids and amino acids inhibit feeding while dopamine, alpha-adrenergic agonists, endogenous opioid peptides and gamma-aminobutyric acid are important appetite stimuli. Naloxone, an opioid inhibitor, inhibits feeding in animals and man.

Dynorphin (a 17-amino acid with leucine-enkephalin at its amino terminal) binds to opioid kappa-receptors to inhibit feeding behavior. A number of peptides, many originally thought to be exclusively of gut origin but now recognized to be produced within the central nervous system (CNS) as well, function in the CNS as neurotransmitters and induce feelings of satiety. Cholecystokinin depresses feeding in both experimental animals and in man [2, 3], although the site of this effect, whether within the CNS or elsewhere, is uncertain. Bombesin, glucagon, calcitonin, thyrotropin-releasing hormone (TRH), corticotropin-releasing factor (CRF), pancreatic polypeptide, somatostatin, gastrin, secretin, neurotensin, substance P and insulin inhibit feeding in experimental animals [1, 4, 5]. However, since, in rats, the satiety effects of glucagon and somatostatin are blocked by abdominal vagotomy, the site of actions of these gut neuropeptides is probably in the periphery rather than in the hypothalamus. However, the satiety effect of bombesin is maintained after vagotomy. Purines can also suppress feeding [1]. *Morley and Levine* [1] postulate that inasmuch as patients with anorexia nervosa are presumably under chronic stress and have relatively elevated plasma cortisol levels, increased CRF activity within the hypothalamus of such patients may contribute to the decreased appetite of this disease [1].

Metabolic Consequences of Malnutrition

There is a phased metabolic-endocrine response to starvation [6]. Body fuels are stored as carbohydrates, proteins and fat; although liver and muscle stores of glycogen and glucose account for only 1,100 cal (4,605 J) in the average adult, they nevertheless are important energy sources for ongoing needs and sudden requirements. Stored in body fat are approximately 135,000 cal (565,218 J) in the average adult, while muscle protein stores may provide 40,000 cal (167,472 J) for use in the calorie-protein depleted state. It is the amount of body protein which limits survival in starvation because of the many important tasks of this nutrient, including body structure, muscle function, enzyme activity, and so forth. In the immediate postabsorptive period, 6–12h after a meal, body energy requirements are met by glycogenolysis (release of glucose primarily from liver glycogen) which supplies glucose for use in cerebral metabolism, and by lipolysis of fat and the metabolism of fatty acids for use by cardiac and striated muscle. Liver glycogen stores are usually depleted by 24-h of fasting, and thereafter carbohydrate requirements are met primarily by gluconeogenesis. Alanine is the principle gluconeogenic amino acid. Glycerol, but not fatty acids, can also be converted to glucose. Lipolysis leads to ketogenesis, i.e. oxidation of free fatty acids in the liver to two carbon ketone acids (beta-hydroxybutyric and acetoacetic acids) which influence acid-base and water homeostasis. In the postabsorptive state serum concentrations of insulin decline and serum concentrations of glucagon increase. Insulin inhibits glycogenolysis and gluconeogenesis and enhances synthesis and storage of glycogen, triglycerides and proteins. Glucagon enhances glycogenolysis, lipolysis and gluconeogenesis. Therefore, the postabsorptive decrease in insulin secretion and increase in glucagon concentrations have additive effects upon the latter three processes. Interestingly, the increase in glucagon values in starvation is apparently due to decreased catabolism rather than increased secretion.

In short-term (3–7 days) starvation, fuel requirements are met by gluconeogenesis, lipolysis, fatty acid oxidation and ketogenesis. This stage is marked primarily by greatly increased gluconeogenesis and mobilization of alanine from muscle protein stores. Late in this phase, ketone acids begin to serve as fuel for brain metabolism. These effects are mediated by the changes in insulin and glucagon secretion cited above. With periods of starvation longer than 7 days, adaptive mechanisms designed to spare protein catabolism appear. There is a decrease in gluconeogenesis from amino acids as fatty acids and ketone bodies provide more energy, particularly for brain metabolism, and inhibit further muscle protein breakdown. Inasmuch as the patient with anorexia nervosa has decreased, but not absent, caloric intake, the stage of starvation and the metabolic-endocrine adaptation thereto may vary within and among patients.

Endocrinologic Response to Malnutrition

In addition to the starvation-induced changes in the secretion of insulin and glucagon previously described, many other hormonal changes occur in this state. Glucagon values, which increase over the first 7–14 days of total starvation, return to basal postabsorptive levels as secretion declines [6].

In the hypocaloric state the rate of conversion of thyroxine (T_4) to triiodothyronine (T_3) decreases, due to a decline in activity of 5′-monodeiodinase activity and thus serum concentrations of total T_3 decline. The decrease in serum T_3 concentrations may be a protective measure to conserve energy stores during periods of low caloric intake. Reverse T_3 levels increase reciprocally. Basal serum concentrations of T_4 and thyrotropin (TSH) are usually normal in patients with anorexia nervosa unless there is very marked protein depletion and lowered concentrations of thyroid-binding globulin (TBG). Serum concentrations of free T_4 are normal in anorexia nervosa, but free T_3 levels are lowered [6]. The free T_4 index (the product of the serum concentration of T_4 times the T_3 resin uptake – a reflection of TBG) is usually normal in anorexia nervosa as is the free T_3 index. The TSH secretory response to TRH may be normal or delayed and prolonged in fasted subjects [7, 8]. Clinically and biochemically the patient with anorexia nervosa has signs of hypothyroidism consistent with the low T_3 levels.

Basal plasma concentrations of cortisol are elevated and its diurnal fluctuation is exaggerated in patients with anorexia nervosa. Elevated plasma cortisol values reflect decreased metabolic turnover as well as increased secretion of this glucocorticoid [6, 9–11]. The urinary excretion of cortisol is often decreased in anorexia nervosa. The metabolism of cortisol is disturbed in the starved state in a manner similar to that observed in hypothyroidism; there is an increased urinary tetrahydrocortisol/tetrahydrocortisone ratio which can be reversed by administration of T_3 [10]. Corticosteroid-binding globulin concentrations are usually normal in anorexia nervosa, suggesting that free cortisol values may be elevated.

Adrenocorticotropic hormone (ACTH)-induced cortisol secretion is usually normal in anorexia nervosa. With prolonged starvation adrenal glucocorticoid secretion may decline and adrenal atrophy occur. In children with protein-calorie malnutrition, autopsy studies have revealed adrenal atrophy [12]. This may be due to decreased hypothalamic-pituitary function rather than to primary adrenal dysfunction. It is essential to remember that the patient with anorexia nervosa may manifest acute adrenal insufficiency. During prolonged fasting plasma renin activity and aldosterone concentrations decline [13].

One of the earliest manifestations of anorexia nervosa in females is disturbance in the menstrual pattern. Amenorrhea and oligomenorrhea may occur even before substantial weight loss has occurred. In patients with anorexia nervosa, as well as in women with simple weight loss [14], there are decreased basal and gonadotropin releasing hormone (GnRH)-induced secretion of luteinizing (LH) and follicle-stimulating (FSH) hormones and decreased plasma concentrations of estradiol [14]. Similar declines in LH, FSH and testosterone concentrations occur in starved adult men [15]. In previously normal women with anorexia nervosa, the 24-hour secretory profile of serum LH reverts to a prepubertal pattern, characterized by very low basal LH levels and no significant change in LH concentration over a 24-hour period [16]. With weight gain, the 24-hour LH profile matures through the stage of adolescence with enhanced nocturnal LH secretion and increased numbers of LH secretory episodes to the mature phase characterized by LH secretory spikes at 60–120 min without diurnal variation. Cyclical secretion of LH and FSH is lost in the patient with anorexia nervosa and can be restored with weight gain, although often weight above that at which the last menstrual period occurred must be achieved before menses resume [17]. In the 'prepubertal', hypogonadotropic state of the adult woman with anorexia nervosa, secretion of LH, FSH and estradiol can be achieved by the intermittent bolus administration of GnRH over several days suggesting that the primary site of failure of the reproductive endocrine system in these patients is in hypothalamic synthesis and/or secretion of GnRH [18]. Peripheral androgen metabolism is disturbed in anorexia nervosa, secondary to the functional hypothyroid state of these subjects as the androsterone/etiocholanolone ratio is low. Although there is increased formation of 2-hydroxyestrone and estriol production from estradiol is reduced in anorexia nervosa, these changes have been attributed to low body weight rather than to functional hypothyroidism [19].

Serum concentrations of growth hormone (GH) tend to increase transiently in fasted subjects while levels of the anabolic effectors of this hormone, the somatomedins, decline. In patients with prolonged starvation involving both protein and energy, GH concentrations are often very high while somatomedin values are low. Somatomedin C concentrations increase in response to the refeeding of both carbohydrates and proteins, and the two foods have additive effects upon the increase in somatomedin C levels which follows refeeding [20]. The regulation of secretion of GH is also aberrant in patients with anorexia nervosa, as it may be in other patients with elevated basal GH concentrations. Thus, glucose may stimulate rather than depress GH levels in anorexia nervosa; TRH and GnRH may also provoke GH secretion in such patients, while in normal subjects these peptides do not do so [21]. Basal prolactin concentrations are normal or slightly elevated in patients with anorexia nervosa, while the prolactin secretory response to TRH may be normal or exaggerated [21, 22]. Plasma and urinary levels of norepinephrine may be elevated during starvation [6].

Patients with anorexia nervosa frequently have difficulty concentrating urine which may be due, in part, to defective osmoregulation of the secretion of arginine vasopressin [23]. These subjects also fail to stabilize body temperature when exposed to cold or heat, further manifestations of the profound hypothalamic dysfunction which accompanies this disorder.

Immunologic Effects of Malnutrition

Malnutrition has deleterious effects upon cell-mediated immunity, the bactericidal activity of white blood cells, complement and secretory immunoglobulin A (IgA) [24], making such patients extremely vulnerable to infection. As noted in chapter 13, the malnutrition that occurs in anorexia nervosa may be different than protein-calorie malnutrition (PCM) since often protein intake is relatively normal. The following is a description of the deleterious effects of PCM on immunological function. Table I in chapter 13 details some of the differences between anorexia nervosa and PCM.

Severe PCM results in thymic involution, decreased lymphoid numbers, cellular depletion within the spleen and lymph nodes and decreased numbers of submucosal plasma cells and intraepithelial lymphocytes. As a result of decreased thymic function, delayed cutaneous hypersensitivity is decreased; it is particularly the helper T cells which are depressed in starvation while there is a moderate decrease in cytotoxic suppressor cells as well. Malnutrition depresses serum concentrations of immunoglobulin G (IgG), immunoglobulin M (IgM) and IgA perhaps by diminishing the interaction of helper T and B lymphocytes. Secretory IgA levels are low in malnourished subjects. There are depressed levels of many complement proteins, particularly C3 and factor B [25]. There may be decreased chemotactic mobility of neutrophils in malnutrition; although bacterial ingestion is normal, intracellular killing capacity is compromised. Many of these immune defects may be due to lack of specific dietary factors, such as folic acid, vitamin A, pyridoxine, zinc and iron, which have quite specific effects on the immune process as well as to the general debilitated state of malnutrition and lack of lipids and protein. Realimentation restores immune function to normal.

References

1 Morley, J.; Levine, A.: The central control of appetite. Lancet *i:* 398–401 (1983).

2 Smith, G.; Gibbs, J.; Jemone, C.; Pi-Junyer, F.X.; Kissileff, H.R.; Thornton, J.: The satiety effect of cholecystokinin: a progress report. Peptides *2:* 57–59 (1981).

3 Pi-Sunyer, X.; Kissileff, H.; Thornton, J.; Smith, G.: C-terminal octapeptide of cholecystokinin decreases food intake in obese men. Physiol. Behav. *29:* 627–630 (1982).

4 Smith, G.: The role of the gut in the control of food intake. Viewpts dig. Dis. *15:* 1–4 (1983).

5 Smith, G.: The peripheral control of appetite. Lancet *ii:* 88–90 (1983).
6 Felig, P.: Starvation; in DeGroot, Endocrinology, pp. 1927–1940 (Grune & Stratton, New York 1979).
7 Burman, K.; Smallridge, R.; Osburne, R.; Dimond, R.; Whorton, N.; Keller, P.; Wartofsky, L.: Nature of suppressed TSH secretion during undernutrition: effect of fasting and refeeding on TSH responses to prolonged TRH infusions. Metabolism *29:* 46–52 (1980).
8 Casper, R.; Frohmen, L.: Delayed TSH release in anorexia nervosa following injection of thyrotropin-releasing hormone (TRH). Psychoneuroendocrinology *7:* 59–68 (1982).
9 Ahsanuddin, K.; Nyeem, R.: Anorexia nervosa: an update. J. Fla med. Ass. *70:* 34–38 (1983).
10 Boyar, R.; Hellman, L.; Roffwarg, H.; Katz, J.; Zumoff, B.; O'Connor, J.; Bradlow, H.; Fukushima, D.: Cortisol secretion and metabolism in anorexia nervosa. New Engl. J. Med. *296:* 190–193 (1977).
11 Walsh, B.; Katz, J.; Levin, J.; Kream, J.; Fukushima, D.; Weiner, H.; Zumoff, B.: The production rate of cortisol declines during recovery from anorexia nervosa. J. clin. Endocr. Metab. *3:* 203–208 (1981).
12 Crim, M.; Munro, H.: Protein-energy malnutrition and endocrine function; in DeGroot, Endocrinology, pp. 1987–2000 (Grune & Stratton, New York 1979).
13 Tuck, M.; Sowers, J.; Dornfeld, L.; Kledzik, G.; Maxwell, M.: The effect of weight reduction on blood pressure, plasma renin activity and plasma aldosterone concentrations in obese patients. New Engl. J. Med. *304:* 930–931 (1981).
14 Vigersky, R.; Andersen, A.; Thompson, R.; Loriaux, D.: Hypothalamic dysfunction in secondary amenorrhea associated with simple weight loss. New Engl. J. Med. *287:* 1141–1145 (1977).
15 Smith, S.; Chhetri, M.; Johanson, A.; Radfar, W.; Migeon, C.: The pituitary-gonadal axis in men with protein-calorie malnutrition. J. clin. Endocr. Metab. *41:* 60–69 (1975).
16 Katz, J.; Boyar, R.; Weiner, H.; Gorzynski, G.; Roffwarg, H.; Hellman, L.: Toward an elucidation of the psychoendocrinology of anorexia nervosa; in Sachar, Hormones, behavior, and psychopathology, pp. 263–282 (Raven Press, New York 1976).
17 Frisch, R.; McArthur, J.: Menstrual cycles: fatness as a determinant of minimum weight for height necessary for their maintenance or onset. Science *185:* 949–951 (1974).
18 Marshall, J.; Kelch, R.: Low dose pulsatile gonadotropin-releasing hormone in anorexia nervosa: a model of human pubertal development. J. clin. Endocr. Metab. *49:* 712–718 (1979).
19 Fishman, J.; Bradlow, H.: Effect of malnutrition on the metabolism of sex hormones in man. Clin. Pharmacol. Ther. *22:* 721–728 (1977).
20 Isley, W.; Underwood, L.; Clemmons, D.: Dietary components that regulate serum somatomedin C concentrations in humans. J. clin. Invest. *71:* 175–182 (1983).
21 Maeda, K.; Kato, Y.; Yamasuchi, N.; Chihara, K.; Ohgo, S.; Iwasaki, Y.; Yoshimoto, Y.; Moridera, K.; Kuromaru, S.; Imura, H.: Growth hormone release following thyrotropin-releasing hormone injection into patients with anorexia nervosa. Acta endocr., Copenh. *81:* 1–8 (1976).

22 Travaglini, P.; Beck-Percoz, P.; Ferrari, C.; Ambrosi, B.; Paracchi, A.; Severgnini, A.; Spada, A.; Faglia, G.: Some aspects of hypothalamic-pituitary function in patients with anorexia nervosa. Acta endocr., Copenh. *81:* 252–262 (1976).
23 Gold, P.; Kaye, W.; Robertson, G.; Ebert, M.: Abnormalities in plasma and cerebrospinal-fluid arginine vasopressin in patients with anorexia nervosa. New Engl. J. Med. *308:* 1117–1123 (1983).
24 Chandra, R.: Nutrition, immunity, and infection: present knowledge and future directions. Lancet *i:* 688–691 (1983).
25 Wyatt, R.; Farrell, M.; Berry, P.; Forristal, J.; Maloney, M.; West, C.: Reduced alternative complement pathway control protein levels in anorexia nervosa: response to parenteral alimentation. Am. J. clin. Nutr. *35:* 973–980 (1982).

10 Multidisciplinary Approach to Treatment and Evaluation

Pauline S. Powers

Introduction

In this chapter, the initial evaluation process utilized at the University of South Florida Eating Disorders Clinic (EDC) will be described. Guidelines found useful for deciding whether or not to hospitalize the patient will be presented. The roles and responsibilities of inpatient and outpatient treatment team members will be reviewed, and factors which interfere with effective and therapeutic team functioning will be addressed. The approach described in this chapter is not intended as an ideal model and is continually evolving as more is learned about treatment.

The unique advantages and limitations of any clinical setting will have important effects on the design and implemention of any treatment program. For example, in our inpatient program, a major limitation is that at the present time there is no psychiatric ward available; thus, we have had to modify the design of our weight-restoration program in such a way that it can be implemented by medical nursing personnel on a pediatric or internal medicine hospital ward where eating and purging behavior cannot be as closely monitored. By contrast, in programs described by *Crisp* [1] and *Russell* [2] a nursing milieu program for weight restoration is utilized; the nursing staff is highly specialized and trained to treat patients with eating disorders. Patients are put to bed and gradually allowed time out of bed as weight is gained at a specified rate; extensive nursing time is required to monitor the patient's behavior. This intense nurse-patient involvement may have some advantages in improving the patient's relationship capacity, but is not feasible in many clinical situations.

Initial Evaluation

At the time of the initial inquiry from the patient, family member, or referring professional, the services provided by the EDC are described, as are the usual fees for the initial evaluation. If the patient is interested, a questionnaire is sent, along with a brochure which reiterates the initial description.

Questionnaire

The questionnaire which we send to patients to complete prior to the initial evaluation is reproduced in the appendix (page 302). Although initially we used separate questionnaires for anorexia nervosa and bulimia, we found that the symptoms of the two conditions so overlapped that we now use one questionnaire. The questionnaire serves several purposes. First, it is designed to obtain factual information quickly and efficiently. When completed it provides individual and family demographic data, diagnostic information, and historical and descriptive data on weight, binge-eating and purging. The questionnaire also includes a typical day's food intake which is part of the nutritional assessment. Also included in the questionnaire are two psychological tests which have been extensively used with anorexia nervosa patients, namely the Eating Attitudes Test [3, 4]. Although there is some question as to the validity of these tests (see chapter 14) the tests have been useful in obtaining preliminary information which can then be clarified in the initial interview. Second, many patients have told us that receiving the questionnaire, with detailed questions about a number of symptoms, has been reassuring, because they have realized they are not alone and that others must have similar problems. However, it is possible that some patients, particularly some anorectic patients who need to see themselves as different or special, decide not to come to the EDC because of the questionnaire. Third, the nature of the questions often prompts patients to remember details of their problems prior to the initial interview, and may make it easier for them to provide adequate histories. Fourth, the questionnaire is used as a screening device; since several professionals devote 2–3 h of their time to the evaluation of 1 patient, or family, it is hoped that requiring a completed questionnaire (which requires about 1 h of the patient's time) will obviate the problem of missed appointments. Fifth, the information obtained by the questionnaire often forms the basis for clinical research or scholarly projects in the EDC.

History and Mental Status Examination

During the initial interivew, a complete psychiatric history is obtained including the history of the eating disorder, the individual, family and cultural factors that facilitated its development, and those factors that promote its maintenance. Many patients who present with symptoms of eating disorders have other psychiatric conditions that are primary, and these need to be identified. In particular, schizophrenia, depression and conversion disorders need to be identified. The eating or purging behavior may be part of another psychiatric disorder (e.g. true anorexia and weight loss are common symptoms of a major depressive disorder). Often, however, there may be an eating disorder co-existing with another psychiatric disorder. At the initial evaluation, it may be difficult to determine how these conditions interact, or if they are but one condition. For example, patients with bulimia may be depressed because of their inability to control their eating, may have more intense bulimic symptoms because they are depressed, or the bulimia itself may represent an atypical depression.

A complete history of possible organic causes of the eating disorder as well as the consequences of the abnormal eating and purging behavior needs to be obtained. An accurate history, in which the diagnostic criteria for anorexia nervosa or bulimia are sought, is the most reliable guide to establishing the diagnosis. The organic conditions which can mimic anorexia nervosa are usually easy to distinguish, and include certain gastrointestinal diseases, various malignancies and a variety of endocrinologic disturbances. These issues are discussed in detail in chapters 12 and 13. Similarly, certain conditions such as the Klein-Levin syndrome, schizophrenia and some neurological conditions (e.g. atypical epilepsy, brain tumors, or severe migraine headaches) may be associated with binge-eating or purging but rarely have the same associated psychological symptoms of guilt after eating, or fear of losing control over eating, and almost always have other signs or symptoms that distinguish them.

A mental status examination is a routine part of the initial evaluation and includes a description of the patient's appearance, behavior, attitude, thought processes, mood and affect, perceptions and sensorium. Sensorium includes orientation (to time, place and person), memory (immediate, recent and remote) and intellectual resources (general information, calculations). Judgment is also assessed as part of the mental status examination and can usually be estimated during the general interview. Various mental defense mechanisms are also noted including denial, rationalization, projection, splitting and intellectualization.

Physical Examination

Table I is the guide used for the physical examination of patients with anorexia nervosa or bulimia. It is important to keep in mind that this is meant only as a guide, and will require significant modification in unusual circumstances.

There are several purposes to this guide. First, it is organized so that the examiner will look for signs of unusual causes of weight loss; e.g. a visual field examination is included to rule out the rare patient who presents with the classic signs and symptoms of anorexia nervosa, but has a suprasellar tumor. Second, the physical examination guide is designed to call the examiner's attention to the signs of semistarvation and the physiological consequences of bingeing, purging, overexercising and unusual eating behavior. The signs of semistarvation might include orthostatic hypotension, acrocyanosis, bradycardia and decreased muscle and fat content. One sign of binge-eating might be parotid gland enlargement. Arrhythmias, subcutaneous emphysema, or buccal erosions may signify the presence of vomiting. For a complete listing of signs and symptoms, see tables II–IV, chapter 13. Failure to gain sufficient weight for puberty to occur may be revealed by delayed breast development or pubic and axillary hair growth as detailed by *Tanner* [5]. Third, certain data from the physical examination are used to complete a nutritional assessment. This information includes anthropometric data (weight, height, fatfold measures, mid-arm circumference), as well as other signs of malnutrition (for example, poor skin turgor and orthostatic hypotension). Table I, chapter 11, lists the components of the nutritional assessment procedure.

Psychological Testing

As noted in chapter 14, no battery of tests have thus far been found routinely useful in the evaluation of patients with anorexia nervosa or bulimia. However, in addition to the Eating Attitudes Test which is included in the questionnaire, we have found it useful to administer a modified version of the Draw-A-Person Test [6] and the Open-Door-Test as clinical estimates for the presence and severity of perceptual and attitudinal disturbances in body image.

The modified Draw-A-Person Test is administered by asking the patient to draw a figure, any figure, and to make it a complete figure, not a stick figure. The examiner notes the time taken to draw the figure as well as the method used. When the figure is complete, the person is asked to draw a person of the sex opposite to the one originally drawn; if the sex of the first drawing is not obvious, the patient is asked its sex and the answer recorded.

Table I. Physical examination guide

Vital signs
Blood pressure ____ lying ____ standing (pediatric cuff ____ regular cuff ____)
Pulse ______ lying ______ standing
Temperature ______
Respiratory rate ______

Anthropometric measures
Weight ______ pounds ______ kilograms (hospital gown)
Height ______ inches ______ centimeters
Frame: Small ______ Medium ______ Large ______
Fatfolds: Triceps ______ (millimeters) Subscapular ______ (millimeters)
Biceps ______ (millimeters) Suprailiac ______ (millimeters)
Left mid-arm circumference (LMAC): ______ (centimeters)

Appearance
Emaciation: Great ______ Moderate ______ Small ______ None ______
Dehydration: Great ______ Moderate ______ Small ______ None ______
Acrocyanosis: Yes (describe) ______________________ No ______
Lanugo: Yes (describe) ______________________ No ______
Yellowish pigmentation: Yes (describe) ______________________ No ______

Head, eyes, ears, nose, throat
Eyes: Extraocular movements ____ Fundus ____ Visual fields by confrontation ____
Conjunctival hemorrhages: Yes ______ No ______
Ears: Is hearing more acute? Yes ______ No ______
Nose ______ Throat (look for pharyngitis) ______
Mouth (buccal erosions): Yes ______ No ______
Dentition (describe): ______________________
Parotid gland enlargement: Yes ______ No ______
Ecchymoses: Yes ______ No ______

Neck
Thyroid palpable: Yes ______ No ______

Chest and lungs (look for ecchymoses and crepitations) ______

Heart and cardiovascular system
Rhythm ______ Rate ______ Pedal edema: Yes ______ No ______
Gallop ______ Murmurs ______

Abdomen
Organomegaly: Yes (describe) ______________________ No ______
Bowel sounds normoactive: No (describe) ______________________ Yes ______
Tenderness: Yes (describe) ______________________ No ______
Stretch marks: Yes (describe) ______________________ No ______

Table I (continued)

Genitourinary
Normal pubic hair distribution: Yes ______ No (describe) ______
Tanner stage(s) of adolescent development: Breast development (stage): ______
Pubic hair (stage) ______ Axillary hair (stage) ______
Pelvic examination:
External genitalia normal: Yes ______ No (describe) ______
Uterus, ovaries, adnexa normal: Yes ______ No (describe) ______

Neurological examination
Cranial nerves including taste recognition normal: Yes ______ No ______
Motor ______ Cerebellum ______
Sensory ______ Reflexes ______

After the second drawing is completed, the patient is asked to draw herself, and after the drawing is complete the patient is asked 'How do you look to yourself?' and the patient's answer is recorded. In addition to the usual uses of the test [6, 7] any difference between the patient's self-sketch and preliminary same sex drawing are noted; differences between the patient's actual size and self-sketch are noted as are any attitudinal disturbances revealed in the patient's description of the self-sketch.

The Open-Door-Test, initially described by *Simonson* [lecture at Conference: Management of Obesity, Johns Hopkins Medical Institutions, February 13–16, 1978], is an office procedure for estimating disturbances in the perceptual aspect of body image. The patient is asked to open a door just wide enough to allow her to pass through unobstructed. Patients who overestimate their size (which is very common among anorectics and bulimics) will often open the door much wider than necessary.

Laboratory Tests

As noted in chapters 12 and 13 there are myriad physiological abnormalities in anorexia nervosa and bulimia. It is time-consuming, expensive and unnecessary to document all the abnormalities known to occur with semistarvation, bingeing and purging. Table II lists the laboratory data recommended on a routine basis for restricting anorectics, anorectics who binge or purge (bulimic anorectics) and bulimic patients at or near normal weight.

Table II. Recommended laboratory evaluation

Organ system	Anorexia nervosa (restricting)	Anorexia nervosa (bulimic)	Bulimia (near normal weight)
Blood	CBC including differential and peripheral smear serum transferrin SMA 18[1] serum amylase	same	same
Genitourinary system	urinalysis urine for culture and sensitivity 24-hour urine for creatinine	same	same
Heart	electrocardiogram posterior-anterior and lateral chest X-ray	same	same
Endocrine	LH FSH thyroid screen AM, PM cortisol	same	omit but add dexamethasone suppression test
Gastrointestinal	upper gastrointestinal roentgenographic study with small bowel follow-through[2]	same but add[3]: lower GI roentgenographic study stool guiaic – 3 samples proctoscopy	upper and lower gastrointestinal roentgenographic studies stool guiaic – 3 samples proctoscopy
Central nervous system	electroencephalogram; computed tomography of head, with and without contrast[2]	same	omit
Immune system	delayed hypersensitivity test to common antigens if below 60% of ideal body weight	same	omit

[1] SMA 18 includes: glucose, BUN, sodium, potassium, chloride, CO_2, albumin, alkaline phosphatase, calcium, cholesterol, CPK, creatinine, total bilirubin, SGOT, LDH, serum iron, total protein, uric acid.
[2] Sometimes optional.
[3] Perform if purging with laxatives has occurred.

Most of the laboratory tests recommended for the restricting anorectic patients are measures of malnutrition. The additional tests recommended for anorectics who binge and/or purge are needed to evaluate damage to the gastrointestinal tract. Certain abnormalities are predictable; for example, a mild normochromic normocytic anemia is to be expected in the emaciated anorectic. However, severe anemia (10 g/100 ml or less) should be thoroughly investigated, including an examination of a bone marrow aspirate.

Certain of the recommended laboratory tests are needed to complete the nutritional assessment. These include a 24-hour urine for creatinine, serum albumin, serum transferrin and delayed hypersensitivity tests to common recall antigens. Because many outpatients will not comply with a 24-hour urine collection, this laboratory data is usually only determined in hospitalized patients. See table II, chapter 11, for details of nutritional assessment.

There are some laboratory tests that are needed only in certain circumstances. An electroencephalogram (EEG) may be indicated if the use of anticonvulsants is under consideration for an anorectic patient with bingeing or purging; however, since a significant percentage of restricting anorectics are known to have nonspecific EEG abnormalities [8], it is not necessary to order an EEG routinely. An upper gastrointestinal roentgenographic series with a small bowel follow-through is usually not necessary for restricting anorectics but nearly always is required if there has been significant purging. Delayed hypersensitivity tests to common recall antigens are usually normal until the patient is 60% below ideal body weight [9].

Case Formulation and Interpretation to Patient and Family

After the initial evaluation there is a team meeting during which the information obtained by various team members is presented. A case formulation is produced which is essentially a hypothesis of the various factors which have contributed to the development of and the maintenance of the disorder. Recommendations for treatment are derived from the case formulation and presented to the patient and family. During this meeting the reasons for the diagnosis are discussed as well as the hazards of continued disturbances in eating behavior. This is usually a critical point in eliciting the cooperation of the patient and often requires significant time (0.5–1 h). After the evaluation, a letter is sent to the patient (and, if suitable, to the family) which describes the reasons for arriving at the diagnosis and the recommendations for treatment. Many patients have been referred by their primary care physician who often becomes an integral part of the treatment team and this physician must be kept informed of the outcome of the evaluation.

Evaluation Team

The initial evaluation requires psychiatric, psychological, nutritional, and physiological data which can be obtained in a variety of ways. Our team includes a psychiatrist, a psychologist, nutritionist and family therapist. The psychiatric history, medical history, mental status examination and physical examination is usually obtained by the psychiatrist or a psychiatric resident under the supervision of a faculty psychiatrist. The psychologist may elicit the psychiatric history and administer psychological tests. A family evaluation is not possible in all situations but, whenever the family is available, even if the patient is emancipated from his or her nuclear family, we ask that the family attend the initial meeting. The approach to the family is described in detail in chapter 5. The nutritionist ensures that a complete nutritional assessment is obtained for each patient; this may require interviewing the patient or family to obtain further information, especially when weight change and reported intake do not match.

Inpatient Treatment of Anorexia Nervosa

Indications for Hospitalization

Chapter 4 lists the major indications for hospitalization of patients with bulimia and they will not be reviewed here. It has been our experience that most patients with anorexia nervosa require hospitalization at some point during treatment [10]. Although certain researchers, notably *Minuchin* et al. [11], have reported favorable results with outpatient family therapy, it may be that many of these patients have good prognostic signs (young age of onset, less weight loss, short duration of illness, absence of binge-eating or purging) and are still in their nuclear families. Ours is a tertiary care center and thus it may be that patients evaluated are more seriously disturbed and therefore more frequently require hospitalization.

Table III lists the major indications for hospitalization. Anorectics who are 30% or more below ideal body weight, or who binge or purge, should be hospitalized. Signs and symptoms of significant malnutrition or the gastrointestinal consequences of binge-eating or purging are also indications for hospitalization. Patients who have lost weight very quickly, even if they have not lost to 25% below their ideal body weight, may nonetheless be in danger. Figure 2 in chapter 11 is a rough guide to estimating the hazard of the weight loss. We have frequently found this diagram helpful in the interpretation to patients and their families.

Table III. Anorexia nervosa: indications for hospitalization

Weight 30% below ideal body weight
Very rapid weight loss (see fig. 2, chapter 11)
Binge-eating or purging
Signs, symptoms or laboratory evidence of significant malnutrition
Gastrointestinal consequences of binge-eating or purging
Duration over 6 months
1 month trial of unsuccessful weight gain attempt as an outpatient
Suicidal
Destructive parent-child relationship

Psychological indications for hospitalization are numerous but specifically include patients who are suicidal or who are in a destructive parent-child relationship. The disorder itself may cause great damage in the parent-child relationship especially if the parents feel particularly guilty; hospitalization may allow the parents a respite during which they can marshall their emotional resources to become a positive influence in the patient's recovery.

Many patients or their families initially refuse hospitalization. This may reflect denial of the severity of the physiological and psychological disturbances. Initially, some patients state they can gain weight outside the hospital on their own or that there is no problem at all. Some families believe they can convince the patient to gain weight. In these situations, it is usually wise to suggest a time-limited trial during which the patient attempts to gain weight gradually, usually 1 lb (0.5 kg) per week. It should be understood that at the end of the outpatient trial (usually no longer than 1 month) if the agreed upon weight has not been achieved, the patient will be hospitalized. It also needs to be agreed that any additional weight loss or the development of certain complications (for example arrhythmias or fainting spells) will mean that the patient is hospitalized immediately.

Inpatient Treatment

The inpatient treatment program is described in detail elsewhere [10] but a brief description follows. A weight restoration program based on operant conditioning principles is utilized; there are thrice-weekly individual psychotherapy sessions and weekly family therapy sessions. The weight restoration program is modified after the one described by *Halmi* et al. [12]. The patient is initially confined to her room with visitors, time out of her room and phone calls contingent on a weight gain of 1 lb (0.5 kg) each 5 days. Failure to gain weight or loss of weight has certain negative consequences chosen with the patient. Table IV is a sample 5-day weight restoration plan individually written with the patient. This particular weight restoration plan is one of many posible approaches and has evolved out of our particular needs and resources.

The individual psychotherapy approach is described in chapter 2 and the principles of family therapy are described in chapter 5.

Inpatient Treatment Team

The treatment team includes a behavior therapist, psychotherapist, a family therapist, a nutritionist, a nurse and a consulting internist or pediatrician. One person, usually the psychiatrist who admits the patient, assumes responsibility for coordinating the interventions with the patient and family. It is important that only one physician write orders to avoid conflict within the team.

The *behavior therapist* negotiates the weight restoration program with the patient, instructs the nurses in the implementation of the program, evaluates the patient's weight progress and incorporates appropriate changes into the program.

The *individual psychotherapist* meets at least thrice weekly with the patient. The reason for dividing responsibility for the behavior program and the psychotherapy is that the anorectic patient is often very angry about the behavior program and may have difficulty relating to the person administering it. As the patient begins to trust the psychotherapist, and as there is improvement in weight, these roles do not need to be as rigidly maintained, and eventually one therapist can monitor weight and provide psychotherapy.

The *family therapist* may be a separate therapist or the behavior therapist or the individual psychotherapist. The choice of team member or members depends on the results of the evaluation of the family transactions.

The *nutritionist* is an essential part of the team and should participate from the beginning in selecting a suitable dietary regimen likely to be acceptable to the patient. Most anorectics obsess about food or have spent considerable time handling food; many want to consult daily or even hourly with the nutritionist. To decrease the patient's obsessions about food and ease the role of the nutritionist, yet still give the patient some food choices, the visits from the nutritionist can be made an integral part of the behavior program.

Table IV. Weight restoration plan. Weighing procedure: Weigh daily in two hospital gowns before consuming food or drink and after voiding. Weigh twice and record average on chart

---

Starting weight ____________ Date ____________

Conditions: In room ____________

Out of room ____________

Meals: Time frame ____________ Place ____________

Observation ____________ Content ____________

Frequency ____________

Special comments: ____________

____

____

Visitors ____________

Phone calls (in ________ out ________)

Mail ____________

Exercise ____________

Dietary consult ____________

Other ____________

Target weight ____________ Date ____________

If target weight is obtained, the following conditions will apply:

In room ____________

Out of room ____________

Meal change ____________

Visitors ____________

Phone calls (in ________ out ________)

Mail ____________

Exercise ____________

Dietary consult ____________

Other ____________

If between *starting weight and target weight:*

____

____

____

If below *starting weight:*

____

____

____

Patient's signature ____________ Date ____________

Signature of person negotiating plan ____________ Date ____________

RN noting above orders ____________ Date ____________

For example, a positive reinforcement for weight gain can be a visit from the nutritionist.

The role of the *nursing staff* is often difficult and may be one of the least rewarding. One of the major advantages of the behavior program is that it gives the nursing staff reasonable and consistent guidelines to follow that may prevent constant unproductive arguments with the patient about food and weight.

The *consulting internist or pediatrician* assists in the evaluation of the patient and follows the patient during the course of treatment. This role is reviewed in detail in chapter 12.

Outpatient Treatment Team

Choice of the treating professional for outpatients depends on the results of the preliminary evaluation and case formulation. For patients with bulimia, family therapy, individual insight-oriented psychotherapy, behavior therapy, or cognitive reeducative therapy, individually or in groups, may be effective in various combinations. Certain medications, especially the monoamine oxidase inhibitors, may be useful as well.

In anorexia nervosa patients who have been hospitalized, follow-up outpatient treatment is necessary. Choice of the primary therapist depends on the quality of the relationship the patient has with each team member. The person to whom the patient has related most closely is selected as the primary outpatient therapist whenever logistically possible. Some patients who have returned to their referring mental health professional have had a very positive relationship with one or more members of the inpatient treatment team and in this situation careful well-coordinated follow-up for a specific part of the therapy (for example, family therapy) may be continued by one or more members of the inpatient team.

Anorexia nervosa patients who are not hospitalized are usually initially in family therapy. With change in the family system, individual issues may emerge that require separate sessions for the patient or certain other family members. Patients who start with individual psychotherapy may later require family therapy or intervention. The professional who works with the patient or family must be flexible in changing to the appropriate modality of treatment as needs dictate. We have also found that periodic team reviews of ongoing treatment are helpful in identifying problems and resolving them early (for example, patients who begin losing weight may require hospitalization) and in providing adequate support to the primary therapist.

References

1 Crisp, A.: A treatment regime for anorexia nervosa. Br. J. Psychiat. *112:* 505–512 (1965).
2 Russell, G.: The management of anorexia nervosa. Symp. Anorexia nervosa and Obesity. R. Coll. Phys. Edinburgh, vol. 42, pp. 44–52 (Constable, Edinburgh 1973).
3 Garner, D.; Garfinkel, P.: The eating attitudes test: an index of the symptoms of anorexia nervosa. Psychol. Med. *9:* 273–279 (1979).
4 Garfinkel, P.; Garner, D.: Anorexia nervosa, a multidimensional perspective (Brunner/Mazel, New York 1982).
5 Tanner, J.: Sequence and tempo in the somatic changes in puberty; in Grumbach, Grave, Mayer, Control of the onset of puberty, pp. 448–470 (Wiley & Sons, New York 1974).
6 Machover, L.: Personality projection in the drawing of the human figure (Thomas, Springfield 1957).
7 Harris, D.: Children's drawings as measures of intellectual maturity (Harcourt, Brace & World, New York 1963).
8 Crisp, A.; Fenton, G.; Scotton, L.: A controlled study of the EEG in anorexia nervosa. Br. J. Psychiat. *114:* 1149–1169 (1968).
9 Pertschuk, M.; Crosby, L.; Barot, L.; Mullen, J.: Immunocompetency in anorexia nervosa. Am. J. clin. Nutr. *35:* 968–972 (1982).
10 Powers, P.; Powers, H.: Inpatient treatment of anorexia nervosa. Psychosomatics (in press).
11 Minuchin, S.; Rosman, B.; Baker, L.: Psychosomatic families: anorexia nervosa in context (Harvard University Press, Cambridge 1978).
12 Halmi, K.; Powers, P.; Cunningham, S.: Treatment of anorexia nervosa with behavior modification. Archs gen. Psychiat. *32:* 93–96 (1975).

11 Role of the Nutritionist

Rebecca Eubanks

Introduction

Although anorexia nervosa and bulimia (or the binge-eating syndrome) are primarily psychiatric disorders, rather than nutritional disorders, nutritional input during evaluation and treatment can add an important dimension to the multidisciplinary approach. The degree of malnutrition, beyond the observed physical appearance of the anorectic patient, can be more accurately determined and defined by a thorough nutritional assessment during the initial evaluation phase. The assessment can then be utilized in choosing among treatment options. During treatment, in conjunction with psychotherapy, the nutritionist can provide individualized counseling, helping the patients establish for themselves a more normal eating pattern, with appropriate food selection, realistic weight goals and a long-term plan for weight maintenance.

Assessment

An assessment of nutritional status should begin with a thorough history. Much of the historical information can be obtained prior to the first interview by questionnaire (appendix, p. 302); these data can then be clarified and completed at the evaluation interview. The history should include information on weight, diet, socioeconomic data, eating attitudes, energy expenditure and medical condition.

The Weight History

The weight history is the patient's own account of her weight from birth to present. A family member's account can be valuable for clarification. The history should include all weights the patient can remember, or alternatively clothing sizes. A flag sign for a nutritional deficiency is a 3-year-old in 1-year-old clothing. Significant events that can be associated with weight change should also be included, such as menarche, graduation from school, marriage, pregnancy, divorce, death or other separation or any other precipitating event associated with weight (for example, a ballet teacher telling a budding ballerina that she needs to lose 5–10 lb [2.3–4.5 kg]. Where there is a weight loss the circumstances should also be noted, such as a successful diet and/or exercise program. Fluctuations shold be noted. Continuous 10–15 lb (4.5–6.8 kg) fluctuations are suggestive of an eating disorder, just as a 25% loss in body weight is currently diagnostic of anorexia nervosa [1]. Reasons for the weight fluctuation should be included, such as an unsuccessful diet, binging and/or purging. Highest weight, lowest weight, usual weight and current weight should be noted; the patient is also asked what she has determined to be her ideal body weight and her weight goal. In a weight history, family background is valuable. If any of the first-degree family members have had a weight problem, it should be determined what measures have been taken to correct the condition and their effectiveness.

From the information collected about weight, a graph can be drawn and all the weights plotted and identified by significant event (fig. 1). The patient's goal, ideal body weight range (discussed later in this chapter), percentage of usual weight, percentage of ideal body weight and net weight loss can also be noted on the graph. A very sharp downward slope indicative of a large weight loss over a short period of time would suggest consideration for hospitalization. *Wilmore,* in his book *Metabolic Management of the Critically Ill* [40] illustrates this concept with sinking ships (fig. 2). The graph can be reviewed with the team to predict prognosis and select treatment, and later plotted to show patient progress from the time of evaluation.

The Diet History

The diet history is a summary of the patient's eating behavior. It includes a typical day's intake, both currently and in the past (premorbid state). The patient is asked to describe her food intake from the time she gets up in the morning until she goes to bed at night plus any additional food consumed after going to bed, such as middle-of-the-night snacks. When interviewing a bulimic, when she binges and what foods trigger her bingeing

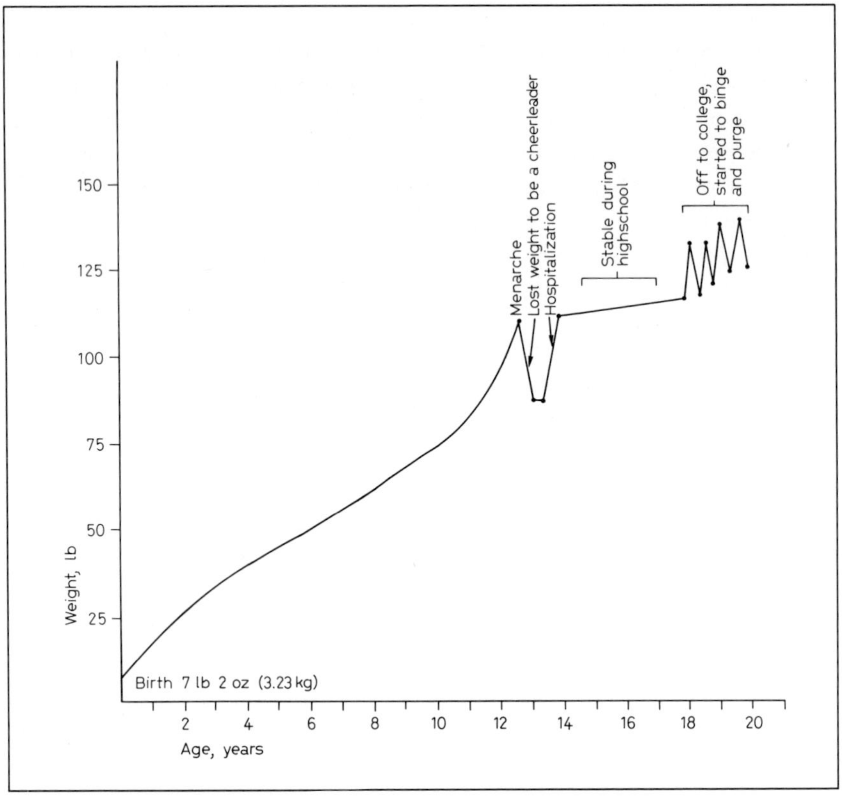

Fig. 1. Historical weight graph drawn from information obtained from the weight history. Patient is a 20-year-old female who was 5 ft 5 inches (165 cm) 125 lb (57 kg) with weight fluctuations from 117 to 130 lb (53–59 kg). Estimated ideal body weight (IBW) 120–130 lb (54.5–59 kg). At time of evaluation, the percentage IBW was 100%.

should be included. The patient can be asked to elaborate on the binge described in the questionnaire. In addition to the actual foods, portion sizes and methods of preparation should be noted; for example, when the patient says she drinks a cold beverage all day long, find out how many empty cans or bottles are left at the end of the day as a step toward determining total intake. If the patient states that she drinks four cups of coffee in the morning, check whether it is plain or with cream and/or sugar. Is there mayonnaise on the sandwich? Are vegetables cooked with butter? Food models can be very valuable for determining portion sizes.

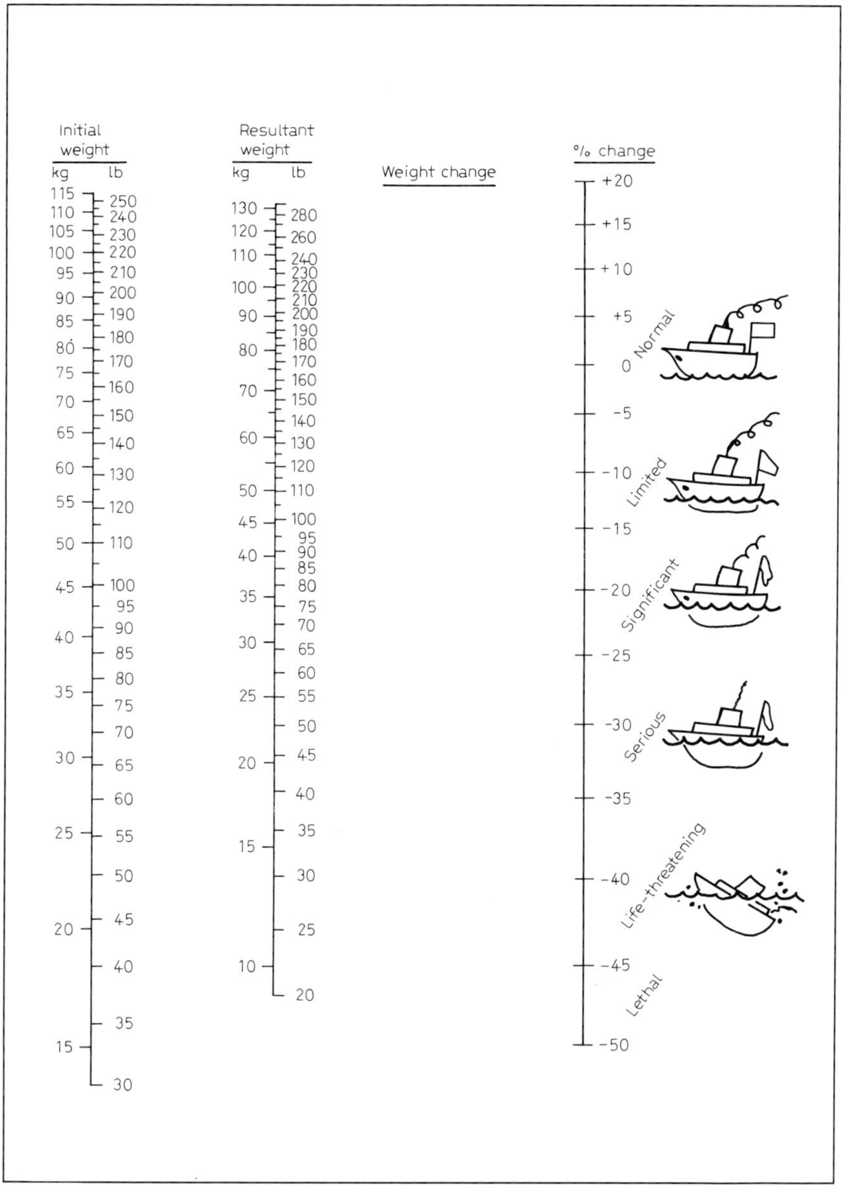

Fig. 2. Locate weight prior to loss on the left scale and present weight on the middle scale. Connect these two points with a straight edge and read the percentage weight loss from the right-hand scale. A rapid weight loss of 25–30% of initial weight is an indication for hospitalization [reprinted with permission from ref. 40].

Whether there is variety or monotony in food selection should be noted. Adequate servings from each of the four food groups should be checked: two servings from the meat group, four servings from the fruit-vegetable group, four servings from the bread-cereal group, and two to three servings from the milk group. Presence or absence of adequate sources of vitamins and minerals should be noted. Target foods are citrus (for vitamin C), milk products (for calcium), orange, yellow, and dark green leafy vegetables (for vitamin A), meat (for iron), and enriched whole grains (for B vitamins). If target foods are noticeably absent and the patient does not take a vitamin-mineral supplement, intake is probably not adequate.

The patient should be questioned concerning any medications or vitamin-mineral supplements that she is currently using; intake of laxatives, diuretics, diet pills and caffeine should be specifically noted. Food allergies, food likes, food dislikes, alcohol intake and smoking should be noted. The extent of the patient's nutritional knowledge should be investigated. If much nutrition information is possessed, is it beneficial, neutral or harmful? Especially note cognitive distortions on which they base their eating habits, such as, 'eating carbohydrates will make me fat'. Anorectics usually have little information on nutrition beyond the caloric content of the foods they eat. Bulimics generally also have very little information on nutrition.

From the diet history, the caloric and nutrient content of the diet can be estimated, using the exchange system published by the American Dietetic Association and the American Diabetes Association [2]. *Bowes and Church* [3], Handbook 456 [4] and Handbook 8 [5] can be used for miscellaneous foods. Caloric value should always be estimated. Protein, carbohydrate and fat should be calculated when any one seems unbalanced in the diet. The current American diet is 48% carbohydrate, 12% protein and 42% fat [6]. The recommended American diet is 55–58% carbohydrate, 12–15% protein and 30% fat [6].

Caloric content will generally be inadequate when compared with estimated caloric needs. A restricting anorectic's typical daily food intake will be both meager and low in calories, which she will accurately describe. Bulimic anorectics, and some bulimics, will describe bingeing and purging as a daily ritual. Others will describe food intakes for a 'good day' (a diet day) and a 'bad day' (a binge day). Their intakes for 'good days' will be both meager and easy to calculate. Their food intakes for 'bad days' will not be as easy to calculate because many are not aware of what and how much they consume during a binge. Also questionable will be the caloric loss during a purge. Some patients will describe beginning a binge with a colorful marker food and only complete the purge when the marker food comes up by vomiting. This marker method is unreliable because contents as far down as the jejunum, where absorption occurs, can be purged by vomiting. Recent studies on purging by laxative abuse have shown only a daily caloric loss of 12% [7].

The carbohydrate content, especially complex carbohydrate (starches), will also usually be inadequate for eating disorder patients. A minimum of 100 g/day (400 kcal/1,680 kJ) of carbohydrate is required to meet the energy needs of the central nervous system [8]. It should be stressed that this figure is a minimum requirement and not a recommendation. 1,200 kcal (5,040 kJ) is the minimum suggested for a daily diet adequate in all nutrients. At this level, 600 kcal (2,520 kJ) or 50%, as a minimum should consist of carbohydrates. Lack of sufficient carbohydrate may precipitate binge behavior in some bulimics, so they alternate starvation with bingeing to fill the deficit. When reviewing a bulimic's diet by the week, carbohydrates will probably be adequate. The anorectic's carbohydrate may add up to the minimum requirement but will be made up primarily of fruits and vegetables and not the complex carbohydrates. A goal during treatment will be reintroduction of complex carbohydrates into the diet.

Recommended protein intake is 0.8–1 g/kg body weight [9]. Anorectics, during the course of their illness, gradually eliminate many protein sources from their diet, leaving chicken and/or fish as the only good protein providers. Bulimics in a binge-starve cycle will more often have adequate levels in their diets when a week's diet is reviewed, binge days making up for inadequate nonbinge days, unless purging is severe.

Fat is essential in the diet and plays an important role in meal satiety. Anorectics shun fat; bulimics may or may not shun fat. One bulimic reported bingeing on mayonnaise by the spoonful. Too little fat in the diet could precipitate a binge by depriving the patient of satiety between meals.

Socioeconomic Data

Invaluable in planning treatment are socioeconomic data, such as education, occupation, living arrangements and facilities, time structure, cultural and religious practices. For example, a patient who fasts as part of a religion may be precipitating a binge physiologically by starvation. Or a college student living in a dormitory may not have cooking facilities. A patient may have a job that does not provide regular meal breaks. Where, when, and with whom meals are taken, who shops, who prepares the meals and how many meals are eaten away from home all help in assessing the patient and in planning treatment.

The Eating Attitudes Test

The eating attitudes test [10] is a psychological test made up of 40 statements suggesting different attitudes about food and food habits. The test is scored using a six-point, forced-choice format; it is used for assessment and as a prognostic index. For the nutritionist, it can become a question list of food habits particular to eating disorders that can be asked if anorexia nervosa or bulimia is suspected. If the patient is not already seeking therapy for an eating disorder, referral for treatment can be made. Sample statements include: 'Avoid eating when I am hungry', 'Enjoy eating meat', and 'Avoid foods with sugar in them'. This test is further discussed in chapter 10.

Energy Expenditure

The assessment should also include a brief account of energy expenditure (past and present), because this information helps determine the prescribed caloric level. In both disorders, some patients can be very, very active. As with food intake, ask for the patient's typical daily activities from getting up in the morning until going to bed at night, including getting up in the middle of the night.

This information can be processed in two ways. First, the energy cost for the day's activities can be calculated using an activity conversion table [11]. The table is a list of activities with energy expenditure factors. The day's activities are assigned to activities in the table, and then calculated individually by weight and time spent. Second, a percentage of basal calories can be added to basal calories based on the amount of muscular work performed. This method requires an educated assessment by the professional. For a sedentary life-style add 20%, for light activity add 30%, for moderate activity add 40% and for heavy activity add 50% to basal calories. The method chosen depends on each particular patient. The first method is more accurate and illustrates for the patient how much energy is spent on different activities. If energy output needs to be reduced, the calculation can be helpful in deciding what activities to delete. The second method is less time-consuming and more valuable when the patient does not have many specific activities. It estimates a useful energy output that can be compared with intake.

Medical History

A medical history is needed to rule out any condition that might be initiating, or contributing to, the malnourished state. For example, fever, infection or pregnancy would increase nutrient needs; chronic blood loss, renal dialysis, malabsorption, diarrhea or vomiting would increase nutrient losses from the body. Chronic disease states, such as diabetes mellitus and arthritis, should also be noted. *Grant* [12, pp. 1–2] lists a more extensive medical outline.

Anthropometric Measurements

Anthropometry provides a measure of the patient's protein and caloric reserves, i.e. her nutritional status. This information is useful for determining nutrition therapy and for patient education topics, such as the value of fat in the body, and why the body needs protein. The measurements most commonly taken are height, weight, frame size, various skinfolds and mid-upper arm circumference, from which mid-upper arm muscle circumference is derived.

It is important to measure height. Anorectics can be manipulative; they may say that they are shorter than they actually are, making their weight seem not quite as low. Emaciated patients may look taller than they really are. Since ideal weight recommendations are based on height and frame size, height measurements should be especially accurate. In anorexia nervosa patients who are beyond the age of usual onset of puberty and have yet to experience the adolescent growth spurt, accurate height becomes part of the baseline data for serial measurements to determine growth, or lack of growth, during treatment.

Weight is best measured in only a gown, not only because of the variability in clothing but also because anorectics can be deceptive. They may hide weights in their pockets, underwear or shoes. To avoid water-loading, weigh them in the morning, upon rising, after voiding. 1.14 liters of water (1 quart) weighs just over 2 lb (0.9 kg). An anorectic determined to lose weight could add an additional glass of water each week or two to mask the continued weight loss and deceive an unobservant family member, or an inexperienced professional. Weight measurement should always be on the same scales, and as accurately determined as possible, especially if it is used as a measure of compliance and as a decisive factor in whether to hospitalize or not. Scales should be routinely checked for calibration.

Frame size measurement aids in determining weight requirement. The most popular tables, the Metropolitan Height and Weight Tables, are listed by height and frame size. For the first time, in their 1983 edition, these tables defined frame size by elbow breadth measurements taken from the National Health and Nutrition Examination Survey 1971–1975, and this information is included in the tables [13]. A quicker rule of thumb for frame size is to grasp the nondominant wrist with the thumb and forefinger of the other hand. If the thumb and forefinger overlap, frame size is small; if they meet, frame size is medium; and if they do not meet, frame size is large. *Grant* [12, pp. 5–7] also provides a method using wrist circumference.

The skinfold and mid-arm circumference measurements require standardized procedures and a trained technician to be used effectively in assessment and treatment. Step-by-step procedures are available [12, pp. 10–14, 14–16]. Generally, measurements for epidemiological surveys are made on the right side; measurements for assessment are made on the left, or nondominant, side [14]. *Burgert and Anderson* [17] found statistically significant differences in some individuals, but no significant differences in a heterogeneous population, when comparing sides of measurement, right versus left. The mid-arm muscle circumference measurement is a derived value using the formula listed in table I. A nomogram has also been developed using this formula for quicker calculation [18].

The triceps skinfold is a measure of the body's energy stores (fat stores). The mid-arm muscle circumference is a measure of the body's protein stores. Several years ago these measurements were compared to a sex-specific standard; no allowances were made for age [19]. Today sex- and age-specific percentile standards are available from the Ten-State Nutrition Survey [20] and the Health and Nutrition Examination Survey [21, 22] calculated from data obtained from a study population more representative of the American population. *Gray and Gray* [23] provide an excellent discussion on the choice of standard.

Both of these measures can be depressed in an emaciated anorectic. *Kovach* [24] reports that 75–80% of anorectics have triceps skinfold values below the fifth percentile, and 80% of patients have arm muscle circumference measurements at or below the fifth percentile. Bulimics tend to have less depressed measurements, and possibly elevated measurements. These measures can be used to modify treatment plans. For example, a normal weight bulimic with elevated triceps skinfold measurement is a candidate for an exercise plan, not a diet.

The sum of the triceps plus biceps, subscapular and suprailiac skinfolds can be translated into percentage body fat [25]. Body fatness will be discussed later in this chapter.

Clinical Evaluation

During the clinical evaluation, the nutritionist will examine the patient for any physical signs suggestive of a nutritional deficiency. This can be incorporated into a physical examination, however, and need not be separate. Any clinical evidence obtained from the examination should be further investigated. Nutritional deficiencies can be primarily detected in the hair, eyes, skin and nails. High-risk signs of possible protein deficiency are usually noted in the hair; it may be lackluster, thin, sparse, falling out or easily plucked, straight when it should be curly, dispigmented or banded (indicated by bands of light and dark pigmentation along the same strand of hair). Enlarged parotid glands and hepatomegaly are also risk signs of possible protein deficiency.

B vitamin deficiency should be considered when any of these conditions are noted: angular stomatitis (bilateral cracks, redness, flaking at corners of the mouth), magenta tongue, atrophic papillae (tongue appears smooth, pale and slick), glossitis (tongue is beefy red, painful, and tastebuds are atrophied), or pellagrous dermatitis (hyperpigmented areas bilaterally on body parts exposed to the sun). Signs of vitamin A deficiency include Bitot spots (grayish-appearing dry spots on conjunctivae), keratomalacia (bilateral softening of all or part of the cornea, eyes becoming a white or yellow gelatinous mass), and conjunctival xerosis (excessive dryness of conjunctivae). Clinical signs of vitamin C deficiency include petechiae, ecchymoses and perifolliculosis (on the abdomen and thighs).

Grant [12, pp. 23–35] includes a complete list of physical abnormalities divided into those of value in nutritional assessment, those that need further investigation, and those not related to nutrition. *Nutrition Today* [26] has a slide series illustrating clinical signs of malnutrition (see chapter 13 for further information).

Laboratory Evaluation

The extent of laboratory work is dependent on the severity of the signs and symptoms noted above (see discussion on laboratory evaluation in chapter 10). If the patient purges by any method, such as vomiting, diuretics, or laxative abuse, the potassium level should be checked. A patient that presents severely malnourished in appearance or by history should be further evaluated, either as an outpatient or as a hospitalized patient. *Blackburn* et al. [27] suggest serum albumin, serum transferrin, lymphocyte count, urinary creatinine and skin testing for immunocompetence. From these parameters the degree of malnutrition and the type of malnutrition (adult marasmus, adult kwashiorkor or a combination) can be specified.

In most anorectic patients, visceral protein (those body proteins other than muscle mass, for example, enzymes and carriers) will generally be within normal limits at the expense of somatic protein (muscle mass) and adipose stores. Serum albumin and serum transferrin will be maintained. Lymphocyte count is usually within the normal range as is immunocompe-

Table I. Nutritional assessment

Preliminary data

Typical day's food intake (appendix)

Anthropometric data (physical examination, chapter 10, table I)
- Height
- Weight
- Frame size
- Mid-upper arm circumference (MAC)
- Fatfold measures (triceps, subscapular, suprailiac, biceps)

Laboratory tests (included in recommended laboratory evaluation, chapter 10, table III)
- 24-hour urine for creatinine (for hospitalized patients)
- Serum albumin (visceral protein)
- Serum transferrin (visceral protein)
- CBC – lymphocyte count
- Delayed hypersensitivity skin testing to common recall antigens[a]

Derived calculations

$$\text{Percentage IBW} = \frac{\text{current weight}}{\text{IBW}} \times 100$$

$$\text{Percentage UBW} = \frac{\text{current weight}}{\text{usual weight}} \times 100$$

$$\text{Percentage predicted weight} = \frac{\text{current weight}}{\text{predicted weight}} \times 100$$
(under 18 years)

Mid-arm muscle circumference = MAC – (TSF × 0.314)

Percentage body fat = triceps + biceps + subscapular + suprailiac
(then compare to nomogram table IV)

$$\text{Creatinine height index} = \frac{\text{actual urinary creatinine}}{\text{expected creatinine}} \times 100^{b}$$

Expected creatinine for females = 18 mg/kg IBW
Expected creatinine for males = 23 mg/kg IBW

$$\text{Total lymphocyte count} = \frac{\text{percentage lymphocytes from CBC} \times \text{WBC}}{100}$$

MAC = Mid-arm circumference; TSF = triceps skinfold; IBW = ideal body weight; UBW = usual body weight; CBC = complete blood count including differential; WBC = white blood count.

[a] Obtained in anorectics who are 60% or less of IBW.

[b] Indirect measure of somatic protein stores.

tence. This state of malnutrition is classified as adult marasmus and results from prolonged starvation. The patient presents emaciated. When these parameters are depleted, indicating a life-threatening marasmus-kwashiorkor combination, the patient should be hospitalized. When laboratory data indicate depletion and the patient with anorexia nervosa is hospitalized, return of laboratory and anthropometric data to normal can be the criterion for improvement, as opposed to weight gain.

Table I is a summary of data collected during the nutritional assessment. Accurate and thorough nutritional assessment defines for the team the degree of malnutrition: whether or not the patient is just at the stage of a dietary deficiency, has progressed to tissue desaturation or metabolic aberrations measured by laboratory analyses, or has progressed to the final stage of physical abnormalities detected by clinical examination. This assessment also modifies treatment options and, finally, provides material for an individualized program during recovery.

Nutritional Aspects of Treatment for Anorexia Nervosa

Goals

Nutritional therapy still remains an adjunct to psychotherapy for the treatment of anorexia nervosa. The goals of nutritional therapy are weight restoration and stabilization to a realistic weight range and normalization of eating habits. The components of these goals include estimation of ideal body weight, estimation of caloric needs, formulation of the diet, a plan for steady weight gain, and a plan for follow-up.

Estimation of Ideal Body Weight

For anorectics, ideal body weight may need to be estimated at the lower ends of ranges. Interim weight goals might also be established. Table II outlines five different methods for estimating ideal body weight. The most popular method for estimating ideal body weight range is the Metropolitan Height and Weight Tables [13]. These tables are based on averages of the insured populations of 25 insurance companies and indicate the weights at which mortality is lowest. The 1983 table weights are higher than the 1959 weights and have received much unfavorable criticism (table III). Many professionals prefer to continue using the old table. Table II lists an estimation from each table for a 20-year-old female, 165 cm tall, with a medium frame. In their January-June 1983 Statistical Bulletin [28], the Metropolitan Life

Table II. Various estimates of ideal body weight

1	Metropolitan height-weight tables [13] 1983 edition: 127–141 lb (57.6–63.9 kg) nude weight 1959 edition: 120–135 lb (54.4–61.2 kg) nude weight
2	Hamwai formula [29] (100 lb/5 ft + 5 lb/1 inch): 100 + 25 = 125 lb (45.36 kg/152.5 cm + 2.25 kg/2.5 cm): 45.36 + 11.34 = 56.7 kg
3	Fogarty center conference on obesity[1] [30] 114–142 lb (51.7–64.4 kg), average 123 lb (55.8 kg) nude weight
4	*Keys* et al. [31] (height in m)^2 × 20.6: 2.72 × 20.6 = 56.0 kg × 2.2 lb/kg = 123 lb nude weight
5	From body fatness (American units are italics): Part A: $\frac{\mathit{125 - (125 \times 0.22)}}{\substack{56.7 - (56.7 \times 0.22)\\ 100 - 22\%}} = \frac{\mathit{125 - 27.5}}{\substack{56.7 - 12.47\\ 78\%}} = \frac{\mathit{97.5}}{\substack{44.23\\ 78\%}} = 56.7\ \text{kg}\ (\mathit{125\ lb})$ Part B: $\frac{\mathit{125 - (125 \times 0.40)}}{\substack{56.7 - (56.7 \times 0.40)\\ 100 - 22\%}} = \frac{\mathit{75}}{\substack{34.02\\ 78\%}} = 43.6\ \text{kg}\ (\mathit{96\ lb})$

Several methods are used to calculate ideal body weight for a 20-year-old female who is 5 ft 5 inches (165 cm), 125 lb (56.8 kg), and a medium frame.
[1] No frame designation.

Insurance Company suggests that it is best to be slender and keep your weight below average weight (which the tables are). What is unclear is whether or not we should maintain our weight at the low end of the suggested range.

The Hamwai Formula [29] for estimating ideal body weight is to allow the height of 5 ft (152 cm) an ideal body weight of 100 lb (45.5 kg) for women and add 5 lb (2.3 kg) for each inch (2.5 cm) over 5 ft (152 cm); add 10% for a large frame and subtract 10% for a small frame (table II). For men, 5 ft (152 cm) has an ideal body weight of 106 lb (48 kg) and 6 lb (2.7 kg) for each additional inch (2.5 cm); again, add or subtract 10% for large or small frame size, respectively. Another table that can be used to determine recommended weight ranges is from the Fogarty Conference on Obesity [30] in 1973. These weight ranges are specific for age, but not frame size, and are somewhat lower than the Life Insurance Tables. Another quick formula developed from data by *Keys* et al. [31] is to square the height in meters and multiply the value by a factor of 20.6 for women and 22.1 for men to obtain needed weight (sample calculation in table II).

Ideal body weight can also be estimated using lean body weight and percentage body fat. Some authors think that *ideal body fatness,* not weight, should be the goal [32, 33]. Body fatness can be determined from the sum of the biceps, triceps, suprailiac and subscapular skinfolds as previously mentioned (table IV). For example (table II, part A), if 22% of body weight is fat for a 20-year-old, 5 ft 5 inches (165 cm), 125 lb (57 kg) female, 27.5 lb (12.5 kg) of her 125 lb (57 kg) is fat and the remaining 97.5 lb (44.5 kg) is lean body mass. Since 22% body weight as fat is a good body fat content for a female (18% for a male), 125 lb (57 kg) is a good ideal body weight. There is disagreement as to how low body fat should be allowed to go in the female and still be healthy. A low body fat in an anorectic or bulimic might suggest a trained body, but more often would suggest a malnourished one where both body fat and lean body mass are inadequate. Too low a body fat has been correlated with amenorrhea. For those with amenorrhea, approximately 17% body fat is necessary before menstruation begins again [34]. A higher body fat (greater than 25–30% in a female) is not an absolute indication for a reduction diet. A patient can be overfat and normal or underweight. In table II, part B, the same female now has a 40% body fat and her calculated ideal body weight is 96 lb (44 kg). This is obviously too low a weight when compared with one of the other methods. Treatment of choice would be an exercise regimen that would increase lean body mass in proportion to body fat.

For children and adolescents up to age 18, the National Center for Health Statistics Growth Charts [35] can be used; these percentile curves are based on large, nationally representative samples of children and reflect a broad consensus of expert opinions.

Estimation of Caloric Needs

Caloric requirements are based on age, height, sex and current weight; the estimate can then be adjusted for weight gain. Table V outlines three different methods requiring various amounts of time and mathematical knowledge for an anorectic and a bulimic. The Mayo Nomogram [36] is accompanied by instructions and, except for the activity factor in column VI, no subjective judgment is required (fig. 3). The choice of percentage for activity should be based on the historical information supplied by the patient and how it translates into the activity factors outlined during the discussion on energy expenditure.

Table III. Comparison of 1959 and 1983 Metropolitan Height and Weight Tables[1]

Height *ft, inches* cm	Weight in *pounds*/kilograms (without clothing)					
	small frame		medium frame		large frame	
	1959	1983	1959	1983	1959	1983
Women						
4′ 9″	*90–97*	*99–108*	*94–106*	*106–118*	*102–118*	*115–128*
145.0	40.8–44.0	44.9–49.0	42.6–48.1	48.1–53.5	46.3–53.5	52.2–58.1
4′ 10″	*92–100*	*100–110*	*97–109*	*108–120*	*105–121*	*117–131*
147.5	41.7–45.3	45.4–49.9	44.0–49.4	49.0–54.4	47.6–54.9	53.1–59.4
4′ 11″	*95–103*	*101–112*	*100–112*	*110–123*	*108–124*	*119–134*
150.0	43.1–46.7	45.8–50.8	45.4–50.8	49.9–55.8	49.0–56.2	54.0–60.8
5′ 0″	*98–106*	*103–115*	*103–115*	*112–126*	*111–127*	*122–137*
152.5	44.4–48.1	46.7–52.2	46.7–52.2	50.8–57.2	50.3–57.6	55.3–62.1
5′ 1″	*101–109*	*105–118*	*106–118*	*115–129*	*114–130*	*125–140*
155.0	45.8–49.4	47.6–53.5	48.1–53.5	52.2–58.5	51.7–59.0	56.7–63.5
5′ 2″	*104–112*	*108–121*	*109–122*	*118–132*	*117–134*	*128–144*
157.5	47.1–50.8	49.0–54.9	49.4–55.3	53.5–59.9	53.1–60.8	58.1–65.
5′ 3″	*107–115*	*111–124*	*112–126*	*121–135*	*121–138*	*131–148*
160.0	48.5–52.2	50.3–56.2	50.8–57.2	54.9–61.2	54.9–62.6	59.4–67.
5′ 4″	*110–119*	*114–127*	*116–131*	*124–138*	*125–142*	*134–152*
162.5	49.9–54.0	51.7–57.6	52.6–59.4	56.2–62.6	56.7–64.4	60.8–68.
5′ 5″	*114–123*	*117–130*	*120–135*	*127–141*	*129–146*	*137–156*
165.0	51.7–55.8	53.1–59.0	54.4–61.2	57.6–64.0	58.5–66.2	62.1–70.
5′ 6″	*118–127*	*120–133*	*124–139*	*130–144*	*133–150*	*140–16*
167.5	53.5–57.6	54.4–60.3	56.2–63.1	59.0–65.3	60.3–68.0	63.5–72.
5′ 7″	*122–131*	*123–136*	*128–143*	*133–147*	*137–154*	*143–16*
170.0	55.3–59.4	55.8–61.7	58.1–64.9	60.3–66.7	62.1–69.9	64.9–74.
5′ 8″	*126–136*	*126–139*	*132–147*	*136–150*	*141–159*	*146–16*
172.5	57.2–61.7	57.2–63.1	59.9–66.7	61.7–68.0	64.0–72.1	66.2–75.
5′ 9″	*130–140*	*129–142*	*136–151*	*139–153*	*145–164*	*149–17*
175.5	59.0–63.5	58.5–64.4	61.7–68.5	63.1–69.4	65.8–74.4	67.6–77.
5′ 10″	*134–144*	*132–145*	*140–155*	*142–156*	*149–169*	*152–17*
178.0	60.8–65.3	59.9–65.8	63.5–70.3	64.4–70.8	67.6–76.7	68.9–78.

[1] Adapted from the 1983 Height and Weight Charts with permission form the Metropolitan Life Insuran
Company.

Table III (continued)

Height *ft, inches* cm	Weight in *pounds*/kilograms (without clothing)					
	small frame		medium frame		large frame	
	1959	1983	1959	1983	1959	1983
Men						
5′ 1″	*105–113*	*123–129*	*111–122*	*126–136*	*119–134*	*133–145*
155.0	47.6–51.3	55.8–58.5	50.3–55.3	57.2–61.7	54.0–60.8	60.3–65.8
5′ 2″	*108–116*	*125–131*	*114–126*	*128–138*	*122–137*	*135–148*
157.5	49.0–52.6	56.7–59.4	51.7–57.2	58.1–62.6	55.3–62.1	61.2–67.1
5′ 3″	*111–119*	*127–133*	*117–129*	*130–140*	*125–141*	*137–151*
160.0	50.3–54.0	57.6–60.3	53.1–58.5	59.0–63.5	56.7–64.0	62.1–68.5
5′ 4″	*114–122*	*129–135*	*120–132*	*132–143*	*128–145*	*139–155*
162.5	51.7–55.3	58.5–61.2	54.4–59.9	59.9–64.9	58.1–65.8	63.1–70.3
5′ 5″	*117–126*	*131–137*	*123–136*	*134–146*	*131–149*	*141–159*
165.0	53.1–57.2	59.4–62.1	55.8–61.7	60.8–66.2	59.4–67.6	64.0–72.1
5′ 6″	*121–130*	*133–140*	*127–140*	*137–149*	*135–154*	*144–163*
167.5	54.9–59.0	60.3–63.5	57.6–63.5	62.1–67.6	61.2–69.9	65.3–73.9
5′ 7″	*125–134*	*135–143*	*131–145*	*140–152*	*140–159*	*147–167*
70.0	56.7–60.8	61.2–64.9	59.4–65.8	63.5–68.9	63.5–72.1	66.7–75.8
5′ 8″	*129–138*	*137–146*	*135–149*	*143–155*	*144–163*	*150–171*
73.0	58.5–62.6	62.1–66.2	61.2–67.6	64.9–70.2	65.3–73.9	68.0–77.6
5′ 9″	*133–143*	*139–149*	*139–153*	*146–158*	*148–167*	*153–175*
75.5	60.3–64.9	63.1–67.6	63.1–69.4	66.2–71.7	67.1–75.8	69.4–79.4
5′ 10″	*137–147*	*141–152*	*143–158*	*149–161*	*152–172*	*156–179*
78.0	62.1–66.7	64.0–68.9	64.9–71.7	67.6–73.0	68.9–78.0	70.8–81.2
′ 11″	*141–151*	*144–155*	*147–163*	*152–165*	*157–177*	*159–183*
80.5	64.0–68.5	65.3–70.3	66.7–73.9	68.9–74.8	71.2–80.3	72.1–83.0
′ 0″	*145–155*	*147–159*	*151–168*	*155–169*	*161–182*	*163–187*
83.0	65.8–70.3	66.7–72.1	68.5–76.2	70.3–76.7	73.0–82.6	73.9–84.8
′ 1″	*149–160*	*150–163*	*155–173*	*159–173*	*166–187*	*167–192*
85.5	67.6–72.6	68.0–73.9	70.3–78.5	72.1–78.5	75.3–84.8	75.8–87.1
′ 2″	*153–164*	*153–167*	*160–178*	*162–177*	*171–192*	*171–197*
88.0	69.4–74.4	69.4–75.8	72.6–80.7	73.5–80.3	77.6–87.1	77.6–89.4
′ 3″	*157–168*	*157–171*	*165–183*	*166–182*	*175–197*	*176–202*
90.5	71.2–76.2	71.2–77.6	74.8–83.0	75.3–82.6	79.4–89.4	79.8–91.6

Table IV. Percentage of body weight as fat [reprinted with permission from ref. 25]

Skinfolds mm	Males, age in years				Females, age in years			
	17–29	30–39	40–49	50+	16–29	30–39	40–49	50+
15	4.8	–	–	–	10.5	–	–	–
20	8.1	12.2	12.2	12.6	14.1	17.0	19.8	21.4
25	10.5	14.2	15.0	15.6	16.8	19.4	22.2	24.0
30	12.9	16.2	17.7	18.6	19.5	21.8	24.5	26.6
35	14.7	17.7	19.6	20.8	21.5	23.7	26.4	28.5
40	16.4	19.2	21.4	22.9	23.4	25.5	28.2	30.3
45	17.7	20.4	23.0	24.7	25.0	26.9	29.6	31.9
50	19.0	21.5	24.6	26.5	26.5	28.2	31.0	33.4
55	20.1	22.5	25.9	27.9	27.8	29.4	32.1	34.6
60	21.2	23.5	27.1	29.2	29.1	30.6	33.2	35.7
65	22.2	24.3	28.2	30.4	30.2	31.6	34.1	36.7
70	23.1	25.1	29.3	31.6	31.2	32.5	35.0	37.7
75	24.0	25.9	30.3	32.7	32.2	33.4	35.9	38.7
80	24.8	26.6	31.2	33.8	33.1	34.3	36.7	39.6
85	25.5	27.2	32.1	34.8	34.0	35.1	37.5	40.4
90	26.2	27.8	33.0	35.8	34.8	35.8	38.3	41.2
95	26.9	28.4	33.7	36.6	35.6	36.5	39.0	41.9
100	27.6	29.0	34.4	37.4	36.4	37.2	39.7	42.6
105	28.2	29.6	35.1	38.2	37.1	37.9	40.4	43.3
110	28.8	30.1	35.8	39.0	37.8	38.6	41.0	43.9
115	29.4	30.6	36.4	39.7	38.4	39.1	41.5	44.5
120	30.0	31.1	37.0	40.4	39.0	39.6	42.0	45.1
125	30.5	31.5	37.6	41.1	39.6	40.1	42.5	45.7
130	31.0	31.9	38.2	41.8	40.2	40.6	43.0	46.2
135	31.5	32.3	38.7	42.4	40.8	41.1	43.5	46.7
140	32.0	32.7	39.2	43.0	41.3	41.6	44.0	47.2
145	32.5	33.1	39.7	43.6	41.8	42.1	44.5	47.7
150	32.9	33.5	40.2	44.1	42.3	42.6	45.0	48.2
155	33.3	33.9	40.7	44.6	42.8	43.1	45.4	48.7
160	33.7	34.3	41.2	45.1	43.3	43.6	45.8	49.2
165	34.1	34.6	41.6	45.6	43.7	44.0	46.2	49.6
170	34.5	34.8	42.0	46.1	44.1	44.4	46.6	50.0
175	34.9	–	–	–	–	44.8	47.0	50.4
180	35.3	–	–	–	–	45.2	47.4	50.8
185	35.6	–	–	–	–	45.6	47.8	51.2
190	35.9	–	–	–	–	45.9	48.2	51.6
195	–	–	–	–	–	46.2	48.5	52.0
200	–	–	–	–	–	46.5	48.8	52.4
205	–	–	–	–	–	–	49.1	52.7
210	–	–	–	–	–	–	49.4	53.0

The equivalent fat content, as a percentage of body weight, for a range of values for the sum of four skinfolds (biceps, triceps, subscapular, and suprailiac) of males and females of different ages.

Table V. Estimation of caloric needs

Method	14.5-year-old: 5 ft 3 inch; 85 lb (160 cm, 38.6 kg)	20-year-old: 5 ft 5 inch, 125 lb (165 cm, 56.7 kg)
Mayo Foundation Nomogram [36] (fig. 3):		
I Weight, lb (kg)	85 (38.6)	125 (56.7)
II Height, inch (cm)	5 ft 3 inch (160 cm)	5 ft 5 inch (165 cm)
III Surface area, m^2	1.25	1.55
IV Age, years	14.5	20
V Basal needs, kcal/day (kJ/day)	1,210 (5,082)	1,380 (5,796)
VI Activity factor, 30%		
VII Total caloric needs, kcal/day (kJ/day)	1,750 (7,350)	1,900 (7,980)
Basal metabolic rate (BMR) + activity + specific dynamic activity (SDA):		
BMR		
Calculation of surface area (Mayo Nomogram), m^2	1.25	1.55
Determination of BMR (table VI), kcal/m^2/h (kJ/m^2/h)	39.2 (165)	35.3 (148)
Surface area × BMR × 24, kcal/day (kJ/day)	1,176 (4,950)	1,313 (5,506)
Activity		
Sedentary +20% Light +30% Moderate +40% Heavy +50% } kcal/day (kJ/day)	353 (1,485)	394 (1,652)
SDA		
10% of (BMR + activity) kcal/day (kJ/day)	153 (643)	171 (716)
Total calorie needs, kcal/day (kJ/day)	1,682 (7,078)	1,878 (7,874)
Recommended dietary allowances [9]:		
Weight (lb) × kcal/lb = kcal/day	85 × 20 = 1,700	125 × 16 = 2,000
Weight (kg) × kJ/kg = kJ/day	38.6 × 185 = 7,141	56.8 × 148 = 8,406

Age, years	kcal/lb/day (kJ/kg/day)	
	male	female
11–14	29 (267)	25 (231
15–18	22 (203)	18 (166)
19–22	20 (185)	16 (148)
23–50	15 (139)	15 (139)

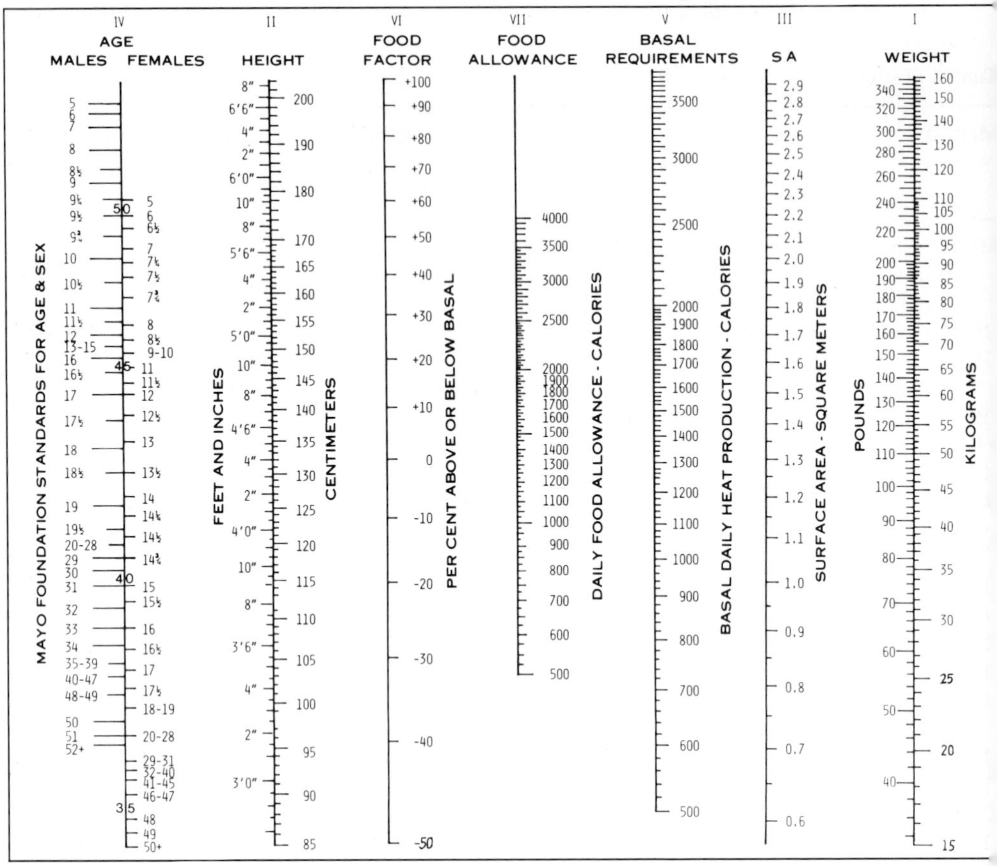

Fig. 3. Food nomogram. Directions: the standards for age are arranged on the basis of the common method of expressing age as of the last birthday. To determine the desired caloric allowance, proceed as follows: (1) Locate the weight on scale I by means of a pin stuck through the eraser of a lead pencil. (2) Place the edge of the ruler against the pin and swing the other end of ruler to the patient's height on scale II. (3) Transfer the pin to the point where the ruler crosses scale III which gives the surface area in square meters (this value need not be read). (4) Holding the ruler against the pin on the surface area scale, swing the left-hand end of the ruler to the patient's standard for age and sex given on scale IV. (5) Transfer the pin to where the ruler now crosses scale V which gives the basal heat production of the patient for 24 h and represents the calories of food required by the fasting patient when resting in bed (basal calories). The calories needed for activity bear a relationship to those demanded for the resting condition. The so-called 'white-collar worker' when at work will need about 50% more than his basal calories. When activity is restricted as in the hospital, the extra calories necessary will range from 10 to 30% of the basal calories. Therefore (6) estimate the percent of calories above the basal and locate this point on scale VI. With the ruler connect this point with the point located previously on scale V, and where the ruler now crosses scale VII read the amount of food calories to be provided by the diet [reprinted with permission from ref. 36]. To convert kcal to kJ, multiply by the conversion factor 4.2.

Table VI. Basal metabolic rate [adapted and printed with permission from ref. 41]

Age years	Males kcal/m²/h (kJ/m²/h)	Females kcal/m²/h (kJ/m²/h)	Age years	Males kcal/m²/h (kJ/m²/h)	Females kcal/m²/h (kJ/m²/h)
3	60.1 (252)	54.5 (229)	26	38.2 (160)	35.0 (147)
4	57.9 (243)	53.9 (226)	27	38.0 (160)	35.0 (147)
5	56.3 (236)	53.0 (223)			
6	54.0 (227)	51.2 (215)	28	37.8 (159)	35.0 (147)
7	52.3 (220)	49.7 (209)	29	37.7 (158)	35.0 (147)
			30	37.6 (158)	35.0 (147)
8	50.8 (213)	48.0 (202)	31	37.4 (157)	35.0 (147)
9	49.5 (208)	46.2 (194)	32	37.2 (156)	34.9 (147)
10	47.7 (200)	44.9 (189)			
11	46.5 (195)	43.5 (183)	33	37.1 (156)	34.9 (147)
12	45.3 (190)	42.0 (176)	34	37.0 (155)	34.9 (147)
			35	36.9 (155)	34.8 (146)
13	44.5 (187)	40.5 (170)	36	36.8 (155)	34.7 (146)
14	43.8 (184)	39.2 (165)	37	36.7 (154)	34.6 (145)
15	42.9 (180)	38.3 (161)			
16	42.0 (176)	37.2 (156)	38	36.7 (154)	34.5 (145)
17	41.5 (174)	36.4 (153)	39	36.6 (154)	34.4 (144)
			40–44	36.4 (153)	34.1 (143)
18	40.8 (171)	35.8 (150)	45–49	36.2 (152)	33.8 (142)
19	40.5 (170)	35.4 (149)	50–54	35.8 (150)	33.1 (139)
20	39.9 (168)	35.3 (148)			
21	39.5 (166)	35.2 (148)	55–59	35.1 (147)	32.8 (138)
22	39.2 (165)	35.2 (148)	60–64	34.5 (145)	32.0 (134)
			65–69	33.5 (141)	31.6 (133)
23	39.0 (164)	35.2 (148)	70–74	32.7 (137)	31.1 (131)
24	38.7 (163)	35.1 (147)	75+	31.8 (134)	
25	38.4 (161)	35.1 (147)			

Caloric needs can also be estimated by determining the basal metabolic rate and adding an activity factor and a factor for specific dynamic effect of food which are those calories required to metabolize daily food intake. The basal metabolic rate is dependent on surface area and age. Surface area can be calculated in the Mayo Nomogram or by other nomograms. Table VI lists the metabolic rates by sex and age in kcal/m^2/h and kJ/m^2/h; intermediate ages can be extrapolated. The rate is then multiplied by the surface area and by 24 h to obtain basal calories for the day. An activity factor is added as discussed previously; and to this total 10% is added for the effect of food (refer to table V for the complete calculation). When using this method for an adult, BMR can be estimated at 1 kcal/kg/h (4.2 kJ/kg/h) for males and 0.9 kcal/kg/h (3.8 kJ/kg/h) for females instead of using the surface area and BMR tables [37].

The easiest and quickest method is weight lb × kcal/lb (kg × kJ/kg) (age-specific) (table V). These figures are adapted from the Recommended Dietary Allowances [9]. The factors provide for increased needs due to growth during the adolescent years based on light-to-moderate activity. Adjustments to these factors would be necessary for a sedentary life-style or heavy activity. Some extrapolation may be required between ages. A drawback to this method is that basal calories are not specified in the calculation. A note of interest is that all three methods discussed above are within 100 kcal (420 kJ) of each other.

Caloric needs for the anorectic during early treatment are based on basal calories unless the patient has routinely been consuming more. Anorectics are in a starvation-adapted state and should not be overfed. It should be noted that fasting and chronic malnutrition lower the basal metabolic rate, so that an anorectic's needs may be overestimated initially, and calculated basal calories will actually be more than basal needs.

Formulation of the Diet

There is no standard diet plan for all patients with anorexia nervosa. The individualized diet must be planned as much as possible with consideration for the patient's past eating habits, likes and dislikes. Six small meals are preferred to three meals because less food is offered at each meal. It is often successful to show the patient an outlined meal day and ask for them to help fill in food choices. Compliance may be better when the choice belongs to the patient.

For some patients, the specific foods and quantities that they should consume need to be outlined. For example, lunch may be specified as one cup macaroni and cheese, one cup salad greens with two teaspoons dressing, one small apple, and 8 oz (240 cm^3) skim milk. If this is necessary, all days between visits need to be planned unless the patient is hospitalized. Other patients will be successful if offered a choice using the exchange system. For example, lunch may be specified as two meat exchanges, two bread exchanges, one vegetable exchange, one fruit exchange, and one milk exchange, and the patient allowed to make the choice of specific foods. Measuring foods gives the patient a sense of control and helps to ensure that the appropriate amount is consumed.

If foods are not measured and the patient chooses portion sizes in relation to her desire for food, intake will often not be adequate.

The planned diet should be checked for nutritional adequacy. Calories should be checked and compared to determined caloric level (usually basal). There should be appropriate balance in the nutrients carbohydrate, protein and fat, or a plan for achieving this balance within a few weeks. Complex carbohydrates may need to be reintroduced slowly. Fat may also need to be reintroduced. If there is little variety in food choices, variety can be encouraged as treatment progresses. If food intake is calculated to be below 1,000 kcal (4,200 kJ) a vitamin-mineral supplement should be included in the regimen.

Daily food diaries should be completed by the patient. These records help the nutritionist assess the progress, address the difficulties and direct the therapy. By providing a written record, diaries encourage compliance with the diet plan and discourage backsliding into old habits such as deficient intake and/or bingeing. The diary can also be used as a meal planner. Daily meals and social situations such as eating out and parties, which might otherwise be difficult, can be preplanned. Usage of the diary should continue until new food habits have become spontaneous.

Severe cases of anorexia nervosa require hospitalization. The goals are still the same, but the diet planning may be modified. The patient may not tolerate food or may be unwilling to consume it. In these instances, formula feeding by mouth (or rarely by nasogastric tube) may have to be utilized until the patient is ready to eat. After the patient has begun to eat, the liquid feedings can then be used as a supplement until calories are increased. Depending on hospital policy, meals may or may not be selected, so the patient's likes and dislikes and food patterns should be given to the kitchen. Diet compliance may be rewarded by allowing a meal choice, or by a visit from the nutritionist. Calorie counts can be ordered to verify a patient's intake. A rapid weight gain is dangerous and should be avoided.

A Plan for Steady Weight Gain

To the anorectic patient, weight gain will be the main issue during treatment. It is therefore important to explain this subject well. At the outset, the composition of weight gain will consist of retention of water through expansion of extracellular water, electrolyte retention and repletion of muscle and liver glycogen stores. This weight gain may be rapid and can occur even at a low caloric level if the patient's pretreatment intake was even less. Weight gain then stabilizes briefly before beginning a steady increase as body fat and protein are stored. It is important to stress composition of weight gain often to the patient. If she does not understand, she may feel 'out of control' with quick weight gain and stop eating for fear that her weight gain will continue at this rate. It should also often be stressed that the gain is not all fat.

During the refeeding, the patient may complain of bloating, water retention, gas pains and constipation. These complaints are usually resolved as food intake increases.

A steady weight gain of 0.5 lb (230 g) per week is a satisfactory gain. Calories in the diet should be increased gradually to allow for the gain. The approach should be individualized. Some patients may prefer to remain at a certain caloric level until there is no further gain before agreeing to increase calories; others will agree to weekly increments of 100–200 kcal (420–840 kJ). Reevaluation of caloric needs as weight is gained can be a valuable tool for encouraging more calories. The diet plan and caloric level are really minimum guidelines for the patient to follow, and more is encouraged. However, most patients consider the plan as maximum guidelines and would eat less before they would eat more than the guidelines.

A rapid weight gain during treatment should be investigated. For example, a recovering anorectic may begin to binge and rapidly gain weight. Events that trigger the bingeing should be discussed and the diet plan arranged to disrupt this behavior. If exercise is allowed during weight gain, the types and allowed time should be planned and extra calories added to the diet. A well-planned and supervised exercise program can improve the quality of the weight gain.

When the patient reaches her weight goal, there should be very little caloric adjustment on the maintenance diet if her gain has been steady and slow. The diet guidelines she has followed during the gain should be fairly established nutritional habits, making weight maintenance an easy goal to achieve.

A Plan for Follow-Up: Nutrition Education

Undoubtedly, the patient up to this stage has received much nutrition information as the weight goal, caloric level, and diet have been planned, weight gain has been explained, and other questions have been answered. The nutritionist can continue to reinforce and elaborate on this information, and field new topics as they arise. A real challenge will be the patient's cognitive distortions or firmly held beliefs that prevent her from making appropriate food selections at times. Statements such as, 'After a certain hour, all that I eat will turn to fat' and, 'I know all my weight gain will go to my thighs' challenge the nutritionist to provide and continually reinforce the facts that make these statements false. Encouraging a trusting relationship will enhance the chances for success in this endeavor.

Nutritional Aspects of Treatment for Bulimia

Goals

The goals of nutritional therapy for bulimia are weight stabilization, weight gain or weight loss to a realistic weight range, and normalization of eating habits. Psychotherapy is necessary to aid in the cessation of the bingeing and purging behavior. Psychotherapy is also the primary focus of treatment, as in anorexia nervosa. The components of treatment are also similar to those for anorexia nervosa and include estimation of ideal body weight, estimation of caloric needs, formulation of the diet, a plan for weight gain or loss, and a plan for follow-up.

Estimation of Ideal Body Weight

The preceding discussion of ideal body weight for anorectics is also applicable to bulimics (table II). What should also be considered is the usual weight of the bulimic prior to the onset of the eating disorder. Was it higher or lower? The setpoint theory of weight control suggests that there may be a weight (determined genetically or during early life) which the body will strive to maintain [38]. A bulimic, therefore, may be unsuccessfully trying to maintain an ideal body weight lower than her setpoint weight. If this seems to be evident, a weight gain may be necessary for weight stabilization. Current thought is that there is probably little that can be done to lower the setpoint with the possible exception of exercise.

Estimation of Caloric Needs

Table V estimates caloric needs for the 20-year-old. Unlike the anorectic at basal needs, the bulimic's caloric needs will include the percentages for activity and digestion of food. These caloric needs will then be adjusted if weight gain or weight loss is needed.

Formulation of the Diet

In addition to the preceding discussion on diet formulation for the anorectic patient, the bulimic's plan will be modified to avoid bingeing. If binges are triggered by certain foods, these foods should be avoided initially. If

Table VII. Tyramine-controlled diet [adapted with permission from ref. 39]

Food groups	Servings daily	Foods to include	Foods to avoid
Milk	as desired	skim, low fat, whole milk, milk-shakes and eggnogs	plain and fruit-flavored yogurts; chocolate-flavored drinks
Meat, fish, poultry, cheese, meat alternates	5–6 oz (142–170 g)	cottage cheese, cream cheese; all meats except those to avoid; peanut butter, dried beans and peas	all cheeses except those allowed; caviar, smoked or pickled fish, beef liver, salami, bologna, peperoni, summer sausage
Egg	3–4 per week	any style	none, except raw
Breads and cereals	4 or more servings	all except those to avoid	bread or crackers containing cheese
Potatoes and alternate	1–2 half-cup servings	all	any prepared with cheese
Vegetables	2 or more half-cup servings	all except those to avoid; include one source high in vitamin A every other day	Italian fava beans (broad beans), eggplant
Fruit and juices	2 or more half-cup servings	all except those to avoid; include 1 vitamin C fruit daily	bananas, figs, raisins
Fat	3 or more servings	all except those to avoid	avocado, sour cream
Sweets and desserts	as desired	sugar, honey, jams and jellies, hard candy, ice cream, sherbet; gelatin desserts made with allowed foods	chocolate in any form
Beverages	as desired	all except those to avoid	wines, ale, beer; excessive coffee, tea, cola drinks (more than 3 cups daily)
Soups	as desired	soups made with foods allowed	soups containing foods to avoid

Indication: This diet is recommended for individuals receiving monoamine oxidase inhibitors (MAOI MAOI prevent the oxidation of tyramine to monoamine oxidase (MAO). Excessive accumulation of tyramine or other pressor amines may cause a severe hypertensive crisis, excruciating headaches, tachycardia or even fatal intracranial hemorrhages.
Description: In this diet, foods containing large amounts of tyramine and dopamine or the bacteria capable of enzymatically converting tyrosine to tyramine are eliminated for patients who are receiving MAOI.
Adequacy: This diet is adequate in the specified nutrients from the 1980 Recommended Dietary Allowance for an adult male and female.

binges are triggered by starvation diets, then a steady daily intake should be stressed. A three-meal plan might be more advantageous for avoiding binges than a six-meal plan. Specific food instructions are again similar to the information listed for anorectics. Some bulimics will need more specific instructions than others.

Nutritional adequacy and variety should also be stressed. A consistent daily diet, if the patient has been on a starvation-binge cycle, should be highly encouraged. As with the anorectic, a reintroduction of complex carbohydrates into the diet will need to be done gradually. Food diaries that note binges and purges aid the nutritionist in planning for future avoidance. In addition to planning meals, bulimics can plan each day to avoid high-risk binge situations.

When bulimics are hospitalized, the reason is often to control purging. Many are currently being given a trial with monoamine oxidase inhibitors (see chapter 4). A tyramine-controlled diet needs to be included in the diet plans for these patients (table VII). Foods to be avoided include chocolate drinks, yogurt, most cheeses, liver, wine, ale, beer, sour cream, and avocado [39].

A Plan for Weight Gain/Loss

For bulimics, the main issue during treatment is cessation of purging and/or bingeing; weight is generally a secondary issue. If it has been decided during evaluation that weight gain is necessary to alleviate symptoms, the composition of weight gain should be explained, even though these bulimics might not be in as malnourished a state as the anorectics. The bulimics can feel out of control and need to be constantly reassured while gaining. Rapid weight gain should be avoided if at all possible. If weight loss is necessary during treatment, the loss should be gradual and the caloric intake adequate enough not to trigger a binge.

The type and amount of exercise among bulimics varies. Excessive exercisers should be curtailed to a healthy amount. Those who do not exercise could be introduced to a healthy regimen. Exercise improves the quality of the weight gain or loss. It can even be scheduled during a high-risk binge period.

Plan for Follow-Up: Nutrition Education

As with the anorectics, the bulimics will have received much nutrition information during the early stages of treatment. The issues to be constantly reinforced include consistent daily intake, including enough carbohydrates at each meal to keep them out of the starvation-binge cycle, and avoidance of foods that trigger bingeing. Bulimics will also have cognitive distortions that inhibit them from being compliant at times. These issues will also need to be resolved.

References

1 American Psychiatric Association: Diagnostic and statistical manual of mental disorders; 3rd ed. (APA, Washington 1980).

2 American Diabetes Association, American Dietetic Association: Exchange lists for meal planning (American Dietetic Association, Chicago 1976).

3 Pennington, J.; Church, H.: Bowes and Church's food values of portions commonly used; 13th ed. (Lippincott, Philadelphia 1979).

4 Adams, C.: Nutritive value of American foods in common units. Agriculture handbook, No. 456 (USDA, Agricultural Research Service, Washington 1975).

5 Consumer and Food Economics Institute: Composition of foods. Agricultural handbook, No. 8 (Science & Education Administration USDA, Washington 1976).

6 Select Committee on Nutrition and Human Needs US Senate: Dietary goals for the United States; 2nd ed.; Stock No. 052-070-04376-8, p. 5 (US Government Printing Office, Washington 1977).

7 Bo-Linn, G.; Santa Ana, C.; Morawski, B.; Fordtran, J.: Purging and calorie absorption in bulimic patients and normal women. Ann. intern. Med. *99:* 14–17 (1983).

8 Guthrie, H.: The role of carbohydrate in a balanced diet, p. 11 (Chocolate Manufacturers Association of the United States of America, McLean 1980).

9 Committee on Dietary Allowances, Food and Nutrition Board: Recommended dietary allowances; 9th ed. (National Academy of Sciences, Washington 1980).

10 Garner, D.; Garfinkel, P.: The eating attitudes test: an index of the symptoms of anorexia nervosa. Psychol. Med. *9:* 273–279 (1979).

11 Mitchell, H.; Rynbergen, H.; Anderson, L.; Dibble, M.: Cooper's nutrition in health and disease; 15th ed., p. 50 (Lippincott, Philadelphia 1968).

12 Grant, A.: Nutritional assessment guidelines; 2nd ed. Seattle 1979.

13 Metropolitan Life Insurance Company Health & Safety Education Division: 1983 Metropolitan height and weight tables, New York (1983).

14 Guidelines for Anthropometric Measurement (Ross Laboratories, Columbus 1981).

15 Murray, R.: Discussion of techniques in anthropometry, part II. Nutr. Support Serv. *2:* 11–14 (1982).

16 Lindner, P.; Lindner, D.: How to assess degrees of fatness (Cambridge Scientific Industries, Cambridge 1973).

17 Burgert, S.; Anderson, C.: An evaluation of upper arm measurements used in nutritional assessment. Am. J. clin. Nutr. *32:* 2136–2142 (1979).

18 Gurney, J.; Jelliffe, D.: Arm anthropometry in nutritional assessment; nomogram for rapid calculation of arm muscle circumference and cross-sectional muscle and fat areas. Am. J. clin. Nutr. *26:* 912–915 (1973).

19 Jeliffe, D.: The assessment of nutritional status of the community. WHO Monogr. *53:* (1966).

20 Frisancho, A.: Triceps skinfold and upper arm muscle size norms for assessment of nutritional status. Am. J. clin. Nutr. *27:* 1052–1058 (1974).

21 Basic data on anthropometric measurements and angular measurements of the hip and knee joints for selected age groups 1–74 years of age, United States, 1971–1975; National Health Survey, Vital and Health Statistics Series No. 219. US Dept of Health and Human Services, Public Health Service, pp. 20–26 (1981).
22 Bishop, C.; Bowen, P.; Ritchey, S.: Norms for nutritional assessment of American adults by upper arm anthropometry. Am. J. clin. Nutr. *34:* 2530–2539 (1981).
23 Gray, G.; Gray, L.: Anthropometric measurements and their interpretation: principles, practices, and problems. J. Am. diet. Ass. *77:* 534–538 (1980).
24 Kovach, K.: The assessment of nutritional status in anorexia nervosa; in Gross, Anorexia nervosa: a comprehensive approach; 1st ed., pp. 69–79 (Collamore Press, Lexington 1982).
25 Durnin, J.; Womersley, J.: Body fat assessed from total body density and its estimation from skinfold thickness: measurements on 481 men and women aged from 16 to 72 years. Br. J. Nutr. *32:* 77–97 (1974).
26 How to diagnose nutritional disorders in daily practice. Teaching Aid. Nutr. today, N.Y. *5* (1969).
27 Blackburn, G.; Bistrian, B.; Maini, B.; Schlamm, H.; Smith, M.: Nutritional and metabolic assessment of the hospitalized patient. J. parent. Nutr. *26:* 11–22 (1977).
28 Metropolitan Life Foundation: Statist. Bull. *64:* 3–9 (1983).
29 American Diabetes Association and American Dietetic Association: A guide for professionals: the effective application of 'exchange lists' for meal planning, p. 17 (Am. Diet. Ass., Chicago 1977).
30 Obesity in Perspective: Fogarty Center Series on Preventive Medicine, vol. 2, p. 3. US Dept of HEW publ. No. (NH)75–708 (1975).
31 Keys, A.; Fidanza, F.; Karvonen, M.; Kimura N.; Taylor, H.: Indices of relative weight and obesity. J. chron. Dis. *25:* 329–343 (1972).
32 Bailey, C.: Fit or fat? pp. 8–16 (Houghton Mifflin, Boston 1978).
33 Seltzer, C.; Mayer, J.: A simple criterion of obesity. Postgrad. Med. *38:* A101–A106 (1965).
34 Frisch, R.; McArthur, J.: Menstrual cycles: fatness as a determinant of minimum weight for height necessary for their maintenance and/or onset. Science *185:* 949–951 (1974).
35 Hamill, P.; Drizd, T.; Johnson, C.; Reed, R.; Roche, A.; Moore, W.: Physical growth: National Center for Health Statistics percentiles. Am. J. clin. Nutr. *32:* 607–629 (1979).
36 Pemberton, C.M.; Gastineau, C.F.: Mayo clinic diet manual: a handbook of dietary practices; 5th ed., p. 282 (Saunders, Philadelphia 1981).
37 Hamilton, E.; Whitney, E.: Nutrition: concepts and controversies; 1st ed., p. 162 (West, St. Paul 1979).
38 Nisbett, R.: Hunger, obesity and the ventromedial hypothalamus. Psychol. Rev. *79:* 433–458 (1972).
39 Diet Manual, The Florida Dietetic Association: Tyramine-controlled diet; in Wiggins, The manual of clinical dietetics (Florida Dietetic Ass., Orlando 1983).
40 Wilmore, D.: The metabolic management of the critically ill; in King, Reemtsma, Reviewing surgical topics; 1st ed., p. 49 (Plenum, New York 1980).
41 Boothby, W.M.: in Spector, Handbook of biological data (Saunders, Philadelphia 1956).

12 Role of the Medical Consultant

Allen W. Root

Introduction

The medical consultant has two major tasks in the management of the patient with anorexia nervosa: (1) to establish or confirm the diagnosis by excluding disorders with which it may be confused, and (2) to assist in nutritional, medical and endocrinologic treatment of the patient (a review of the regulation of appetite, the metabolic consequences of malnutrition, the endocrinologic responses to malnutrition and the immunologic effects of malnutrition is contained in chapter 9). It is usually the primary care physician who is first consulted by the patient or the family of the patient for weight loss, growth retardation, sexual immaturity or regression of secondary sexual characteristics, and who must exclude disease which might produce these symptoms and adduce positive evidence for the diagnosis of anorexia nervosa. Thereafter, this physician must assist the patient and family into the therapy of this disorder, serving as the liaison between the psychiatrist skilled in the management of this disease and the patient. Not infrequently the suggested diagnosis of anorexia nervosa is not accepted by the patient, in which case it is the primary physician's responsibility to assist the patient into its acceptance. Depending upon individual circumstances the primary physician may serve as the medical contact for patients who are unable to accept psychiatric care at least until such acceptance is forthcoming. However, with increasing frequency this writer is impressed by the patient who, after being informed of the diagnosis of anorexia nervosa, actually seems relieved, and even states that he or she had 'suspected' it or that the diagnosis of anorexia nervosa had been suggested by family members or close friends.

Diagnosis of Anorexia Nervosa

Differential Diagnosis

Weight loss may be: (1) the consequence of inadequate intake of calories and other nutrients due to socioeconomic deprivation, psychological illness, or systemic or endocrinologic diseases; (2) associated with decreased absorption of food due to diseases of the gastrointestinal tract, pancreas, or hepatobiliary system; (3) due to excessive caloric utilization, or (4) due to calorie loss prior to metabolism. Since amenorrhea is almost always observed in females with anorexia nervosa, one must consider the differential diagnosis of this symptom, which includes disorders of the central nervous system, hypothalamus, pituitary, or ovaries. Interestingly, there is an association between anorexia nervosa and gonadal dysgenesis (Turner's syndrome) and the two entities may coexist [1]. In children and adolescents anorexia nervosa may present as growth retardation or failure to thrive and thus the differential diagnosis of this problem must also include anorexia nervosa. The causes of weight loss are enumerated in table I.

Evaluation of the Patient with Weight Loss

The diagnosis of anorexia nervosa is established both by the presence of specific criteria (morbid fear of becoming obese, disturbed body image, weight loss of 25% from ideal body weight, refusal to maintain a minimal safe body weight, no other psychiatric illness to account for weight loss and two of the following: amenorrhea, bradycardia, overactivity, bulimia, or purging) and by the absence of specific identifiable systemic or endocrinologic disease. Since it is to the family practitioner, internist or pediatrician to whom the patient with anorexia nervosa will often initially present, rather than to the psychiatrist, it is imperative that the primary physician consider the diagnosis of anorexia nervosa in all patients with weight loss and in children with a subnormal growth pattern and/or failure to gain weight [2].

Evaluation begins with a thorough history, seeking symptoms of a specific systemic or endocrinologic disease. In children data regarding patterns of linear growth, weight gain and sexual development should be sought. One inquires systematically about general symptoms (malaise, unexplained fevers, fatigue), and symptoms specifically related to each system (central nervous, gastrointestinal, cardiorespiratory, genitourinary, musculoskeletal, integumentary and endocrinologic). A detailed dietary history is obtained, although the validity of this history may be suspect. In patients with anorexia

Table I. Causes of weight loss

- Inadequate caloric intake
  - Socioeconomic deprivation
  - Psychological dysfunction
    - Intrinsic: anorexia nervosa
    - Extrinsic: abuse
  - Systemic disease
    - Inflammatory systemic lupus erythematosus, rheumatoid arthritis, dermatomyositis
    - Neoplastic
    - Central nervous system
      - Hypothalamic: tumor, trauma, inflammation
      - Hyposmia, hypogeusia: zinc deficiency, lead poisoning
      - Neuromuscular: myasthenia gravis
    - Gastrointestinal system
      - Structural – esophageal stricture, diverticulum, fistula
      - Functional – achalasia, chalasia, scleroderma, esophagitis
      - Inflammatory – chronic inflammatory bowel disease, chronic hepatitis
    - Cardiorespiratory system
      - Congenital/acquired heart disease
      - Respiratory insufficiency – cystic fibrosis
    - Genitourinary system
      - Chronic renal insufficiency, acidosis
    - Endocrinologic
      - Hypoadrenalism
      - Hypopituitarism
      - Hypercalcemia (hyperparathyroidism, sarcoid, vitamin D intoxication)

- Decreased caloric absorption (malabsorption)
  - Gastroenteropathies
    - Celiac disease
    - Infiltrative disease
  - Pancreatic insufficiency
    - Cystic fibrosis
    - Chronic alcoholism
    - Schwachman-Diamond syndrome
  - Hepatobiliary disease

- Excessive caloric utilization
  - Hyperthyroidism
  - Dissociation of oxidative phosphorylation
    - Intrinsic
    - Toxic

- Excessive caloric loss (urine or stool)

nervosa, the menstrual pattern is carefully documented in relation to the change in weight. In children and adolescents with anorexia nervosa, the presenting complaint may be poor growth, delayed adolescent sexual maturation and failure to gain weight, rather than weight loss [2]. One must be alert to such clues in order to elicit those positive findings consistent with anorexia nervosa. The history should also identify positive criteria for diagnosis of anorexia nervosa. The physical examination complements the historical review by seeking signs of physical or systemic illness, and by documenting the state of nutrition. Laboratory studies which are useful in eliminating systemic disease and providing baseline data are outlined in table II. Once systemic disease has been excluded and the diagnosis of anorexia nervosa established, treatment is initiated.

The Role of the Consultant in the Treatment of Anorexia Nervosa

The consultant has three tasks in the treatment of the patient with anorexia nervosa: (1) to convince the patient of the diagnosis; (2) to supervise the medical aspects of nutritional rehabilitation, and (3) to provide long-term medical follow-up. When the diagnosis of anorexia nervosa has been established, the consultant initiates treatment by detailing for the patient the method of diagnosis, assuring them that no other identifiable disease has been overlooked. The initial discussion after diagnosis is critically important. If the patient accepts the diagnosis and the family assumes a positive supportive role, then specific treatment can be initiated with a high probability of success. If the patient or family denies the diagnosis, treatment becomes a great deal harder. It is the task of the initial consultant to present the diagnosis in such a manner as to permit its acceptance by the patient with consequent positive entrance into specific therapy. An honest, straightforward but sympathetic statement relating the diagnosis is usually helpful in facilitating acceptance.

Subsequently the consultant supports the psychiatrist in the management of the patient with anorexia nervosa. Either the consultant or the psychiatrist assumes the primary responsibility for nutritional rehabilitation of the patient; such rehabilitation is the primary objective of initial management and must be accomplished either with or without the acquiescence and cooperation of the patient. Hypovolemia, hypotension and dehydration require immediate treatment. If an attempt at behavior modification is

Table II. Laboratory studies for the evaluation of weight loss

Blood count	to determine if hemoglobin concentrations and white cell count and morphology are normal
Sedimentation rate	frequently elevated in patients with chronic inflammatory bowel disease, collagen–vascular and other inflammatory illnesses
Urinalysis	to rule out urinary tract infection, and to evaluate urinary concentrating and acidification ability
Chemical studies	to document acid base balance, hypo- or hyperelectrolytemia, hypoalbuminemia, hypercalcemia, hyperuricemia, azotemia, hypophosphatemia, abnormalities of enzyme activity or bilirubin levels; to document intestinal fat absorption by measuring plasma levels of vitamins A and E, or determining fat balance by measuring excretion of fat in the stool while the patient is ingesting known amount of fat
Endocrinologic studies	thyroid function (T_4, free T_4, T_3RIA, reverse T_3, T_3RU, or TSH), somatomedin C, GH provocative and suppressive tests, cortisol, ACTH, LH, FSH, estradiol, testosterone, and prolactin measures as indicated in individual patients; somatomedin C and T_3 concentrations increase as nutritional status improves
Chest X-ray	to rule out tuberculosis or other chronic pulmonary disease
Bone age	to determine growth potential (in children and adolescents)
Skull X-ray or CAT scan of the head	in selected patients with symptoms of central nervous system involvement (such scans may reveal cerebral atrophy in patients with anorexia nervosa) [3]
Upper GI series with small bowel follow-through	seeking abnormalities of deglutition, obstruction and inflammatory bowel disease (inflammatory bowel disease may be a difficult diagnosis to establish [4], requiring repetitive roentgenographic examinations of the intestinal tract and direct inspection)

T_4 = Thyroxine; T_3 = triiodothyronine; T_3RIA = triiodothyronine by radioimmunoassay; T_3RU = triiodothyronine resin uptake; TSH = thyroid-stimulating hormone; GH = growth hormone; ACTH = adrenocorticotropic hormone; LH = luteinizing hormone; FSH = follicle-stimulating hormone; CAT = computerized axial tomography; GI = gastrointestinal.

unsuccessful in securing patient cooperation and willing oral ingestion of adequate calories, then nutrition must be administered by nasogastric intubation or by peripheral hyperalimentation. Chronic, severe starvation impairs muscle function (particularly the respiratory muscles, which may compromise cardiorespiratory function), leads to adrenal failure and increases susceptibility to infection. The consultant should be prepared for these catastrophic complications with appropriate therapeutic planning.

Initial nutritional rehabilitation should begin with lower than optimal intake of calories, proteins, carbohydrates and electrolytes, because too rapid increase in intravascular volume may result in acute congestive heart failure in a patient with an impaired cardiovascular system. Monitoring of body weight, blood pressure, heart rate, fluid intake and urine output is critically important at this point. Usually caloric intake can be increased to optimal levels within 7–14 days after initiation of treatment. The excess caloric requirements (above maintenance amounts) for weight gain in patients with anorexia nervosa is approximately 7,500 cal/kg (31,500 kJ/kg) of weight gained [5] and is inversely related to the degree of weight loss of the patient at the initiation of nutritional rehabilitation [6]. Thus, the closer the patient's weight approaches her standard weight, the more extra calories that are required for weight gain (see chapter 11). Once a treatment program involving both nutritional and psychiatric components has become successfully established the consulting physician should maintain periodic contact with the patient in order to assure her of the consulting physician's genuine interest and concern.

Monitoring the biochemical aspects of nutritional rehabilitation (increasing serum concentrations of proteins, T_3, somatomedin C, restoration of immune function and so forth) is of interest, but in the majority of patients is not essential. However, not initially, but after weight recovery, sex hormonal replacement therapy may be considered in certain young women. In these subjects 3–6 months of cycling with estrogen/progestin may be beneficial. On occasion the consulting physician may assume primary responsibility for managing the medical and nutritional aspects of care while the psychiatrist assumes responsibility for the other aspects of care. Each consultant/psychiatrist team must determine which treatment regimen is best suited to the achievement of the overall therapeutic goals for the individual patient. Certainly these roles change from patient to patient and also from time to time in the treatment of the same patient.

The consultant often finds that he (she) has developed good rapport with the family of the patient and can support the entrance of the entire family into family therapy which complements the individual therapy of the patient. Since anorexia nervosa is a chronic disease, the consultant must be prepared to follow these patients for prolonged periods, offering supportive and medical care as appropriate for the individual situation.

References

1 Kron, L.; Katz, J.; Gorzynski, G.; Werner, H.: Anorexia nervosa and gonadal dysgenesis. Further evidence of a relationship. Archs gen. Psychiat. *34:* 332–335 (1977).

2 Root, A.; Powers, P.: Anorexia nervosa presenting as growth retardation in adolescents. J. adolesc. Hlth Care *4:* 25–30 (1983).

3 Nussbaum, M.; Shenker, I.; March, J.; Klein, M.: Cerebral atrophy in anorexia nervosa. J. Pediat. *96:* 867–869 (1980).

4 Kulig, J.; Siqueira, L.: Diagnosis of anorexia nervosa in the adolescent male. J. adolesc. Hlth Care *4:* 31–34 (1983).

5 Russell, G.; Mezey, A.: An analysis of weight gain in patients with anorexia nervosa treated with high calorie diets. Clin. Sci. *23:* 449–461 (1962).

6 Walker, J.; Roberts, S.; Halmi, K.; Goldberg, S.: Caloric requirements for weight gain in anorexia nervosa. Am. J. clin. Nutr. *32:* 1396–1400 (1979).

13 Therapeutic Use of Symptoms, Signs and Laboratory Data

Pauline S. Powers

Introduction

As physicians, psychiatrists are in a unique position to be able to use symptoms, physical findings and laboratory tests in a way that can facilitate psychotherapy. As noted in chapter 12, family physicians and other medical specialists can also be helpful in utilizing this information in assisting the family and the patient overcome the denial that is so common among eating disorder patients. In this chapter, common errors in the therapeutic utilization of these findings will be briefly outlined. The implications of the semistarvation studies of *Keys* et al. [1] for understanding anorexia nervosa will be discussed. Then, the common symptoms, signs and laboratory findings that result from semistarvation, abnormal food intake and purging behavior will be reviewed. The physiological abnormalities that occur during weight restoration, or when bingeing and purging behavior is relinquished, will be presented. The abnormal findings that remain after weight is restored and eating patterns are normalized will be reviewed in the light of the potential for relapse.

In this chapter, terms familiar to laymen are used (e.g. pounds and degrees Fahrenheit) to demonstrate the psychotherapeutic usefulness of conveying physiological information to the patient. As described in chapter 10, the preliminary evaluation at the University of South Florida Eating Disorders Clinic includes a detailed medical and psychiatric history, mental status examination, physical examination and selected laboratory tests. After the evaluation, the diagnosis is presented to the patient, along with the positive findings that confirm the diagnosis. The reasons for excluding other diagnoses are reviewed and the signs and symptoms of the patient's malnutrition are described. The mortality rate of anorexia nervosa is estimated to be 6–10% without treatment [2, 3], and more than half these deaths are due to the consequences of starvation, purging and electrolyte disturbances. With treatment, mortality may be reduced to approximately 2–4% [4, 5]. These mortality figures and the very significant morbidity of prolonged malnutrition are reviewed with the patient.

Common Errors

Medicine has a tendency to divide mind and body. Psychiatrists and other physicians need to resist this tendency. The eating disorders are examples of complex biopsychosocial disorders that require an integrated view of the person in the context of the family and social system. The following examples illustrate errors resulting from a unidimensional view of the patient.

One common error is that some patients in the early stages of anorexia nervosa have been told by their doctors that the weight loss is a minor problem that will be outgrown. Although it is probably true that there are a few patients who have a spontaneous recovery, it is unlikely. Of the first 50 anorectic patients seen at the Eating Disorders Clinic at the University of South Florida [5], only 1 is known to have recovered her weight without treatment. This clinic is a tertiary referral center, and patients seen may have a poorer prognosis than patients who are initially seen by primary care physicians. However, for most patients, inappropriate early reassurance facilitates denial and may lengthen the time until psychiatric intervention occurs, during which time additional weight may be lost. Prognosis worsens with both increasing length of time prior to weight restoration [6] and with greater weight loss [7–9]. Thus, early intervention may significantly improve long-term outcome. Similarly, patients who have not yet lost 25% of their ideal body weight (IBW), but who have other symptoms (morbid fear of obesity, preoccupation with food, binge-eating or purging), should receive treatment. As noted in chapter 2, the biological solution (starvation) may become an autonomous process, especially if the condition persists and, thus, treatment should not be withheld until the patient meets the strict DSM III weight criteria.

The second common error is to overlook significant symptoms, signs or abnormal laboratory tests. For example, many patients have not been weighed, or care is not taken to determine accurate, repeated weights. Many anorectic patients are deceitful about their weight, particularly initially, if they suspect that the therapist is only interested in weight gain. In this situation, the patient may sew weights into underclothing, or change the weight recorded by the nurse. A patient referred to our clinic drank several liters of water prior to her weigh-in, and when weighed unexpectedly was 10 lb (4.5 kg) lighter than on scheduled weigh-in days. Many patients who voluntarily report that they have been vomiting or abusing laxatives or diuretics (all of which can cause electrolyte abnormalities) have not been asked about symptoms of hypokalemia (for example, weakness, gastrointestinal disturbances, palpitations, or difficulty concentrating). Assisting the patient to recognize the relationship between certain behavior (for example, binge-eating) and a physiological consequence (for example, parotid gland enlargement) can be one step in reuniting the mind-body dichotomy that is usually an integral part of the eating disorder.

Semistarvation Studies and Anorexia Nervosa

In the last few years it has been recognized that many of the signs and symptoms of anorexia nervosa are not specific to the condition, but are the consequence of semistarvation. The studies in the 1940s by *Keys* et al. [1] were designed to evaluate the biological consequences of semistarvation. Many physiological and cognitive findings were noted that recently have been recognized as identical to anorexia nervosa (e.g. fatigue, decreased fat stores, and obsessive preoccupation with food). However, it is important to remember that in those studies, and in the experience of many victims of famine or concentration camps, the malnutrition is essentially a combination of deficient protein and too few calories (protein-calorie malnutrition, PCM). Marasmus is essentially a type of PCM. Kwashiorkor is another type of malnutrition, in which protein is deficient, although caloric intake is near normal levels. Most anorectics decrease total caloric intake and eliminate carbohydrates and fats, but often maintain a near normal protein intake and may take vitamin supplements.

It has been suggested that PCM, kwashiorkor, marasmus and anorexia nervosa are all on a continuum, with varying degrees of protein and calorie deficits [10]. This may be the case but it is important to recognize that there are certain well-documented differences between PCM and anorexia nervosa. Table I illustrates certain of these differences. Although a normochromic, normocytic anemia and a mild leukopenia occur in PCM [1] and anorexia nervosa [11, 12], anorectics characteristically have acanthocytes (spur cells) on peripheral smear, and the bone marrow of anorexia nervosa patients reveals an accumulation of an amorphous acid mucopolysaccharide [12]. This finding may be specific to anorexia nervosa, and may reflect the relatively selective elimination of carbohydrates and fats. Similarly, patients with PCM characteristically are prone to viral and bacterial infections [13], and have low serum protein, low serum transferrin and a low total lymphocyte count. By contrast, the majority of patients with anorexia have a normal total body lymphocyte count, and more than half have normal serum protein and serum transferrin [14]; anorectics are also relatively immune to viral diseases

Table I. Selected similarities and differences

PCM (protein-calorie malnutrition)	Anorexia nervosa
Normochromic, normocytic anemia [1]	same plus acanthocytes and an acid mucopolysaccharide in bone marrow [11, 12]
Decreased serum protein and transferrin [13]	majority have normal serum protein [14]
Cell-mediated immunocompetence impaired [13]	normal in most patients [10, 14]
Susceptible to viral and bacterial infections [13]	relatively immune to viral infections [15]
Elevated plasma cortisol; diminished cortisol metabolism rates [16]	elevated plasma cortisol; diminished cortisol metabolism rates [17]
Abnormal DST [16]	abnormal DST [18]; may be more common among bulimic anorectic subgroup [19]
With weight gain cortisol production rates rise [16]	with weight gain cortisol production rate falls [17]
Elevated plasma GH [20]	elevated plasma GH [21]
Amenorrhea [22]	amenorrhea earlier than in externally imposed starvation in about one third of patients [23]
Decreased LH and FSH [22]	decreased LH and FSH [24]
Normal or low cholesterol [25]	elevated cholesterol [26–28]
Decreased concentrating capacity of kidney reverses with vasopressin [29]	decreased concentrating capacity of kidney not reversed with vasopressin [30]
Obsessions about food, compulsive handling of food, dreams about food, slow rate of eating [1]	similar but also morbid fear of obesity [2]

DST = Dexamethasone suppression test; LH = luteinizing hormone; FSH = follicle-stimulating hormone; GH = growth hormone.

until late in the course. *Pertschuk* et al. [15] note that only with severe weight loss (i.e. weight below 60% of IBW) did anergy become the rule in anorectic patients (reflecting the loss of cellular immunity). Another difference between PCM and anorexia nervosa is that anorectics have elevated cholesterol levels [26, 27]; the reason for this finding is unknown, but may be due to repeated bouts of bingeing [28]. Another difference between PCM and anorexia nervosa is that the reduced concentrating capacity of the kidneys that occurs in both states of starvation is reversible with vasopressin in PCM, but is not in anorexia nervosa [29, 30].

Although our understanding of the differences between various types of malnutrition remains sketchy, it seems likely that specific abnormalities may occur if carbohydrates and fats are preferentially eliminated. Chapter 9 describes certain of the metabolic pathways that are affected with different types of malnutrition.

Initial Symptoms, Signs, and Laboratory Data

Tables II–IV illustrate possible connections between symptoms, signs and certain laboratory tests, and the types of behaviors utilized by patients. Not all patients will have all symptoms, and not all physical signs or abnormal laboratory tests will be present in all patients. These abnormalities will not all be reviewed in the following discussion, but several examples of ways in which the information can be utilized therapeutically to assist the patient to reunite mind and body will be described. The tables are not divided into anorexia nervosa and bulimia, because the same symptoms and signs can occur in either condition. However, since, by definition, patients with bulimia are not as underweight as anorexia nervosa patients, signs and symptoms of semistarvation (table II) are probably less common in this group.

The symptoms, signs and laboratory data have been divided into tables by the postulated usual cause: semistarvation (table II), abnormal food intake (table III) or purging behavior (table IV). Certain symptoms can have multiple causes: e.g. convulsions can occur in restricting anorexia nervosa patients who diet and fast and have developed hypoglycemia as a result [31]; patients who have purged, using very large quantities of laxatives, may also develop convulsions due to hyponatremia [32]. Similarly, enlarged parotid glands usually occur in patients who chronically vomit [33], but may also occur during severe malnutrition without purging, or in patients who binge [34]. Thus, the tables are meant as preliminary guides to understanding symptoms, so that their meanings can be discussed with patients.

Table II. Semistarvation: relationship to initial symptoms, signs, and laboratory data

Symptom	Signs	Related laboratory data
Fatigue	low body weight	anemia; anisocytosis, poikilocytosis [12]; acanthocytes or spur cells [12]; bone marrow: decreased iron stores [38]; acid mucopolysaccharide [12, 38]; hypoplasia [38]
	decreased muscle stores	decreased LMAC [36]; increased SGOT [39]; abnormal muscle function and possible selective atrophy type II fibers [40]
Dry skin	emaciation	low T_3 syndrome: decreased peripheral conversion of T_4 to T_3 [41]
Light-headedness; syncope	dehydration; – orthostatic hypotension (pulse rises and BP falls on standing) – decreased skin turgor	low T_3 syndrome; decreased LMAC
	– bradycardia	cardiac findings [42, 43]
Palpitations	arrhythmias	abnormal exercise tests [42]; EKG: ST–T wave abnormalities and/or arrhythmias [43]; decreased cardiac performance [44]; decreased LV mass (small heart on chest X-ray) [42]; serum electrolyte disturbances [32]; decreased total body K^+ [30]
Cold intolerance	hypothermia decreased fat content acrocyanosis	abnormal responses to heat and cold stresses [37]; skinfold measures less than 15th percentile [36]
Swollen ankles or generalized swelling	edema	? central hypothalamic abnormality: reversal of normal (< 1.0) CSF/plasma vasopressin and abnormal osmoregulation vasopressin [45]; peripheral renal abnormality: decreased concentrating capacity kidneys [37]; occasionally low serum albumin [46]

Table II (continued)

Symptom	Signs	Related laboratory data
Females: amenorrhea, loss of libido	fat content less than 17% [35]	'immature' LH secretory pattern [47, 48]; low estrogens [24]; decreased LH and FSH [24]; monthly cycling LH and FSH absent [24]; no response to clomiphene citrate [48]
Females: dyspareunia	pelvic examination: hypoestrogenic vaginal changes [49]	low estrogens
Males: impotence; loss of libido		low testosterone [50]; decreased LH and FSH [51]
Hair growth	lanugo on face and upper torso	decreased protein [1]
Sleep disturbance		increased plasma cortisol [17]; partial failure of suppression with dexamethasone [52]; abnormal sleep EEGs [53]; decreased prolactin during sleep [54]
Noise sensitivity [1]	hyperacusis	
Early satiety; postprandial discomfort; bloating; constipation	occasionally in chronically ill – moderate hepato-splenomegaly	delayed gastric emptying [55]; increased SGOT and other liver enzymes [39]
Abdominal pain	rarely, symptoms pancreatitis: tenderness, fever, decreased bowel sounds	elevated serum amylase [56–58]; various findings on X-ray examination: duodenal dilatation [59]; mild nonobstructive jejunal dilatation [60]
Anorexia	weight loss	decreased zinc [61]; elevated serum carotene [61]
Poor taste recognition	hypogeusia, especially for bitter and sour tastes	decreased plasma zinc [61]

Table II (continued)

Symptom	Signs	Related laboratory data
Short stature	below 5th percentile on Tanner charts [62, 63] or NCHS charts [65]; delayed pubertal developmental	normal alkaline phosphatase during growth spurt [66]; delayed bone age [64, 67]; occasionally Turner's syndrome [68]
Fewer viral infections [69]		intact cellular immunity lost when 60% below IBW [15]
Mood changes:		
– euphoria		increased endorphins [70];
– depression		abnormal DST [52, 71] and occasionally blunted TSH response to TRH [19]
Cognitive: poor concentration, obsessions, compulsions about food	multiple signs may be related: dehydration, bradycardia, hypotension, etc.	cognitive disturbances on psychological tests (chapter 9) [72]; hypoglycemia [31]; hypokalemia and hyponatremia [32]; abnormal CT scans – atrophy and enlarged sulci ('pseudoatrophy') and enlarged ventricles [73]
Convulsions	generalized or atypical seizure activity	hyponatremia [32]; hypoglycemia and low circulating insulin, increased insulin sensitivity, increased insulin binding to monocytes [31]; EEG abnormalities – abnormal background activity, unstable response to hyperventilation, occasional epileptiform paroxysmal dysrhythmia [74]

BP = Blood pressure; CSF = cerebrospinal fluid; DST = dexamethasone suppression test; FSH = follicle stimulating hormone; IBW = ideal body weight; LH = luteinizing hormone; LMAC = left mid-arm circumference; LV = left ventricle; NCHS = National Center for Health Statistics; SGOT = serum glutamic oxaloacetic transaminase; T_3 = triiodothyronine; T_4 = thyroxine; TRH = thyrotropin-releasing hormone; TSH = thyroid-stimulating hormone.

Semistarvation

Common symptoms of starvation include fatigue, light-headedness or syncope, amenorrhea and feeling cold when others are warm. Although the connection between these symptoms and the patient's emaciated state may seem apparent to the treating physician, the patient and family often do not recognize these connections. This may reflect the patient's psychological

Table III. Abnormal food intake: initial symptoms, signs, and laboratory data

Symptom	Signs	Related laboratory data
Binge behavior		
Toothache	dental caries from high carbohydrate intake [75]	X-ray findings
Swollen painless cheeks	parotid gland enlargement [34]	benign biopsy [76]
Abdominal pain	abdominal tenderness, change in bowel sounds	gastric dilatation or perforation on radiologic studies of upper gastrointestinal tract [77]
Stretch marks (from quick weight changes)	stria distensae	
No symptoms		elevated cholesterol [26–28]
Unusual eating or drinking behavior		
Salt restriction	seizures	hyponatremia [32, 78]; abnormal EEG [78]
Polyuria and polydipsia (water intoxication)		low specific gravity of urine; decreased concentrating capacity kidneys [37]
Ingestion carotene-containing foods (all green vegetables)	yellowish skin tone, especially soles and palms	carotinemia [61]: in addition to increased intake, there may also be acquired defect in carotene metabolism

defense mechanism of denial, as well as the patient's tendency to ignore or misinterpret information arising from bodily states. However, the patient and family often benefit from being taught these connections. The following case vignette illustrates that multiple factors, including lack of knowledge, may contribute to the patient's erroneous conclusions.

Table IV. Purging behavior: initial symptoms, signs, and laboratory data

Symptom	Signs	Related laboratory data
Vomiting, laxative abuse and diuretics		
Palpitations	arrhythmias	abnormal electrolytes, especially hypokalemia [30, 32] or hypochloremic alkalosis [32]; abnormal EKG, etc. (see under *Malnutrition,* table II)
Bloody diarrhea from laxative abuse – usually Correctol[1] [83]	multiple signs including dehydration, bradycardia, hypotension, anemia, etc.	increased creatinine phosphokinase [56]; fluid and electrolyte disturbances; positive stool guiaic
Bruises over knuckles	ecchymoses (from repeated vomiting)	
Mouth pain	buccal erosions from regurgitated hydrochloric acid [75]	
Dry mouth, worse with anticholinergic medications	xerostomia [80]	buffering capacity, pH, quantity and quality of saliva are decreased [80]
Tooth sensitivity to heat, cold and acidic substances	perimolysis – loss of enamel and dentin on lingual surfaces of teeth [75]	
Red eyes	conjunctival hemorrhages	results from increased intrathoracic pressure from vomiting
Bruises on face and neck	ecchymoses	results from increased intrathoracic pressure from vomiting
Shortness of breath	pneumothorax or pneumo-mediastinum or subcutaneous emphysema [84]	results from increased intrathoracic pressure from vomiting

Table IV (continued)

Symptom	Signs	Related laboratory data
Overexercise		
Fatigue	dehydration; bradycardia	increased creatinine phosphokinase due to muscle breakdown; decreased muscle and fat content
Amenorrhea		see *Malnutrition;* women runners without anorexia: luteinizing hormone response to gonadotropin-releasing hormone is increased compared to normal or decreased response of anorectics [85]

[1] Correctol laxatives made by Plough, Inc., Memphis, Tenn., include phenolphthalein and dioctyl sodium sulfosuccinate.

Ms. K. had lost from 120 lb (54.5 kg) to 86 lb (39 kg). She was a straight A student, and presented with a chief complaint that she could not concentrate on her studies. She interpreted this symptom as evidence that she was a lazy, incompetent person. The relationship between her difficulty in concentration and her state of semistarvation was discussed with her in the initial evaluation, and became one of the primary reasons she was willing to be hospitalized for a weight restoration program. She was also frequently depressed and, although this undoubtedly worsened her capacity to concentrate, the therapeutic focus was on the relationship to her starved state.

Clarifying the relationship between a symptom (e.g. light-headedness or syncope), a sign (e.g. orthostatic hypotension) and behavior (e.g. failure to eat and consequent weight loss) can be therapeutically useful.

Helen weighed 80 lb (36 kg) at 5 feet 6 inches (168 cm) and felt light-headed, with morning headaches. In the hospital she took a very hot shower and fainted. The nurse immediately took her lying and standing blood pressure and pulse, to confirm the fall in blood pressure and rise in pulse. The nurse explained to Helen that she already had orthostatic hypotension due to her severe weight loss, and that the hot water had caused blood to pool in the periphery, worsening the hypotension and causing her to faint. The response of the nurse helped the patient begin to correlate certain body states (light-headedness, headaches and fainting) and her behavior (continued refusal to eat).

Certain signs can be utilized effectively in encouraging the patient to consider treatment. Although a decreased fat content is the goal of anorectics, many are unaware that a certain fat content, probably 17%, is required for regular menstrual periods to occur [35]. Some patients welcome amenorrhea, either because it symbolizes a return to a childlike state, or because menses were painful or frightening. But there are other patients who want normal hormonal functioning, menses and reproductive capacity.

Ms. M. who had had anorexia nervosa for many years, married and wanted to have children. She was able to gain weight and increase fat content when her gynecologist explained the connection between fat content and fertility. The theory that a critical fat content is needed for the maintenance of menses and restoration of fertility was understood by this patient and was therapeutically useful.

Another common sign is a decrease in somatic muscle stores [36]. Since some patients rationalize that excessive exercise and weight loss are in fact healthy, it is occasionally useful to describe the loss of muscle content. As discussed in chapter 11, muscle content by percentile for height can be determined using the Lange skinfold calipers, the left mid-arm circumference (LMAC) and standard reference tables.

Cold intolerance (graphically demonstrated by anorectics wearing heavy clothing in summer) is a common symptom, and is reflected in low temperatures – often below 97 °F (36 °C) – on physical examination. This is due to decreased fat stores (demonstrated on physical examination by dramatically low tricep skinfold measurements), but may also reflect hypothalamic dysfunction. *Mecklenburg* et al. [37] demonstrated that 5 anorectics failed to shiver in response to cold stress, and had an abnormal decrease in core temperature. These researchers note that the primary motor center for shivering is in the posterior hypothalamus, under inhibition of the anterior hypothalamic thermosensitive cells. Thus, the cold intolerance may reflect both a central (hypothalamic) dysfunction, as well as a peripheral abnormality (loss of insulating fat tissue). Both of these abnormalities are probably the consequence of semistarvation.

Bradycardia is a common sign in anorexia nervosa. Patients may identify their low pulse as evidence of good health and fitness; this is an example of a cognitive distortion. While it is true that athletes have lower pulse rates and may be more fit than controls, a low pulse rate can have multiple meanings, only one of which is 'fitness'.

Abnormal Food Intake

Other symptoms, signs and abnormal laboratory data are related to binge-eating, or unusual eating, or drinking behavior (table III). Prolonged bouts of bingeing can result in swollen parotid glands [34] and various gastrointestinal symptoms (e.g. bloating and abdominal pain). Patients with very quick weight changes may have stretch marks. Swollen ankles are a symptom of peripheral edema with diverse causes. Bingeing on high carbohydrate foods, or the purposeful ingestion of large quantities of salt to prevent or shorten hospitalization can result in generalized, or pedal, edema.

Purging Behavior

Purging behavior includes vomiting, laxative abuse and, rarely, diuretic abuse [5]. Use of diuretics, in patients who utilize other methods of purging as well, can result in a quick depletion of potassium, and be particularly dangerous. Exercise may be overused as a method of 'getting rid' of consumed calories and, thus, overexercise has been included as a method of purge behavior. *Yates* et al. [79] have recently shown that certain male runners have psychological similarities to classic female anorectic patients. Table IV lists the common symptoms, signs, and laboratory data in patients who purge.

Vomiting can result in mouth pain, due to buccal lesions caused by erosion from hydrochloric acid in regurgitated stomach contents [80]. Prolonged vomiting can result in pharyngitis, esophagitis, gastritis, or esophageal laceration and produce hematemesis [81]. Repeated increases in intra-abdominal or intrathoracic pressure from vomiting can result in bruises on the face and neck (ecchymoses), and red eyes (conjunctival hemorrhages).

Laxative abuse can be particularly severe, and we have seen patients who consume several hundred at a time and must be hospitalized for treatment of overdose. Rectal bleeding and various lower gastrointestinal lesions from repeated laxative abuse may occur. Patients are often under the misapprehension that the use of laxatives will 'get rid of it (the food)' and are often surprised to learn that a recent study has shown that even with a huge laxative intake (up to 50 laxatives a day), only 12% of the calories consumed are lost [82].

Palpitations may occur in the patient with electrolyte disturbances. Some restricting anorectics, but particularly patients who purge (whether they are normal weight or severely underweight), are prone to electrolyte imbalance. Restricting anorectics may have a total body deficiency of potassium [30] and thus develop arrhythmias. Patients who purge by vomiting or laxative abuse may develop hypokalemia and may be particularly prone to cardiac arrhythmias. These patients frequently have a compensatory hypochloremic alkalosis [32]. These electrolyte disturbances probably account for the occasional sudden death of bulimic or anorectic patients. The hazards posed by these findings are much more readily accepted since the death in 1982 of singer Karen Carpenter (who probably died due to an arrhythmia secondary to hypokalemia, after gaining weight quickly in an unmonitored situation).

Subtle Symptoms: Failure to Grow in Height and Weight

Certain symptoms may be subtle indications of anorexia nervosa. 4 patients have been described with delayed adolescent development and lifelong histories of slow height and weight growth [67]. *Pugliese* et al. [63] have recently described 17 similar patients from families in which thinness was a virtue. Characteristically, these patients have not lost weight, but rather have failed to gain weight and height as expected. There may be no body image disturbance, no evidence of semistarvation, and most do not appear to be relentlessly pursuing even greater thinness. The only major psychological similarity in this group is a conflict about growing up.

One short, underweight, teenage boy said he did not want to grow up, because then he would need new motorcycle boots that his family could not afford. This statement symbolized both his own fear of growing up and a genuine recognition that his father, an unemployed lawyer, was unable to support him in his emerging independence, either financially or emotionally.

Many of these 'atypical anorectics' (so called for lack of a better term) are not only at low percentile levels on the height-weight charts, but also are in very early stages of pubertal development [63] and have delayed bone ages [67]. It is often useful to review with the patient that the growth spurt in height occurs only during a certain age span (usually prior to age 21), and that for optimal growth in height to occur, nutritional intake must increase (and/or exercise must decrease). Unlike typical anorectic patients, it has been our experience that these teenagers understand and integrate this information by increasing food intake. Many are particularly gratified by increases in height, and have accepted increases in weight without terror.

Asymptomatic Abnormal Laboratory Tests

Certain laboratory abnormalities are asymptomatic. For example, liver enzymes may be mildly elevated [56], but there are often no symptoms, and no signs on physical examination, although rarely, late in the course of anorexia nervosa, there may be hepatosplenomegaly. There may be a decreased concentrating capacity of the kidney with no signs or symptoms [37]. Certain abnormal neuroendocrine tests, the dexamethasone suppression test (DST) and the thyrotropin-releasing hormone (TRH) test, that had been thought to be specific for endogenous depression, have been found to be abnormal in normal weight bulimics [19] and some anorectics [71].

Elevated cholesterol levels are asymptomatic. However, it is often helpful to inform the patient of this finding. Most patients associate elevated cholesterol levels with being fat, and are surprised to learn that with weight restoration, cholesterol levels usually return to normal [28].

Symptoms Rarely Reported

Some symptoms may be considered advantageous and, thus, not reported. These symptoms may be among several factors which serve to maintain the disorder. Amenorrhea, relative immunity to viral diseases and euphoria during the initial phase of weight loss are often welcomed by the patient.

Amenorrhea has been reported to occur prior to significant weight loss in one third to one half of patients [23]. This finding has been the basis for speculation that there is a preexisting physiological abnormality (perhaps in the hypothalamus) that predisposes to the development of anorexia nervosa. Although it is the author's opinion that there probably are physiological risk factors for anorexia nervosa, it is also well-known that psychological stress can cause amenorrhea [86]. Although the neurohormonal abnormalities of stress-related amenorrhea in normal weight women are only poorly understood, there are similarities to the endocrine abnormalities in anorexia nervosa. Anorectics are known to have four well-documented abnormalities of the hypothalamic pituitary ovarian axis [17]. First, plasma and urinary gonadotropins (LH and FSH) are low in the face of low plasma estrogens. Second, monthly cycling of gonadotropins is absent. Third, clomiphene (an anti-estrogen agent) does not result in an increase in LH. Fourth, the circadian pattern of LH release is absent. *Boyar* et al. [47] have reported on the arrest, or regression (i.e. 'immaturity'), of the 24-hour secretory pattern of LH. This is an interesting finding in terms of one postulated psychodynamic etiology of anorexia nervosa. This theory posits that weight loss allows the teenage girl to regress psychologically and physically, thus avoiding the tasks of adolescence, including the development of heterosexual relationships; the regression of LH patterns to pubertal or prepubertal levels has been seen as one biological expression of this regression.

Amenorrhea can also occur in women who run, but who do not have anorexia nervosa. One major neurohormonal difference is that the administration of gonadotropin-releasing hormone (GnRH) to these runners results in an increase in LH compared to anorectics, who usually have a diminished (or occasionally a normal) response [85].

Anorexia nervosa patients have a *relative immunity to viral infections* at low weights. Although this observation was reported years ago [69], it has only recently been studied [10, 11, 15]. Unlike PCM where infection, both bacterial and viral, is common and cellular immunity is impaired [13], patients with anorexia nervosa apparently have intact cellular immunity until their weight falls to 60% of IBW [15]. Furthermore, there is an enhanced proliferative lymphocyte response to mitogenic stimulation which may account for the apparent enhanced immunity to viral disease.

Many anorectics describe themselves as *euphoric* with initial weight loss, an experience which may facilitate continued efforts to lose weight. *Kaye* et al. [70] have found elevated cerebral spinal fluid (CSF) levels of endogenous opioid peptides (expressed as beta-endorphin equivalents) in underweight anorectics compared to normal controls; the opioids were lower after weight restoration. Another group of patients with chronic anorexia nervosa (but not seriously underweight) had normal levels of CSF opioid activity. Since the endogenous opioids may be one group of neurotransmitters involved in the regulation of eating behavior, this finding may have important implications, especially for the psychopathophysiology of the condition.

Signs and Symptoms during Weight and Eating Normalization

It is often helpful to tell the patient who is about to undertake a weight restoration program that gaining weight is difficult, partly because the person wants to remain thin, and partly because any change in weight homeostasis is difficult. *Sims* et al. [87] found that subjects who attempted to gain 25% above their usual weight were more emotional and less active physically. Many recovering anorectics are dysphoric, with frequent crying spells and irritability. The factors that contribute to this mood change are multiple, but probably include a decline in endorphins, emotional stress related to relinquishing a previously effective defense mechanism (e.g. starvation) and the physiological stress of altering a homeostatic weight.

We have noted that many patients complain of fatigue. After 1 young woman gained back more than half the weight she had lost, she was so tired she could not lift her head off the pillow. This lethargy is perplexing to the patient, who may complain that he or she felt fine before gaining weight and now is exhausted. Warning the patient prior to weight gain that these symptoms can occur may promote cooperation with the treatment plan. We postulate that the factors which promote feelings of fatigue are present at the nadir of weight loss (i.e. mild anemia, low weight, decreased muscle stores and electrolyte imbalance), but that the physical feeling is denied; with improvement in capacity to identify internal sensations and feeling states, the patient becomes aware of the fatigue.

There are many other symptoms experienced during weight restoration. Table V itemizes some of these. Some are to be expected; others are harbingers of serious complications from the weight gain. Most patients complain of gastrointestinal symptoms, including fullness, bloating, or abdominal cramping. Although these symptoms sometimes are used by patients to avoid weight gain, anorectics at low and restored weights have delayed gastric emptying which may account for some of these symptoms [55]. Metoclopramide, which improves gastric emptying, can often provide some relief [90]. There have been many reports of serious complications of the gastrointestinal system, especially with treatment protocols in which quick weight gain is encouraged, or nasogastric (NG) tube feedings utilized. The major complications noted have been acute gastric dilatation and perforation [77, 91].

With weight gain, there is a return of hypothalamic pituitary activity in a definite sequence which recapitulates puberty [89]. Patients may develop

Table V. Signs and symptoms during weight restoration

Mood changes related to decline in endorphins [70]
Fatigue
Decreased physical activity [87]
Gastrointestinal symptoms: fullness, bloating, cramps (may be due to delayed gastric emptying) [55]
Unmasked electrolyte disturbances after hydration (e.g. tetany from low calcium or arrhythmias from hypokalemia)
Loss of viral immunity
Generalized or pedal edema may be 'refeeding' edema or sign of serious complication
Signs and symptoms of congestive heart failure – quick weight gain, edema, shortness of breath, rales, gallop [88]
Signs and symptoms of pulmonary emboli – chest pain, hemoptysis
Quick weight gain – from relinquishing various purging techniques and consequent decrease in loss of fluids and electrolytes
Acne, breast enlargement, menstrual cramping – return of hypothalamic pituitary activity which recapitulates puberty [89]
Abdominal pain – acute gastric dilatation or perforation especially with nasogastric feedings [77]

acne, breast enlargement, and finally menses. Prior preparation for these events can be helpful.

Quick weight gain, after purging is relinquished, or during weight restoration, can be alarming to the patient, who often interprets this occurrence as evidence that weight gain will be uncontrollable. In some underweight patients who have the low triiodothyronine syndrome [41], the quicker-than-predicted weight gain may be due to the relative hypometabolism during a period of high calorie intake. However, a more frequent cause of quick weight gain is a correction of the initial dehydration that occurs in anorectics and purging bulimics. Patients who purge with laxatives commonly lose 4–6 liters per day of fluid and electrolytes while actual calorie loss is less than 12% of consumed calories [82]. Each liter of fluid weighs about 2.2 lb (1 kg). If the patient stops losing 6 liters of fluid per day by stopping laxative use, there may be a weight gain of 12–13 lb (5.4–6 kg) in a very short span of time. This is hazardous, both psychologically and physiologically. The patient may erroneously conclude that the only way to prevent massive obesity is to continue laxative abuse. In purging anorectics, who are already severely depleted nutritionally, quick weight gain may pose additional stress to an already impaired cardiac function. Congestive heart failure has been reported during the recovery phase of anorexia nervosa [88]. Recently, we have seen a patient who gained 20 lb (9 kg) on intravenous feedings, then developed chest pain and had multiple pulmonary emboli on lung scan.

Dehydration which is present initially may mask certain electrolyte and hematologic abnormalities. These may become apparent when the patient is rehydrated. For example, we have seen 1 patient who developed tetany when she was rehydrated; her calcium level dropped as her plasma volume increased after relinquishing use of laxatives. Hypokalemia may become more apparent after the patient is rehydrated.

Physiological Abnormalities in Anorectics after Weight Restoration

Although it has usually been predicted that the physiological abnormalities present at the lowest weight would return to normal with adequate weight gain, this is not strictly accurate. Table VI lists physiological abnormalities which do not necessarily return to normal, even with weight gain.

Since it is not known what factors result in relapse, these remaining physiological abnormalities may be of great importance. Patients with these abnormalities may require more intensive follow-up. Similarly, patients who

Table VI. Physiological abnormalities remaining after weight restoration

Symptoms	Signs or laboratory data
Potentially reversible	
Erratic menses	normal biphasic response of LH estrogen not restored [92]
Infertility even if above 95% of IBW [95]	24-hour secretory pattern of LH often not normal [93]; failure of *L*-dopa to produce prompt rise in GH continues
Bloating, fullness, cramps	delayed gastric emptying [55]
Swollen cheeks	parotid gland enlargement [34]
Sleep disturbance	reduction tonic and phasic components of REM sleep [78, 99]
Subtle cognitive effects	abnormalities on neuropsychological tests [72]
Yellowish soles and palms	carotinemia [100]
Edema	erratic release of vasopressin [45]
Irreversible	
Short stature	early closure of epiphyses [67]
Dental caries	X-ray findings [75]
Blindness	optic atrophy
Intractable diarrhea	? exocrine pancreatic disease [58]

recover, both physiologically and psychologically, and who later undertake even modest weight loss regimens, should probably be closely monitored, since they may be more vulnerable to the development of the physiological mechanisms which, in combination with potent psychological factors, promote the disorder.

Potentially Reversible

Some anorectics who regain to their prior weight do not have a return of regular menses [92–94]. Probably some of these patients continue abnormal eating practices, or purge, but there may be some weight-restored patients who eat normally, but still fail to menstruate regularly. Possibly this is because there is an underlying hypothalamic abnormality, or possibly there has been irreversible hypothalamic pituitary or ovarian damage caused by the malnutrition.

Reproductive capacity of weight-recovered anorectics may be impaired. Some women who recover to their original weight may still be more than 5% below IBW by the Metropolitan Height-Weight Tables (see chapter 11). *Bates* et al. [95] have shown that women who are 85–95% of their IBW may experience fertility problems; willingness to gain to within 5% of IBW resulted in spontaneous conception in 73%. One study of anorexia nervosa has shown that more than half the patients with anorexia nervosa were more than 5% below IBW before weight loss began [5]. Thus, restoration of weight to premorbid levels may be inadequate to establish fertility. This can be a particularly difficult problem, even for women without eating disorders, since the current female shape considered ideal is probably more than 5% below the IBW noted in the Metropolitan Height-Weight Tables. It is proposed that one criterion of physiological health in a woman is capacity to conceive. A necessary minimum fat content for fertility is probably 17% [35], and it may be that for a significant percentage of women the minimum is greater than 17%.

Certain gastrointestinal signs and symptoms may remain even after weight restoration and normalization of eating patterns. Some patients with bingeing may continue to have parotid gland enlargement even after bingeing and purging are relinquished [34]. Some patients with anorexia nervosa continue to have delayed gastric emptying for months after weight is restored [55].

Irreversible Changes

There may be several irreversible changes secondary to starvation. Prolonged malnutrition can result in optic atrophy and blindness, as in a 53-year-old woman treated in our clinic. More commonly, short stature can result when patients are nutritionally deprived throughout the adolescent growth spurt [67]. Dental caries from binge-eating carbohydrates are irreversible [75]. 1 patient with exocrine pancreatic disease from laxative abuse has been reported [58]. In our clinic, we have seen 1 patient with intractable diarrhea who abused huge quantities of laxatives for years; exocrine pancreatic disease was diagnosed.

Suspected Remaining Abnormalities

In another category are abnormalities that are suspected to remain for some time, perhaps permanently, after weight gain, or after normalization of eating patterns. In this category are abnormalities noted on computerized tomography of the head which reveal enlarged ventricles and sulci (termed 'pseudoatrophy' by some authors) which sometimes return to normal with weight gain [96] but not invariably [97]. Although cardiac function after weight gain has not been rigorously investigated, animal models of starvation [98] suggest that the abnormalities present during starvation are not completely reversed until several months after attainment of normal weight and eating patterns.

Conclusion

There are many symptoms, signs, and abnormal laboratory tests that occur in anorexia nervosa and bulimia. The physician who evaluates and treats patients with eating disorders is in a unique position to utilize these findings to facilitate treatment. Since many patients experience a mind-body dichotomy (yet paradoxically are exquisitely sensitive to any change in their body), reeducative treatment methods that assist the patient in reuniting thoughts, feelings and bodily sensations can be particularly effective. During the evaluation, anorectics characteristically deny awareness of any problem; tactful confrontation of the patient and family with the signs and symptoms of malnutrition may allow the denial to be partially relinquished. During treatment, some of the terror of weight gain, and of certain bodily changes, can be averted if the patient understands the meaning of certain symptoms and signs.

References

1 Keys, A.; Brozek, J.; Henschel, A.; Michelsen, O.; Taylor, H.: The biology of human starvation (University of Minnesota Press, Minneapolis 1950).
2 Bruch, H.: Eating disorders, pp. 377–387 (Basic Books, New York 1973).
3 Hsu, L.; Crisp, A.; Harding, B.: Outcome of anorexia nervosa. Lancet *i:* 61–65 (1979).
4 Garfinkel, P.; Moldofsky, H.; Garner, D.: The outcome of anorexia nervosa. Significance of clinical features, body image and behavior modification; in Vigersky, Anorexia nervosa, pp. 315–329 (Raven Press, New York 1977).
5 Powers, P.; Powers, H.: Inpatient treatment of anorexia nervosa. Psychosomatics (in press).
6 Crisp, A.; Kalucy, R.; Lacey, J.; Hardin, B.: The long-term prognosis in anorexia nervosa: some factors predictive of outcome; in Vigersky, Anorexia nervosa, pp. 55–65 (Raven Press, New York 1977).

7 Halmi, K.; Brodland, G.; Loney, J.: Prognosis in anorexia nervosa. Ann. intern. Med. *78:* 907–909 (1973).
8 Morgan, H.; Russell, G.: Value of family background and clinical features as predictors of long-term outcome in anorexia nervosa: four-year follow-up study of 41 patients. Psychol. Med. *5:* 355–371 (1975).
9 Seidensticker, J.; Tzagournis, M.: Anorexia nervosa – clinical features and long-term follow-up. J. chron. Dis. *21:* 361–367 (1968).
10 Golla, J.; Larson, L.; Anderson, C.; Lucas, A.; Wilson, W.; Tomasi, T.: An immunological assessment of patients with anorexia nervosa. Am. J. clin. Nutr. *34:* 2756–2762 (1981).
11 Bowers, T.; Eckert, E.: Leukopenia in anorexia nervosa. Lack of increased risk of infection. Archs intern. Med. *138:* 1520–1523 (1978).
12 Mant, M.; Faragher, B.: The hematology of anorexia nervosa. Br. J. Haemat. *23:* 737–749 (1972).
13 Chandra, R.: Nutrition, immunity, and infection: present knowledge and future directions. Lancet *i:* 688–691 (1983).
14 Casper, R.; Chatterton, R.; Davis, J.: Alterations in serum cortisol and its binding characteristics in anorexia nervosa. J. clin. Endocr. Metab. *49:* 406–411 (1979).
15 Pertschuk, M.; Crosby, L.; Barot, L.; Mullen, J.: Immunocompetency in anorexia nervosa. Am. J. clin. Nutr. *35:* 968–972 (1982).
16 Beitens, I.; Zowarski, A.; Migeon, C.; Graham, G.: Adrenal function in normal infants and in marasmus and kwashiorkor. J. Pediat. *86:* 302–308 (1975).
17 Walsh, B.: The endocrinology of anorexia nervosa. Psychiat. Clin. N. Am. *3:* 299–312 (1980).
18 Doerr, P.; Fichter, M.; Pirke, K.; Lund, R.: Relationship between weight gain and hypothalamic pituitary adrenal function in patients with anorexia nervosa. J. Steroid Biochem. *13:* 529–537 (1980).
19 Gwirtsman, H.; Roy-Byrne, P.; Yager, J.; Gerner, R.: Neuroendocrine abnormalities in bulimia. Am. J. Psychiat. *140:* 559–563 (1983).
20 Pimston, B.; Barbezat, G.; Hamsen, J.; Hansen, J.; Murray, P.: Studies on growth hormone secretion in protein calorie malnutrition. Am. J. clin. Nutr. *21:* 482–487 (1968).
21 Casper, R.; Davis, J.; Pandey, G.: The effect of nutritional status and weight changes on hypothalamic function tests in anorexia nervosa; in Vigersky, Anorexia nervosa, pp. 137–147 (Raven Press, New York 1977).
22 Zubiran, S.; Gomez-Mont, F.: Endocrine disturbance in chronic human malnutrition. Vitams Horm. *2:* 97–130 (1953).
23 Katz, J.; Weiner, H.: The aberrant reproductive endocrinology of anorexia nervosa; in Weiner, Mahofer, Stunkard, Brain, behavior and bodily disease, pp. 165–180 (Raven Press, New York 1981).
24 Russell, G.; Loraine, J.; Bell, E.; Harkness, R.: Gonadotropin and estrogen excretion in patients with anorexia nervosa. J. psychosom. Res. *9:* 79–85 (1965).
25 Lisch, H.; Bolzano, K.; Herbst, M.; Sailers, S.; Sandhofer, F.; Braunsteiner, H.: Effect of body weight changes on plasma lipids in patients with primary hyperlipoproteinemia. Atherosclerosis *19:* 477–484 (1974).
26 Crisp, A.; Blendis, L.; Pawan, G.: Aspects of fat metabolism in anorexia nervosa. Metabolism *17:* 1109–1118 (1968).

27 Mordasini, R.; Klose, G.; Greten, H.: Secondary type II hyperlipoproteinemia in patients with anorexia nervosa. Metabolism *27:* 71–79 (1978).

28 Blendis, L.; Crisp, A.: Serum cholesterol levels in anorexia nervosa. Post-grad. med. J. *44:* 327–330 (1968).

29 Klahr, S.; Alleyne, G.: Effects of chronic protein-calorie malnutrition on the kidney. Kidney int. *3:* 129–141 (1973).

30 Fohlin, L.: Body composition, cardiovascular and renal function in adolescent patients with anorexia nervosa. Acta paediat. scand., suppl. 268, pp. 1–20 (1977).

31 Soman, V.; Felig, P.: Insulin binding to monocytes and insulin sensitivity in anorexia nervosa. Am. J. Med. *68:* 66–72 (1980).

32 Elkington, J.; Huth, E.: Body fluid abnormalities in anorexia nervosa and undernutrition. Metabolism *8:* 376–403 (1959).

33 Hasler, J.: Parotid enlargement: a presenting sign in anorexia nervosa. Oral Surg. *53:* 567–573 (1982).

34 Watt, J.: Benign parotid swellings: a review. Proc. R. Soc. Med. *70:* 483–486 (1977).

35 Frisch, R.: Food intake, fatness and reproductive ability; in Vigersky, Anorexia nervosa, pp. 149–161 (Raven Press, New York 1977).

36 Kovach, K.: The assessment of nutritional status in anorexia nervosa; in Gross, Anorexia nervosa (Collamore Press, Lexington 1982).

37 Mecklenburg, R.; Loriaux, D.; Thompson, R.; Andersen, A.; Lipsett, M.: Hypothalamic dysfunction in patients with anorexia nervosa. Medicine, Baltimore *523:* 147–159 (1974).

38 Myers, T.; Perkerson, M.; Wittner, B.; Granville, N.: Hematologic findings in anorexia nervosa. Conn. Med. *45:* 14–17 (1981).

39 Garfinkel, P.; Garner, D.: Anorexia nervosa: a multidisciplinary perspective, pp. 319–320 (Brunner/Mazel, New York 1982).

40 Russell, D.; Prendergast, P.; Darby, P.; Garfinkel, P.; Whitwall, J.; Jeejeebboy, K.: A comparison between muscle function and body composition in anorexia nervosa: the effect of refeeding. Am. J. clin. Nutr. *38:* 229–237 (1983).

41 Moshang, T.; Utiger, R.: Low tri-iodothyronine euthyroidism in anorexia nervosa; in Vigersky, Anorexia nervosa (Raven Press, New York 1977).

42 Gottdiener, J.; Gross, H.; Henry, W.; Borer, J.; Ebert, M.: Effects of self-induced starvation on cardiac size and function in anorexia nervosa. Circulation *58:* 425–433 (1978).

43 Thurston, J.; Marks, P.: Electrocardiographic abnormalities in patients with anorexia nervosa. Br. Heart J. *36:* 719–723 (1974).

44 Kalager, T.; Brubakk, D.; Bassoe, H.: Cardiac performance in patients with anorexia nervosa. Cardiology *63:* 1–4 (1978).

45 Gold, P.; Kaye, W.; Robertson, G.; Ebert, M.: Abnormalities in plasma and cerebrospinal fluid arginine vasopressin in patients with anorexia nervosa. New Engl. J. Med. *308:* 1117–1123 (1983).

46 Berkman, J.; Weir, J.; Kepler, E.: Clinical observations on starvation edema, serum protein and the effect of forced feeding in anorexia nervosa. Gastroenterology *9:* 357–390 (1947).

47 Boyar, R.; Katz, J.; Finkelstein, J.; Kapen, S.; Weiner, H.; Weitzman, E.; Hellman, L.: Anorexia nervosa: immaturity of the 24-hour luteinizing hormone secretory pattern. New Engl. J. Med. *291:* 861–865 (1974).

48 Marshall, J.; Fraser, T.: Amenorrhea in anorexia nervosa: assessment and treatment with clomiphene citrate. Br. med. J. *iv:* 590–592 (1971).
49 Warren, M.: Weight loss and responsiveness to LH-RH; in Vigersky, Anorexia nervosa, pp. 189–198 (Raven Press, New York 1977).
50 Ischmail, A.; Harkness, R.: Urinary testosterone excretion in men in normal and pathological conditions. Acta endocr., Copenh. *56:* 469–480 (1967).
51 Beaumont, P.: Anorexia nervosa in male subjects. Psychother. Psychosom. *18:* 365–371 (1970).
52 Walsh, B.; Katz, J.; Levin, J.; Kream, J.; Fukushima, D.; Hellman, L.; Weiner, H.; Zumoff, B.: Adrenal activity in anorexia nervosa. Psychosom. Med. *40:* 499–506 (1978).
53 Nell, J.; Merikangas, J.; Foster, F.; Merikangas, K.; Spiker, D.; Kupfer, D.: Waking and all-night EEGs in anorexia nervosa. Clin. Electroenceph. *11:* 9–15 (1980).
54 Kalucy, R.; Crisp, A.; Chard, T.; McNeilly, A.; Chen, C.; Lacey, J.: Nocturnal hormonal profiles in massive obesity, anorexia nervosa and normal females. J. psychosom. Res. *20:* 595–604 (1976).
55 Holt, S.; Ford, M.; Grant, S.; Heading, R.: Abnormal gastric emptying in primary anorexia nervosa. Br. J. Psychiat. *139:* 550–552 (1981).
56 Nordgren, L.; Scheele, C. von: Hepatic and pancreatic dysfunction in anorexia nervosa: a report of two cases. Biol. Psychiat. *12:* 681–686 (1977).
57 Schoettle, U.: Pancreatitis: a complication, a concomitant or a cause of an anorexia nervosa-like syndrome. J. Am. Acad. Child Psychiat. *18:* 384–390 (1979).
58 Zurbrügg, L.: A puzzling triad: anorexia nervosa, high sweat electrolytes and indication of partial exocrine pancreatic insufficiency. Helv. paediat. Acta *38:* 149–158 (1983).
59 Scobie, B.: Acute dilation of the stomach in patients with anorexia nervosa (Abstract). Aust. N.Z. J. Med. *2:* 335 (1972).
60 Haller, J.; Slovis, T.; Baker, D.; Berdon, W.; Silverman, J.: Anorexia nervosa – the paucity of radiological findings in more than 50 patients. Pediatr. Radiol. *5:* 145–147 (1977).
61 Casper, R.; Kirschner, B.; Sandstead, H.; Jacob, R.; Davis, J.: An evaluation of trace metals, vitamins and taste function in anorexia nervosa. Am. J. clin. Nutr. *33:* 1801–1808 (1980).
62 Tanner, J.; Whitehouse, R.: Clinical longitudinal standards for height, weight, height velocity, weight velocity and stages of puberty. Archs Dis. Childh. *51:* 170–179 (1976).
63 Pugliese, M.; Lifshitz, F.; Grad, G.; Fort, P.; Marks-Katz, M.: Fear of obesity: a cause of short stature and delayed puberty. New Engl. J. Med. *309:* 513–518 (1983).
64 Lacey, J.; Crisp, A.; Hart, G.; Kirkwood, B.: Weight and skeletal maturation – a study of radiological and chronological age in an anorexia nervosa population. Post-grad. med. J. *55:* 381–385 (1979).
65 Hamill, P.; Drizd, T.; Johnson, C.; Reed, R.; Roche, A.; Moore, W.: Physical growth: National Center for Health Statistics percentiles. Am. J. clin. Nutr. *32:* 607–629 (1979).
66 Doering, E.: The role of the primary care physician in the diagnosis and management of anorexia nervosa; in Gross, Anorexia nervosa, pp. 15–25 (Collamore Press, Lexington 1982).
67 Root, A.; Powers, P.: Anorexia nervosa presenting as growth retardation in adolescents. J. Adolesc. Hlth Care *4:* 25–30 (1983).

68 Pitts, F.; Guze, S.: Anorexia nervosa and gonadal dysgenesis (Turner's syndrome). Am. J. Psychiat. *119:* 1100–1102 (1963).
69 Dally, P.: Anorexia nervosa (Heinemann, London 1969).
70 Kaye, W.; Pickar, D.; Naber, D.; Ebert, M.: Cerebrospinal fluid opioid activity in anorexia nervosa. Am. J. Psychiat. *139:* 643–645 (1982).
71 Gwirtsman, H.; Gerner, R.: Neurochemical abnormalities in anorexia nervosa; similarities to affective disorders. Biol. Psychiat. *16:* 991–995 (1981).
72 Halmi, K.; Hamsher, K.; Benton, A.: Neuropsychological predictors in anorexia nervosa. Syllabus and scient. Proc. 133rd Meet. Am. Psychiat. Ass., San Francisco 1980, p. 327.
73 Kohlmeyer, K.; Lehmkuhl, G.; Poutska, F.: Computed tomography of anorexia nervosa. AJNR *4:* 437–438 (1983).
74 Crisp, A.: Sleep, activity, nutrition and mood. Br. J. Psychiat. *137:* 1–7 (1980).
75 Hellstrom, I.: Oral complications in anorexia nervosa. Scand. J. dent. Res. *85:* 71–86 (1977).
76 Levin, P.; Falko, J.; Dixon, K.; Gallup, E.; Saunders, W.: Benign parotid enlargement in bulimia. Ann. intern. Med. *93:* 827–829 (1980).
77 Bruch, H.: Death in anorexia nervosa. Psychosom. Med. *33:* 135–144 (1971).
78 Crisp, A.; Fenton, G.; Scotton, L.: A controlled study of the EEG in anorexia nervosa. Br. J. Psychiat. *114:* 1149–1169 (1968).
79 Yates, A.; Leehey, K.; Shisslak, C.: Running – an analogue of anorexia. New Engl. J. Med. *308:* 251–255 (1983).
80 Brady, W.: The anorexia nervosa syndrome. Oral Med. *50:* 509–516 (1980).
81 Gross, M.: Bulimia; in Gross, Anorexia nervosa, pp. 153–161 (Collamore Press, Lexington 1982).
82 Bo-Linn, G.; Santa Ana, C.; Morawski, S.; Fordtran, S.: Purging and calorie absorption in bulimic patients and normal women. Ann. intern. Med. *99:* 14–17 (1983).
83 Krejs, G.; Fordtran, J.: Diarrhea; in Sleisenger, Fordtran, Gastrointestinal disease; 3rd ed. (Saunders, Philadelphia 1983); cited in Bo-Linn, G.; Santa Ana, C.; Morawski, B.; Fordtran, S.: Purging and calorie absorption in bulimic patients and normal women. Ann. intern. Med. *99:* 14–17 (1983).
84 Al-Muffy, N.; Bevan, D.: A case of subcutaneous emphysema, pneumomediastinum and pneumoretroperitoneum associated with functional anorexia. Br. J. clin. Pract. *31:* 160–161 (1977).
85 Fears, W.; Glass, A.; Vigersky, R.: Role of exercise in the pathogenesis of the amenorrhea associated with anorexia nervosa. J. Adolesc. Hlth Care *4:* 22–24 (1983).
86 McCormick, W.: Amenorrhea and other menstrual symptoms in student nurses. J. psychosom. Res. *19:* 131–137 (1975).
87 Sims, E.; Goldman, R.; Gluck, C.; Horton, E.; Kelleher, P.; Rowe, D.: Experimental obesity in man. Trans. Ass. Am. Physns *81:* 153–170 (1968).
88 Powers, P.: Heart failure during treatment of anorexia nervosa. Am. J. Psychiat. *139:* 1167–1170 (1982).
89 Donovan, B.; Van Der Werfften Bosch, J.: Physiology of puberty. Monographs of the Physiological Society (Arnold, London 1965).
90 Moldofsky, H.; Jeuniewig, N.; Garfinkel, P.: Preliminary report on metoclopramide in anorexia nervosa; in Vigersky, Anorexia nervosa (Raven Press, New York 1977).

91 Kline, C.: Anorexia nervosa: death from complications of ruptured gastric ulcer. Can. J. Psychiat. *24:* 153–156 (1979).

92 Wakeling, A.; Souza, V. De; Beardwood, C.: Assessment of the negative and positive feedback effects of administered estrogen on gonadotropin release in patients with anorexia nervosa. Psychol. Med. *7:* 397–405 (1977).

93 Katz, J.; Boyar, R.; Roffwarg, H.; Hellman, L.; Weiner, H.: LHRH responsiveness in anorexia nervosa: intactness despite prepubertal circadian LH pattern. Psychosom. Med. *39:* 241–251 (1977).

94 Sherman, B.; Halmi, K.; Zamudio, R.: LH and FSH response to gonadotropin-releasing hormone in anorexia nervosa: effect of nutritional rehabilitation. J. clin. Endocr. Metab. *41:* 135–142 (1975).

95 Bates, G.; Bates, S.; Whitworth, N.: Reproductive failure in women who practice weight control. Fert. Steril. *37:* 373–378 (1982).

96 Enzmann, D.; Lane, B.: Cranial computed tomography in anorexia nervosa. J. Comput. assist. Tomogr. *1:* 410–414 (1977).

97 Nussbaum, M.; Shenker, I.; Marc, J.; Klein, M.: Cerebral atrophy in anorexia nervosa. J. Pediat. *96:* 867–869 (1980).

98 Abel, R.; Paul, J.: Failure of short-term nutritional convalescence to reverse the adverse effects of protein calorie malnutrition in dogs. Am. Heart J. *97:* 733–744 (1979).

99 Foster, F.; Kupfer, D.; Spiker, D.: EEG sleep in anorexia nervosa. Sleep Res. *5:* 143 (1976).

100 Lucas, A.: On the meaning of laboratory values in anorexia nervosa. Mayo Clin. Proc. *52:* 748–750 (1977).

14 Psychological Testing and Eating Disorders

Judith C. Knight, Susan C. Litton

Introduction

Before reviewing the literature on psychological testing with eating-disorder patients, several problem areas need to be addressed. The first is the confusion in the field concerning the concept and diagnosis of anorexia nervosa and other eating disorders. Despite the seeming uniformity of symptoms, there is controversy over whether or not anorexia nervosa exists as a discrete disorder, or if it is a variation of some other illness. There is not even agreement of opinion regarding the various features considered essential to warrant the diagnosis [1]. Further confusion surrounds the question of whether or not anorexia nervosa is a discrete syndrome or a continuum of behaviors [2]. The idea of a continuum is supported by the existence of two groups of anorectics – those who maintain emaciated conditions by starving versus those who accomplish this goal by cycles of binge-eating and purging. The picture is further complicated by the occurrence of the same binge/purge/fast cycle in normal-weight individuals. According to DSM III, such a person would be diagnosed as having bulimia. Various authors, however, have developed different terms to describe such patients. *Russell* [3] sees bulimia as a variant of anorexia nervosa and, therefore, uses the term 'bulimia nervosa'. *White and Boskind-White* [4] also subscribe to the notion that bulimia and anorexia nervosa are variations of the same syndrome. But they use the term 'bulimarexia' for normal-weight individuals. In addition to the difficulty created by using non-standardized terminologies, there is also a lack of agreement concerning criteria for diagnosis. Even in a descriptive stage of research this confusion makes comparisons between studies tedious and often impossible.

Effects of Starvation

Another problem in reviewing this literature and making sense of the results comes from the potentially confounding factor of starvation and, more broadly, dietary chaos. Various clinicians have tested patients who were emaciated or who were vomiting frequently and have made assumptions about the patients' premorbid personalities. There is evidence to suggest that avitaminosis and semistarvation alone can lead to disorders which may warrant psychiatric diagnoses [5–10]. Therefore, caution must be exercised in the interpretation of such test results.

For example, lack of thiamine has been demonstrated to lead to ideas of persecution, mental confusion and memory loss [5]. Restricted riboflavin has been shown to produce significant changes on five MMPI subscales (Hs, D, Hy, Pd, Ma) [9]. Similarly, ascorbic acid deficiency has been shown to produce such behavioral changes as listlessness, lassitude, weakness and aversion to work. A study withholding ascorbic acid from subjects found that, as their deficiency progressed, their scores on the MMPI 'neurotic triad' scales (Hs, D and Hy) became more elevated [10].

In a series of studies conducted at the University of Minnesota, prolonged reduction of caloric intake resulted in such marked personality change that the authors referred to the resulting state as an 'experimental neurosis' [7, 11]. In these studies, a group of young men, screened for physical and psychological health, was maintained on a semistarvation diet for 120 days. As the starvation progressed, marked elevations on the MMPI 'neurotic triad' scales became apparent [11]. An item analysis revealed no fundamental differences between the kind of answers given by the semistarved subjects and those given by a group of physically normal psychoneurotic patients [12]. It was concluded that these semistarved men suffered from actual, though reversible, personality disturbances. Additionally, these men were found to manifest obsessional thoughts of food, irritability and depression, decrease in self-initiated activities, loss of sexual drive and social introversion. With the exception of decrease in activity levels, these are the same characteristics often exhibited by anorexia nervosa patients.

The Minnesota experiments and the vitamin deficiency studies raise a critical question concerning the relationship of nutritional distress to anorexia nervosa. It is generally recognized that one of the principal reasons why most types of such illness are considered to be functional or 'psychological' in nature is that no physical etiology has been shown to produce the disorder. This may not be the case. *Garfinkel and Garner* [1] maintain that meaningful psychotherapy cannot occur until the symptoms of starvation and dietary chaos are alleviated. This may also hold true for the testing of these patients.

Although not as readily apparent, nutritional deficiencies and/or starvation effects may also present a problem in interpreting the test results of normal or overweight bulimics. In addition to physiological imbalances which result from poor nutrition and frequent vomiting, starvation may also be a factor in the emotional status of these individuals. According to set-point theory [13], normal or overweight persons may be in a state of semi-starvation with reference to their own physiology [13–16]. In such cases, the results of psychological testing may be affected.

Other Confounding Variables

Age and duration of illness are two additional factors which make comparisons of studies using psychological testing difficult. It is likely that an adolescent with a recent onset of illness presents a different psychological profile from an older or more chronically ill individual. Although some researchers, for example *Strober* [2], are sensitive to this issue and control for age and chronicity by careful patient selection or by statistical means, others do not attend to these factors. Some studies have also failed to report the sex of their subjects.

The fact that anorectics tend to deny their illness also poses problems for test interpretation. Denial is most likely to influence self-report measures which have high face validity.

Two additional confounding factors may be hospitalization and the timing of test administration. Obviously, a person who is hospitalized is in a very different situation from one who is being treated as an outpatient. For those patients who are hospitalized, testing done early in the stay is more likely to be affected by anxiety, starvation and dietary chaos. Therefore, it is critical that the timing of administration be reported. Again, although some researchers have designed their research with consideration of these threats to validity, others have not.

Finally, several general problems arise when comparing studies which utilize psychological tests. One of these occurs when comparing studies using different tests which purport to measure the same trait. If the findings from a number of studies using different measures of a characteristic converge, the level of confidence in the conclusions is heightened. If, on the other hand, disparate results are achieved, it is not clear whether there is a validity problem or whether only certain samples have the trait in question. Other problems arise due to: (1) the use of different scoring systems or cut-off scores, (2) the subjective element involved in interpreting projective tests, and (3) the use of shortened or modified tests.

Overview of Uses of Psychological Testing

Due to the problems already mentioned, it is difficult to reach definitive conclusions when reviewing the literature on psychological testing with eating-disorder patients. Also, until recently, few such studies were available. However, there is no longer a shortage of research in this area. Over 50 articles employing psychological tests now exist. Although most investigators have studied anorectics rather than normal or overweight bulimics, the research on both populations is increasing. There are four major ways in which tests have been used with anorectics and bulimics: in descriptive studies, comparison studies, outcome studies and as screening devices. Psychological tests have also been used to attempt to provide information on the personalities of parents of patients with eating disorders.

The earliest use of testing was to provide descriptive information. These researchers have simply administered psychological tests to anorectics or bulimics and reported their findings. A variety of tests has been employed in these studies, and the findings are useful in that they provide initial information for understanding the dynamics of such patients.

In addition to the descriptive studies, there is a large number of comparison studies in the eating-disorder literature. Anorectics and bulimics have been compared to one another, to other types of psychiatric patients, and to normal controls. Results from these studies, having more heuristic value, will lead to clarification of the relationship of eating disorders to other psychiatric illnesses. In addition, they will help define the relationships among the various eating disorders.

The third major use of psychological testing in the literature is in outcome studies. Tests have been used to evaluate treatment techniques, as well as to provide information about personality variables which might be helpful in predicting outcome.

Tests have also been used as screening devices to determine treatment group membership. In this way, a test score is used as a selection criterion. Although there are inherent problems involved in using tests to screen for low base-rate disorders [17], such instruments can be useful adjuncts to other assessment techniques. It is also possible to use tests to divide a large group of patients into smaller, more homogeneous groups before administering treatments.

Studies using psychological tests and body image measures with anorectics and bulimics are presented in table I. Investigations focusing primarily on measuring body image distortions are not included, unless other types of psychological tests have been used, since an excellent review of these articles already exists [1]. Also excluded are clinical descriptions of testing results such as those provided by *Bruch* [18] and *Selvini-Palazzoli* [19] which do not provide enough data to allow for meaningful interpretations, and studies whose primary purpose was test validation, for example *Stunkard* [16], *Crisp* et al. [20], *Garner and Garfinkel* [21], *Garner* et al. [22, 23], *Gormally* et al. [24], *Hawkins and Clement* [25] and *Slade* [26]. Interviews or questionnaires which were primarily demographic in nature or which are not readily available are not listed.

Descriptive Studies

Anorexia Nervosa

In spite of the fact that many of the populations surveyed have included rather heterogeneous groups of anorectics and the fact that the criteria for defining the population have varied across studies, several personality factors have been described with some degree of consistency. In general, anorectics seem to report high levels of personal disturbance [27], introversion [28–30], depression [30–34] and obsessiveness [29, 30, 32]. Additionally, there are indications of neurotic tendencies [29, 30], anxiety [27, 30, 32] and somatic complaints [30, 32]. It has also been suggested that anorectics may be overly submissive and masochistic [31].

Although some reports have described anorectics as being emotionally labile, for example *Wagner and Wagner* [35], the type and/or degree of emotions displayed may not be an accurate reflection of true feelings [36]. It has been noted that low emotionality scores on the Eysenck Personality Inventory tend to correlate with high MMPI Lie scores, thus suggesting that some anorectics may deny the extent of their emotions [28]. Intelligence levels reported have tended to be average or above average, but there is a fair amount of variability in IQ scores, for example *Smart* et al. [29], *Palmer* et al. [36], *Pierloot* et al. [37] and *Sours* [38].

Table I. Studies using psychological tests with anorectics and/or bulimics

Reference	Type of patient[1]		Type of test[2]	
	anorectic	bulimic	personality and/or intelligence	eating disorder and/or body image
Allerdissen et al., 1981 [65]		28	BDI; Picture Frustration Test; Locus of Control Scale	
Ben-Tovim et al.,1979 [74]	12-r 9-b		EPI; Hostility and Direction of Hostility Questionnaire	
Beumont, 1977 [45]	17-r 14-b		EPI; 16PF; LOI	
Bhanji and Mattingly, 1981 [49]	10-r 10-b		CCEI	
Boskind-Lodahl and White, 1978 [75]		26	16PF	Body Cathexis Test
Button and Whitehouse, 1981 [76]	14-ns			EAT
Casper et al., 1980 [46]	56-r		MMPI; HSCL, Raskin Mood Scale	SABS; AAS; S&R
Casper et al., 1979 [77]	79-ns			AAS; S&R
Crisp and Bhat, 1982 [32]	100-ns		CCEI	
Crisp et al., 1979 [28]	27-ns		EPI	
Dunn and Ondercin, 1981 [66]		23	16PF; Rotter: Marlowe-Crowne; Bem Sex Role Inventory	Compulsive Eating Scale
Eckert et al., 1982 [33]	105-ns		MMPI; HSCL; Raskin Mood Scale	SABS; AAS; S&R
Falk and Halmi, 1982 [55]	40-ns		HSCL; Raskin Mood Scale	SABS; PRSAN; S&R
Garner, 1981 [53]	115-ns		BDI; Rotter (modified)	EAT; Restraint Scale; G&H; Body Dissatisfaction Questionnaire

Table I (continued)

Reference	Type of patient[1]		Type of test[2]	
	anorectic	bulimic	personality and/or intelligence	eating disorder and/or body image
Garner et al., 1976 [63]	18-ns		EPI; Rotter (modified)	G&H; S&R
Goldberg et al., 1977 [67]	44-ns		HSCL; Raskin Mood Scale; Interpersonal Manipulativeness Scale	SABS; AAS; Situational Discomfort Scale; PRSAN; S&R
Gomez and Dally, 1980 [27]	30-r 12-b		EPI; Symptom-Sign Inventory; Life Events Schedule	
Halmi et al., 1979 [71]	81-ns		HSCL	SABS; AAS
Hendren, 1983 [34]	84-ns		MMPI	
Hsu and Crisp, 1980 [48]	66-r 14-b		CCEI	
Johnson and Berndt, 1983 [42]		80	Weissman Social Adjustment Scale	Eating Problems Inventory
Johnson et al., 1982 [43]		316	HSCL	Eating Disorders Questionnaire; Eating Problems Questionnaire
Leon et al., 1979 [52]	33-ns		MAC Scale of MMPI	
Litton, 1981 [unpublished]		4	MMPI; WAIS; LOI; Rorschach; Comrey Personality Scale; Bender Gestalt Test; House-Tree-Person Drawings; Kahn Test of Symbol Arrangement	
Norman and Herzog, 1983 [50]	10-r 15-b	14	MMPI	
Orleans and Barnett, 1983 [31]	6-b	4	MMPI	
Palmer et al., 1952 [36]	5-b		TAT; Rorschach, Wechsler-Bellevue	

Table I (continued)

Reference	Type of patient[1]		Type of test[2]	
	anorectic	bulimic	personality and/or intelligence	eating disorder and/or body image
Pierloot and Houben, 1978 [40]	31-ns		MMPI; Rorschach; locus of control questionnaire; an IQ measure (not specified)	S&R; Askevold
Pierloot et al., 1975 [37]	12-r 20-b		WAIS (or Progressive Matrices); Amsterdam Biographic Questionnaire; MMPI; TAT	
Pillay and Crisp, 1977 [60]	11-ns		EPPS; Hysteroid Obsessoid Questionnaire; Fear Survey Schedule; Social Questionnaire	
Pillay and Crisp, 1981 [78]	13-r 10-b		CCEI; Social Questionnaire; Social Situations Questionnaire; WAIS	
Pyle et al., 1981 [44]		30	MMPI	
Rollins and Piazza, 1981 [68]	30-r 5-b		BDI	Anorexia Scale
Rost et al., 1982 [64]		34	Sex Role Attitude; Sex Role Behavior; Sex Role Locus of Control	
Small et al., 1981 [57]	14-ns		MMPI; WAIS-Verbal	
Small et al., 1982 [58]	27-ns		WAIS (WISC-R); Rorschach	
Smart et al., 1976 [29]	22-ns		EPI; 16PF; LOI; Progressive Matrices	

Table I (continued)

Reference	Type of patient[1]		Type of test[2]	
	anorectic	bulimic	personality and/or intelligence	eating disorder and/or body image
Solyom et al., 1982 [47]	6-r 9-b		LOI; Maudsley Personality Inventory; Manifest Anxiety Scale; Fear Survey Schedule	
Sours, 1969 [38]	4-ns		MMPI; TAT; Family Relations Indicator; Human Figure Drawings; Imbedded Figure Test; Object Scoring Test; Bender Gestalt Test; Wechsler; Rorschach	Secord Body Cathexis Test
Stonehill and Crisp, 1977 [30]	39-r 6-b		MHQ (CCEI); EPI	
Strober, 1980 [2]	14-r 8-b		HSCL; CPI; EPI; LOI; Marlowe-Crowne	
Strober, 1981 [39]	65-ns		MMPI; WISC-R	G&H; Fisher Body Distortion Questionnaire
Strober, 1981 [56]	50-ns		Cattell High School Personality Questionnaire	
Strober, 1981 [69]	22-r 22-b		Moos Family Environment Scale; Short Marital Adjustment Test	Askevold; PRSAN; SABS
Strober, 1982 [54]	30-ns		Norwicki-Strickland Locus of Control Scale	PRSAN; Askevold
Strober and Goldenberg, 1981 [51]	13-r 7-b		Rorschach	
Strober et al., 1982 [70]	parents of 35-r and 35-b		MMPI	

Table I (continued)

Reference	Type of patient[1]		Type of test[2]	
	anorectic	bulimic	personality and/or intelligence	eating disorder and/or body image
Sugarman et al., 1982 [62]	12-ns		Rorschach	
Thompson and Schwartz, 1982 [59]	26-ns		BDI; HSCL (5 scales); WAIS-Information Subtest; Weissman Social Adjustment Scale (4 subscales)	EAT
Wagner and Wagner, 1978 [35]	3-ns		Rorschach	
White and Boskind-White, 1981 [4]		14	CPI	Body Cathexis Test (modified)
Wingate and Christie, 1978 [61]	15-ns		Es scale of MMPI	Askevold

[1] r = Restricting anorectic;
b = bulimic anorectic;
ns = not specified.

[2] AAS = Anorectic Attitude Scale
Askevold = image marking technique of body size estimation
BDI = Beck Depression Inventory
CCEI = Crown-Crisp Experiential Index
CPI = California Psychological Inventory
EAT = Eating Attitudes Test
EPI = Eysenck Personality Inventory
EPPS = Edwards Personal Preference Schedule
Es Scale = Ego Strength Scale
G&H = Glucksman and Hirsch distorting photograph technique of body size estimation
HSCL = Hopkins Symptom Checklist
LOI = Leyton Obsessional Inventory
MAC Scale = MacAndrew Scale
Marlowe-Crowne = Marlowe-Crowne Social Desirability Scale
MHQ = Middlesex Hospital Questionnaire (an early version of the CCEI)
MMPI = Minnesota Multiphasic Personality Inventory
Progressive Matrices = Raven's Standard Progressive Matrices
PRSAN = Psychiatric Rating Scale for Anorexia Nervosa
Rotter = Internal-External Locus of Control Scale
SABS = Slade Anorectic Behavior Scale
S&R = Slade and Russell movable caliper technique of body size estimation
16PF = Sixteen Personality Factor Questionnaire
TAT = Thematic Apperception Test
WAIS = Wechsler Adult Intelligence Scale
WISC-R = Wechsler Intelligence Scale for Children, Revised.

Two studies which have attempted to find personality variables which distinguish anorectics who have severe body image distortions from those who do not have produced mixed results. One study found that both size estimation and subjective sense of body distortion were associated with elevation on scales Hs, Pt and Sc of the MMPI [39]. The second study found no significant correlation between findings generated from the MMPI or the Rorschach and two measures of body image distortion [40].

Bulimia

It is more difficult to draw conclusions concerning trends in personality dynamics in bulimics since there are fewer data on this population. Bulimics have been found to have rather poor overall adjustment. In fact, their scores on the Social Adjustment Scale [41] were similar to those of a normative group of female alcoholics [42]. Concerning psychiatric symptomatology, one study found that bulimics received scores on the Hopkins Symptom Checklist which were generally comparable to non-clinical controls [43]. The only significant differences were found on the Interpersonal Sensitivity and Depression Scales. The authors noted, however, that although the bulimics appeared rather normal, this may be misleading, since most of the distress of this population is related to food and/or body weight, and these areas are not generally tapped by standard psychological tests.

Additional indication of impairment has been reported from MMPI data. Specifically, bulimics have been found to have significant elevations (greater than 70) on the Pd, D, Pt and Sc scales [44]. Also, *Orleans and Barnett* [31] have reported bulimics as having low Mf scores coupled with high scores on the Pd and Pa scales and indicate that the valley configuration formed by these three scales suggests passivity and masochism.

Based on data from complete psychological test batteries, bulimic patients were described as having unsatisfactory interpersonal relationships, identity disturbances (including body image distortions and low self-esteem) and difficulty in experiencing and/or expressing certain emotions in appropriate ways. High degrees of obsessionality were also revealed [*Litton,* unpublished].

Comparison Studies

Comparisons among Eating Disorder Subtypes

There are many studies which compare bulimic anorectics with restricting anorectics. Problems arise in trying to make comparisons across studies in that some investigators have distinguished between these two groups based solely on the presence of periodic binges, whereas others use purging as the main diagnostic factor. In spite of this difficulty, however, the findings across studies are surprisingly consistent.

Much attention has been focused on the relative degrees of extroversion between the two types of anorectics. Although most studies have found bulimic anorectics to be more extroverted than restricting anorectics [2, 27, 45, 46], there is one study that found the opposite [47]. There is also indication that normal-weight bulimics may be more extroverted than bulimic anorectics [31]. It seems that the presence of bulimia, regardless of the patient's weight, is more likely to be associated with extroversion.

The possibility of extroversion in bulimic anorectics is especially intriguing in light of the fact that they have also been found to be socially phobic [32, 48]. It has been suggested that this combination of sociability in conjunction with a fear of socializing may be indicative of an intense emotional turmoil within this group [48].

Along these lines, several studies have found bulimic anorectics to be more anxious than restricting anorectics [32, 46, 48, 49]. In fact, one group of researchers noted that, in contrast to bulimic anorectics, restricting anorectics showed little overt distress [46]. One study, however, found no significant differences between the two groups on an anxiety measure [27], and another found restricting anorectics to be more anxious than bulimic anorectics [45]. In the latter study, bulimic anorectics did not differ significantly from normals in terms of anxiety.

Concerning levels of depression, most studies report bulimic anorectics to be more depressed than either restricting anorectics [46, 48–50] or normal-weight bulimics [31, 50]. However, two other studies have not found a significant difference among anorectics on this variable [27, 32]. Similarly, one study failed to find any difference in the level of somatic complaints [32], whereas others have found bulimic anorectics to have higher somatic scores [46, 48, 49].

There is considerable confusion concerning obsessive symptomatology. *Crisp and Bhat* [32] found no differences between groups on this measure. *Hsu and Crisp* [48] found bulimic anorectics to be more obsessive, but *Gomez and Dally* [27] reported the opposite. *Beumont* [45] found that although both groups were more obsessive than normals, restricting anorectics were more so.

Group differences in hysterical tendencies are also not clear in the literature. Although two studies reported bulimic anorectics as having higher hysteria scores [46, 48], other groups of researchers found no difference on this measure [27, 32].

As might be expected, bulimic anorectics have been found to have poorer impulse control than restricting anorectics [2, 46, 50]. Additionally, *Norman and Herzog* [50] found that both bulimic anorectics and normal-weight bulimics had substantially elevated Pd scales on the MMPI, and that these scores were significantly higher than those of the restricting anorectics. Other differences reported between restricting and bulimic anorectics are that restricting anorectics are more independent [45] and manic [27], whereas bulimic anorectics are more neurotic [27], have more boundary disturbances [51], greater interpersonal sensitivity and more feelings of guilt [46].

Four remaining studies belong in this category because they make comparisons among various subtypes of eating disorder patients. *Leon* et al. [52] compared anorectics (both types) with obese persons, as well as with smokers and control groups using the MacAndrew (MAC) Scale of the MMPI. They found no significant differences among obese, normal and anorectic patients on this measure. Furthermore, bulimic anorectics did not receive scores which were different from restricting anorectics.

Garner [53] compared anorectics who markedly overestimated body size to a group of anorectics who did not. He found that the marked overestimators displayed more anorectic symptoms, had a more external locus of control, were more depressed and anxious, exhibited more physical anhedonia and had greater dissatisfaction with their bodies. He concluded that marked body image overestimation was correlated with a poor prognosis and disturbance in psychological functioning.

Strober [54] found that anorectics who had an external locus of control showed greater denial of illness, lack of impulse control, fear of weight change, rigidity of self-imposed controls, use of purgatives and body image distortion than those who had an internal locus of control. Also, those who scored higher on measures of internal locus of control gained weight more rapidly during treatment.

Finally, *Falk and Halmi* [55] did a 1-year follow-up comparison of treated anorectics of similar weights who were either menstruating or amenorrheic. They found that amenorrheic patients, regardless of weight, had significantly more anorectic attitudes and behaviors than menstruating patients. Furthermore, those in the former group were more likely to overestimate their body size and show more obsessive behaviors. The authors suggested that the recovery of menses may be a significant marker indicating a true recovery from anorexia.

Comparisons of Eating Disorder Patients to Other Psychiatric Patients

There are several studies which have compared test results of eating disorder patients with matched groups of other psychiatric patient populations or with normative test results from such patients. The most frequent comparison has been between anorectics and depressed patients, but anorectics have also been compared to patients having schizophrenia, obsessive-compulsive disorders, phobias, conduct disorders and antisocial or other personality disorders.

In comparison to depressed patients, anorectics have been found to have lower scores on tests measuring phobias, somatic complaints and depression [31]. The same authors reported that anorectics were less anxious than depressed patients, but another investigator found the opposite to be true [56]. Anorectics have also been found to have more boundary disturbances on the Rorschach, and to produce responses emphasizing the solidity of object boundaries more often than depressed patients [51]. *Strober* [54] compared anorectics with groups of conduct-disorder patients, depressed patients and normal adolescents. He found that anorectics scored higher on measures of internal locus of control than any of the other groups. Compared to depressed and personality-disordered patients, anorectics have been found to be more responsible and seeking of social appraisal, and to have more obsessive symptoms, self-control, conformance and intellectual efficiency. Anorectics also displayed less social presence, psychological mindedness and flexibility than the other groups [2]. Similar findings emerged when comparing anorectics with depressed patients and antisocial patients [56]. Here, anorectics were found to have more self-control (also in regard to emotionality), conformance, submissiveness and conscientiousness than the other groups. Anorectics were also reported as being more timid, shy and stimulus-avoiding than the others, as well as having less stable self-images.

Comparisons of anorectics and schizophrenics have revealed more similarities than differences on psychological testing. One team of investigators found no significant difference between the two groups on mean MMPI scores [57]. However, closer examination revealed differences in the ordering of the scale elevations and in the amount of variability within each scale. Both anorectics and schizophrenics have also been found to produce Rorschachs which are suggestive of disturbed thought processes [58]. Those differences which have been found between the two groups are that anorectics have higher IQs, better organizing abilities, more depression and more awareness of their need for affection than do schizophrenics [58].

Anorectics have been compared and found to be similar to obsessive patients in terms of obsessive symptoms and traits, as well as in the tendencies in both groups toward introversion, neuroticism and anxiety [47]. When compared to phobic patients [31], anorectics have been found to be less phobic. Comparisons between anorectic and personality-disordered patients show anorectics to be more depressed and less neurotic, hostile and extraverted than the latter group [2].

One study comparing bulimic patients with other patients (using normative test results from the other groups) found bulimics to have less impairment in social adjustment than acutely depressed populations, but more impairment than normals [42]. However, this somewhat surprising finding may have been a reflection of the fact that the bulimic sample was comprised of self-selected volunteers who had written to an eating disorder center to request information. Since these individuals may have been desirous of receiving treatment, it is possible that they overreported their symptoms.

Comparisons of Eating Disorder Patients to Normal Controls

Compared to normals, anorectics have been found to be more anxious, somatizing and depressed [32, 59]. They also are reported to have more obsessive symptoms [32, 60], less ego strength [61], more disturbances in boundaries between self and other [62] and more introversion, shyness, and self-effacing behaviors than control groups [60, 63].

Some interesting contradictions exist which may serve to elucidate the inner turmoil of an anorectic individual. For example, although one study found that anorectics who had recently attained target weights had more fears and sensitivities than did normal controls, they also reported that the anorectics were much less likely to display their emotions [60]. Also, although anorectics displayed greater fears of social isolation, they received higher social avoidance and lower heterosexuality scores, both of which often characterize someone who is afraid to mix with others. Anorectics were also found to have low dominance and high abasement needs, suggestive of a submissive stance. However, this trait, coupled with a need for perfectionism, suggests an individual who has definite ideas about the way things should be but is not able to take control in order to effect changes. Finally, although anorectics have been reported as having fears of hostility [60], they have also been characterized as being hostile [59].

There are three studies which have compared bulimics (non-anorectic) to normals. *Rost* et al. [64] found that both the sex role attitudes and the sex role behaviors in bulimic women were less liberated than in controls. Also, bulimic women reported discrepancies between their sex role attitudes and behaviors (with attitudes being more liberated than actual behaviors) whereas normal women did not. Additionally, it was found that bulimics experienced a greater sense of external and fatalistic control of their sex role attitudes and behaviors than did normal women.

Other researchers report that bulimics, when compared to normal populations, are more depressed, blame others less frequently and depend more on persons whom they regard as superior [65]. The same study found that bulimics reported less pleasure in sex than did normals and felt this would improve if they were thinner.

A final study compared 'high compulsive eaters' with 'low compulsive eaters' using the extreme scores on a compulsive eating scale to differentiate the two groups [66]. Although it is reasonable to presume that the 'high compulsive eaters' may have fit the category of bulimia, the nature of the criteria used to define the groups makes it impossible to ascertain this with certainty. Nevertheless, high compulsive eaters were found to have greater inner tension, a greater need for approval and more suspiciousness than the normal group. They were also less emotionally stable, more external in locus of control and had self-ideals which were more masculine in nature.

Outcome Studies

Several studies have correlated results from psychological tests with various outcome criteria in an effort to determine potential prognostic variables. All of these studies pertain to anorectic populations.

Two studies have focused on personality variables which correlate with weight gain. Although one group of investigators found that weight gain was positively correlated with a decrease in depression [33], another team did not find a significant relationship between these two variables [67]. The latter study found weight gain to be negatively correlated with denial, psychosexual immaturity, body size overestimation and sleep disturbance. Hyperactivity and hunger were positively related to weight gain.

Personality variables which correlate with return to normal weight are not necessarily predictive of eventual outcome. *Crisp* et al. [28] found that although normal body weight restoration was associated with a significant shift away from introversion, there was no relationship between introversion and overall outcome 7–9 years later. In contrast, however, *Gomez and Dally*

[27] found that increased extroversion correlated with favorable outcome at 6-, 18- and 36-month follow-ups.

Hsu and Crisp [48] found that positive outcome was associated with lower initial scores on scales measuring anxiety, phobias, obsession, somatic complaints and depression, and with higher initial scores on hysteria. Similarly, *Pierloot* et al. [37] reported that positive outcome was predicted by lower initial scores on neuroticism, schizophrenia, infantile regression, passivity, sexual repression and lower overall MMPI profiles, but by higher initial scores on self-defensiveness. In contrast, however, two other studies either found no significant predictors of outcome, or inconsistent predictors (i.e. predictive on one type of outcome measure, but not on another) [31, 68].

Family Studies

Three studies have made special attempts to provide personality profiles on parents of anorectics. The first is a descriptive study in which findings of normal MMPI profiles in the parents contradicted the author's clinical impressions [38]. The author suggested that this may have been reflective of the parents' tendencies to hide feelings of self-doubt and insecurity, and to stress status, social recognition and approval.

The remaining studies compare parents of restricting anorectics with those of bulimic anorectics. *Strober* [69] found that parents of bulimic anorectics exhibited more marital discord, more emotional distance from their children, more psychiatric morbidity and more physical health problems than did parents of restricting anorectics. Similarly, *Strober* et al. [70] also reported greater indication of pathology among parents of bulimic anorectics.

Eating Disorder Measures

Several tests have been designed in recent years which specifically assess eating problems. The purpose of such tests is generally either to aid in diagnosing eating disorders or to provide qualifying or quantifying information about the specific behaviors involved. In an effort to measure responses to various inpatient treatment regimens, *Slade* [26] developed the Anorexic Behavior Scale. This instrument taps three categories of anorectic behavior: resistance to eating, methods of disposing of food and overactivity. All items are judged by the nursing staff as to whether or not a particular behavior has been displayed by the patient. Inter-rater reliability was reported to be 0.90.

A 63-item measure of anorectic behaviors and attitudes was developed by *Halmi* et al. [71]. Although also designed for inpatient assessment, the Anorectic Attitude Scale differs from the Anorexic Behavior Scale in that it is to be completed by the patient. The Anorectic Attitude Scale covers nine question areas: denial, psychosexual immaturity, appetite, interpersonal control, thin body idea, hypothermia, compulsivity, hyperactivity and purgatives. The items are rated on a four-point scale ranging from 'not at all' to 'extremely'. A face-valid scale such as this should be interpreted cautiously, due to the denial which is common among anorectics. *Halmi* et al. [71] used this scale in conjunction with *Slade's* [26] Anorexic Behavioral Scale. In this way, it was possible to compare the patient's ratings with those of the staff.

Various questionnaires have been developed to assess the behavioral parameters of eating disorders. *Herman and Mack* [14] introduced the term 'restrained eating' as a way to identify a pattern of habitual dieting to control body weight. To measure the degree of eating restraint, they developed a five-item questionnaire which has subsequently been revised and extended several times [15, 16, 72].

Since there are no accepted criteria for determining the amount of food necessary to qualify as a binge-eating episode, *Hawkins and Clement* [25] developed a nine-item self-report Binge Scale Questionnaire to measure subjective perception of uncontrolled excessive eating. This questionnaire quantifies several important factors of bingeing, such as frequency, duration and rate of eating.

A similar type of instrument has been developed by *Gormally* et al. [24] to assess binge-eating severity among obese persons. Two scales, a 16-item Binge Eating Scale and an 11-item Cognitive Factors Scale, were designed to tap the behavioral manifestations of the binge as well as the thoughts surrounding the binge episode. Such information has been used to individualize obesity treatment.

Dunn and Ondercin [66] developed still another measure of uncontrolled excessive eating and called it the Compulsive Eating Scale. This 32-item scale assesses emotional states related to food and eating and provides information on weight, weight control and eating binges.

Orleans and Barnett [31] believe that assessment and treatment of bulimic behavior has to begin with a clear definition of the individual's maladaptive eating patterns. Accordingly, they developed an 11-item Personal

Data Questionnaire to provide a preliminary functional analysis of bingeing and purging habits. This questionnaire is useful in gathering information regarding the antecedents and consequences of the bingeing and purging behavior, ratings of changes in motivation, and descriptions of past attempts to overcome the pattern. The authors suggest using the results to develop an individualized self-monitoring protocol for baseline and treatment assessments.

In an effort to quantify a broad range of symptoms common in anorexia nervosa, *Garner and Garfinkel* [21] developed a 40-item self-report questionnaire. The Eating Attitudes Test (EAT) asks subjects to rate items on a six-point scale ranging from 'always' to 'never'. The items are summed for a total score. The authors found that 30 was the cut-off score which maximally differentiated anorectics from normal weight students [1, 21]. A discriminant function analysis showed the EAT to be 91% accurate in classifying the two groups. The authors make it clear that although the EAT may be used for screening purposes, the diagnosis of anorexia nervosa should only be made on the basis of a clinical evaluation. They also suggest that the EAT may serve as an index of improvement, since recovered anorectics obtain normal scores [21]. An abbreviated 26-item version of the EAT is also available [22].

Garner et al. [23] observed that the existing eating disorder scales were designed either for inpatient use, for example *Slade* [26], *Halmi* et al. [71], or for assessing specific behavioral parameters of eating disorder patients [14, 16, 21, 24, 25, 66, 73]. Based on this observation and their growing conviction that eating disorders are multidimensional, they developed the Eating Disorder Inventory (EDI). The EDI is a 64-item self-report measure designed for the assessment of psychological and behavioral traits common in anorexia nervosa and bulimia. It consists of eight subscales: drive for thinness, bulimia, body dissatisfaction, ineffectiveness, perfectionism, interpersonal distrust, interoceptive awareness and maturity fears. The authors caution against using the EDI as a screening device. Tests of this type are useful and appropriate as an adjunct to, rather than a substitute for, clinical judgment.

Conclusions

The widespread interest in eating disorders evidenced both in lay and scientific circles has been followed by an enormous growth of research in this area. Although much of the literature prior to 1980 was descriptive in nature, those studies have laid the groundwork for research with more stringent experimental control. Many of the early studies focused on finding the composite personality profile of the eating-disorder patient. Given the similarities across cases of the symptoms in these syndromes, it is tempting to assume that these patients are a homogeneous group with respect to underlying dynamics or premorbid personalities. The more recent literature is beginning to challenge this myth of uniformity.

Researchers, as well as clinicians, have begun to account for the potentially confounding physiological factors that are inherent in studying and/or treating patients with anorexia nervosa or bulimia. *Garfinkel and Garner* [1] have done a great deal towards increasing awareness of eating disorders as multidimensional disorders with a strong physiological component. Many of the typical behavioral symptoms and personality characteristics exhibited by these patients may be directly related to the effects of starvation or dietary chaos. Although tests administered during this time may be used to provide an assessment of current functioning, they should not be relied upon for assumptions about premorbid personality. Similarly, treatments should not be planned around such test results, since many of the symptoms may diminish or disappear entirely once a physiological balance has been restored. Researchers using psychological tests for the purpose of treatment evaluation should also be cognizant of this potential confounding variable.

Although some statements regarding the general personality characteristics and functioning of anorectics and bulimics can now be made with a reasonable degree of confidence, there are many unanswered questions. For example, there is still debate over whether eating disorder patients can be divided into discrete categories or whether they fall along a continuum [32, 45, 46, 50, 74]. Similarly, there are differences in opinion as to the relationship between eating disorders and other disorders, such as depression, and phobic, hysterical, obsessive-compulsive and borderline personality disorders [2, 31, 32, 47, 51, 54, 56–58]. Also, information regarding premorbid personality traits is scarce. However, if the quality as well as the quantity of research continues to grow at the rate it has over the past few years, these, as well as other questions, may be answered.

References

1 Garfinkel, P.; Garner, D.: Anorexia nervosa: a multidimensional perspective (Brunner/Mazel, New York 1982).

2 Strober, M.: Personality and symptomatological features in young, nonchronic anorexia nervosa patients. J. psychosom. Res. *24:* 353–359 (1980).

3 Russell, G.: Bulimia nervosa: an ominous variant of anorexia nervosa. Psychol. Med. *9:* 429–448 (1979).
4 White, W.; Boskind-White, M.: An experiential-behavioral approach to the treatment of bulimarexia. Psychotherapy *18:* 501–507 (1981).
5 Peterman, R.; Goodhart, R.: Current status of vitamin therapy in nervous and mental disease. J. clin. Nutr. *2:* 11–21 (1954).
6 Weinberg, J.; Mandel, H.; Miller, G.: The relationship between various dietary factors and MMPI sub-scales: implications for clinical practice. J. clin. Psychol. *35:* 880–886 (1979).
7 Keys, A.; Brozek, J.; Henschel, A.; Mickelsen, O.; Taylor, H.L.: The biology of human starvation (University of Minnesota Press, Minneapolis 1950).
8 Watson, G.: Vitamin deficiencies in mental illness. J. Psychol. *43:* 47–63 (1957).
9 Sterner, R.; Price, W.: Restricted riboflavin: within-subject behavioral effects in humans. Am. J. clin. Nutr. *26:* 150–160 (1973).
10 Kinsman, R.; Hood, J.: Some behavioral effects of ascorbic acid deficiency. Am. J. clin. Nutr. *24:* 455–464 (1971).
11 Schiele, B.; Brozek, J.: Experimental neurosis resulting from semistarvation in man. Psychosom. Med. *10:* 31–50 (1948).
12 Brozek, J.; Erickson, N.: Item analysis of the psychoneurotic scales of the MMPI in experimental starvation. J. consult. Psychol. *12:* 403–411 (1948).
13 Nisbett, R.: Hunger, obesity, and the ventromedial hypothalamus. Psychol. Rev. *79:* 433–453 (1972).
14 Herman, C.; Mack, D.: Restrained and unrestrained eating. J. Personality *43:* 647–660 (1975).
15 Herman, C.; Polivy, J.; Pliner, P.; Threlkeld, J.; Munic, D.: Distractability in dieters and non-dieters: an alternative view of 'externality'. J. Personality soc. Psychol. *36:* 536–548 (1978).
16 Stunkard, A.: Restrained eating: what it is and a new scale to measure it; in Croff, James, Van Itallie, The body weight regulatory system: normal and disturbed mechanisms, pp. 243–251 (Raven Press, New York 1981).
17 Williams, P.; Hand, D.; Tarnopolsky, A.: The problem of screening for uncommon disorders – a comment on the eating attitudes test. Psychol. Med. *12:* 431–434 (1982).
18 Bruch, H.: Eating disorders (Basic Books, New York 1973).
19 Selvini-Palazzoli, M.: Self-starvation (Aronson, New York 1978).
20 Crisp, A.; Jones, G.; Slater, P.: The Middlesex Hospital Questionnaire: a validity study. Br. J. med. Psychol. *51:* 269–280 (1978).
21 Garner, D.; Garfinkel, P.: The eating attitudes test: an index of the symptoms of anorexia nervosa. Psychol. Med. *9:* 273–279 (1979).
22 Garner, D.; Olmstead, M.; Bohr, Y.; Garfinkel, P.: The eating attitudes test: psychometric features and clinical correlates. Psychol. Med. *12:* 871–878 (1982).
23 Garner, D.; Olmstead, M.; Polivy, J.: Development and validation of a multidimensional eating disorder inventory for anorexia nervosa and bulimia. Int. J. Eating Disord. *2:* 15–34 (1983).
24 Gormally, J.; Black, S.; Daston, S.; Rardin, D.: The assessment of binge eating severity among obese persons. Addict. Behav. *7:* 47–55 (1982).
25 Hawkins, R.; Clement, P.: Development and construct validation of a self-report measure of binge-eating tendencies. Addict. Behav. *5:* 219–226 (1980).

26 Slade, P.: A short anorexic behavior scale. Br. J. Psychiat. *122:* 83–85 (1973).

27 Gomez, J.; Dally, P.: Psychometric rating in the assessment of progress in anorexia nervosa. Br. J. Psychiat. *136:* 290–296 (1980).

28 Crisp, A.; Hsu, L.; Stonehill, E.: Personality, body weight and ultimate outcome in anorexia nervosa. J. clin. Psychiat. *40:* 332–335 (1979).

29 Smart, D.; Beumont, P.; George, G.: Some personality characteristics of patients with anorexia nervosa. Br. J. Psychiat. *128:* 57–60 (1976).

30 Stonehill, E.; Crisp, A.: Psychoneurotic characteristics of patients with anorexia nervosa before and after treatment and at follow-up 4–7 years later. J. psychosom. Res. *21:* 187–193 (1977).

31 Orleans, C.; Barnett, L.: Bingeing and purging: guidelines for behavioral assessment and treatment; in Hawkins, Fremouw, Clement, Binge-eating: theory, research and treatment (Springer, New York, in press).

32 Crisp, A.; Bhat, A.: 'Personality' and anorexia nervosa – the phobic avoidance stance. Psychother. Psychosom. *38:* 178–200 (1982).

33 Eckert, E.; Goldberg, S.; Halmi, K.; Casper, R.; Davis, J.: Depression in anorexia nervosa. Psychol. Med. *12:* 115–122 (1982).

34 Hendren, R.: Depression in anorexia nervosa. J. Am. Acad. Child Psychiat. *22:* 59–62 (1983).

35 Wagner, E.; Wagner, D.: Similar Rorschach patterning in three cases of anorexia nervosa. J. Personality Assess. *42:* 426–432 (1978).

36 Palmer, J.; Mensh, I.; Matarazzo, D.: Anorexia nervosa: case history and psychological examination data with implications for test validity. J. abnorm. Psychol. *8:* 168–173 (1952).

37 Pierloot, R.; Wellens, W.; Houben, M.: Elements of resistance to a combined medical and psychotherapeutic program in anorexia nervosa. Psychother. Psychosom. *26:* 101–117 (1975).

38 Sours, J.: The anorexia nervosa syndrome: phenomenologic and psychodynamic components. Psychiat. Q. *43:* 240–256 (1969).

39 Strober, M.: The relation of personality characteristics to body image disturbances in juvenile anorexia nervosa: a multivariate analysis. Psychosom. Med. *43:* 323–330 (1981).

40 Pierloot, R.; Houben, M.: Estimation of body dimensions in anorexia nervosa. Psychol. Med. *8:* 317–324 (1978).

41 Weissman, M.; Bothwell, S.: Assessment of social adjustment by patient self-report. Archs gen. Psychiat. *33:* 1111–1115 (1976).

42 Johnson, C.; Berndt, D.: Preliminary investigation of bulimia and life adjustment. Am. J. Psychiat. *140:* 774–777 (1983).

43 Johnson, C.; Stuckey, M.; Lewis, L.; Schwartz, D.: Bulimia: a descriptive survey of 316 cases. Int. J. Eating Disord. *2:* 3–16 (1982).

44 Pyle, R.; Mitchell, J.; Eckert, E.: Bulimia: a report of 34 cases. J. clin. Psychiat. *42:* 60–64 (1981).

45 Beumont, P.: Further categorization of patients with anorexia nervosa. Austral. N.Z. J. Psychiat. *11:* 223–226 (1977).

46 Casper, R.; Eckert, E.; Halmi, K.; Goldberg, S.; Davis, J.: Bulimia: its incidence and clinical importance in patients with anorexia nervosa. Archs gen. Psychiat. *37:* 1030–1035 (1980).

47 Solyom, L.; Freeman, R.; Miles, J.: A comparative psychometric study of anorexia nervosa and obsessive neurosis. Can. J. Psychiat. *27:* 282–286 (1982).

48 Hsu, L.; Crisp, A.: The Crown-Crisp Experiential Index (CCEI) profile in anorexia nervosa. Br. J. Psychiat. *136:* 567–573 (1980).

49 Bhanji, S.; Mattingly, D.: Anorexia nervosa: some observations on 'dieters' and 'vomiters', cholesterol and carotene. Br. J. Psychiat. *139:* 238–241 (1981).

50 Norman, D.; Herzog, D.: Bulimia, anorexia nervosa and anorexia nervosa with bulimia: a comparative analysis of MMPI profiles. Int. J. Eating Disord. *2:* 43–52 (1983).

51 Strober, M.; Goldenberg, I.: Ego boundary disturbance in juvenile anorexia nervosa. J. clin. Psychol. *37:* 433–438 (1981).

52 Leon, G.; Kolotkin, R.; Korgeski, G.: MacAndrew Addiction Scale and other MMPI characteristics associated with obesity, anorexia and smoking behavior. Addict. Behav. *4:* 401–407 (1979).

53 Garner, D.: Body image in anorexia nervosa. Can. J. Psychiat. *26:* 224–227 (1981).

54 Strober, M.: Locus of control, psychopathology and weight gain in juvenile anorexia nervosa. J. abnorm. Child Psychol. *10:* 97–106 (1982).

55 Falk, J.; Halmi, K.: Amenorrhea in anorexia nervosa: examination of the critical body weight hypothesis. Biol. Psychiat. *17:* 799–806 (1982).

56 Strober, M.: A comparative analysis of personality organization in juvenile anorexia nervosa. J. Youth Adol. *10:* 285–295 (1981).

57 Small, A.; Madero, J.; Gross, H.; Teagno, L.; Leib, J.; Ebert, M.: A comparative analysis of primary anorexics and schizophrenics on the MMPI. J. clin. Psychol. *37:* 733–736 (1981).

58 Small, A.; Teagno, L.; Madero, J.; Gross, H.; Ebert, M.: A comparison of anorexics and schizophrenics on psychodiagnostic measures. Int. J. Eating Disord. *1:* 49–56 (1982).

59 Thompson, M.; Schwartz, D.: Life adjustment of women with anorexia nervosa and anorexic-like behavior. Int. J. Eating Disord. *1:* 47–60 (1982).

60 Pillay, M.; Crisp, A.: Some psychological characteristics of patients with anorexia nervosa whose weight has been newly restored. Br. J. med. Psychol. *50:* 375–380 (1977).

61 Wingate, B.; Christie, M.: Ego strength and body image in anorexia nervosa. J. psychosom. Res. *22:* 201–204 (1978).

62 Sugarman, A.; Quinlan, D.; Devenis, L.: Ego boundary disturbance in anorexia nervosa: preliminary findings. J. Personality Assess. *46:* 455–461 (1982).

63 Garner, D.; Garfinkel, P.; Stancer, H.; Moldofsky, H.: Body image disturbances in anorexia nervosa and obesity. Psychosom. Med. *38:* 327–336 (1976).

64 Rost, W.; Neuhaus, M.; Florin, I.: Bulimia nervosa: sex role attitude, sex role behavior and sex-related locus of control in bulimarexic women. J. psychosom. Res. *26:* 403–408 (1982).

65 Allerdissen, R.; Florin, I.; Rost, W.: Psychological characteristics of women with bulimia nervosa (bulimarexia). Behav. Anal. Modif. *4:* 314–317 (1981).

66 Dunn, P.; Ondercin, P.: Personality variables related to compulsive eating in college women. J. clin. Psychol. *37:* 43–49 (1981).

67 Goldberg, S.; Halmi, K.; Casper, R.; Eckert, E.; Davis, J.M.: Pretreatment predictors of weight change in anorexia nervosa; in Vigersky, Anorexia nervosa (Raven Press, New York 1977).

68 Rollins, N.; Piazza, E.: Anorexia nervosa: a quantitative approach to follow-up. J. Am. Acad. Child Psychiat. *20:* 167–183 (1981).
69 Strober, M.: The significance of bulimia in juvenile anorexia nervosa: an exploration of possible etiologic factors. Int. J. Eating Disord. *1:* 28–43 (1981).
70 Strober, M.; Salkin, B.; Burroughs, J.; Morrell, W.: Validity of the bulimia restricter distinction in anorexia nervosa: parental personality characteristics and family psychiatric morbidity. J. nerv. ment. Dis. *170:* 345–351 (1982).
71 Halmi, K.; Goldberg, S.; Casper, R.; Eckert, E.; Davis, J.: Pretreatment predictors of outcome in anorexia nervosa. Br. J. Psychiat. *134:* 71–78 (1979).
72 Herman, C.; Polivy, J.: Anxiety, restraint and eating behavior. J. abnorm. Psychol. *84:* 666–672 (1975).
73 Halmi, K.; Falk, J.; Schwartz, E.: Binge-eating and vomiting: a survey of a college population. Psychol. Med. *11:* 697–706 (1981).
74 Ben-Tovim, D.; Marilov, V.; Crisp, A.: Personality and mental state (PSE) within anorexia nervosa. J. psychosom. Res. *23:* 321–325 (1979).
75 Boskind-Lodahl, M.; White, W.: The definition and treatment of bulimarexia in college women – a pilot study. J. Am. Coll. Hlth Ass. *27:* 84–97 (1978).
76 Button, E.; Whitehouse, A.: Subclinical anorexia nervosa. Psychol. Med. *11:* 509–516 (1981).
77 Casper, R.; Halmi, K.; Goldberg, S.; Eckert, E.; Davis, J.: Disturbances in body image estimation as related to other characteristics and outcome in anorexia nervosa. Br. J. Psychiat. *134:* 60–66 (1979).
78 Pillay, M.; Crisp, A.: The impact of social skills training within an established inpatient treatment programme for anorexia nervosa. Br. J. Psychiat. *139:* 533–539 (1981).

15 Group Therapy for Anorexia Nervosa

Michael S. Maher

Introduction

The utility of group therapy in the treatment of primary psychiatric illness, as well as psychosomatic illness, is well established [1–3]. Homogeneous groups have been found to offer a variety of advantages [4] and have been utilized effectively in the treatment of psychosomatic illness [1]. This chapter will consider prior reports of group therapy in the treatment of anorexia nervosa, as well as our experience. The problems of utilizing group therapy, and for what specific goals, will also be considered.

The descriptive diagnostic criteria of anorexia nervosa as specified in DSM III [5] or *Feighner* et al. [6] are quite clear. However, there are many factors, both psychological and physiological, which are highly significant in anorexia nervosa that have yet to be characterized. Anorexia nervosa can exist as a self-limited disorder of relatively brief duration with little apparent residual psychiatric symptomatology. Conversely, it may remain as a severe illness which persists for years and has a high mortality rate [7]. Anorexia nervosa may be a final manifestation of a complex variety of social, psychological and physiological factors. In view of the diverse characteristics of anorexia nervosa, various treatment modalities, including group psychotherapy, have been proposed.

During the planning process for the group described in this paper, it was postulated that certain characteristics of anorexia nervosa, which are especially difficult to deal with in individual and family therapy, might lend themselves well to treatment in groups (e.g. denial of illness and social isolation). *Yalom* [4] has identified a number of curative factors in groups, among which several have been noted as perhaps being particularly relevant to the treatment of anorexia nervosa in homogeneous groups. These factors include cohesiveness, universality, instillation of hope and family reenactment. Many patients feel extremely frustrated that well-meaning family, friends and, occasionally, professionals implore them to eat, as if it were a simple matter of choice; it was anticipated that even the least insightful of the anorectic group members would understand the futility of the 'just eat' approach and thus facilitate the sense of group cohesiveness. Since groups with homogeneity along a broad spectrum of variables tend to be more cohesive, it was anticipated that the group could tolerate greater change. It was hypothesized that the sense of universality experienced in a group of patients with similar symptoms would be therapeutic; i.e. early group interactions might provide opportunities to discuss similar symptoms and feelings and thus diminish the patient's social isolation. Anorectics have body image distortions, which are resistant to objective, reality-based interventions by professionals. Since anorexia nervosa patients usually perceive others accurately, it was anticipated that the comparison of conflicting perceptions within the context of a group might provide opportunities for improved reality testing. In view of the high frequency of depression in anorectics, the instillation of hope was postulated to be an important curative factor. The prominence of family dynamics in the symptom formation as well as the importance of family therapy in the overall treatment of anorexia nervosa suggested that family reenactment might be particularly significant in the patient who is physically, but not psychologically, separated from her family.

It must be noted that group psychotherapy, as well as any other treatment modality, must be considered in the context of the patient's overall condition. Particularly important as a prerequisite for successful psychotherapy of any variety is the patient's nutritional and physiological status. Thus, the patients included in all the groups described in this chapter were not more than 15–20% below ideal body weight.

Reports of Group Therapy for Anorexia Nervosa

There is little research reported in the literature of group therapy in the treatment of anorexia nervosa. The literature on the use of group therapy in the treatment of other eating disorders, including bulimia (see chapter 16) and obesity [8], is more extensive. However, even this is largely directed toward obesity.

Report of Huerta

Optimistic results are reported by *Huerta* [9] in the outpatient group therapy of anorectics. She describes an open-ended group in which patients participate weekly for 8–12 weeks, and then less often. She describes a very high level of cohesiveness early in the group, and reports [9, p. 117] that 'a large proportion of patients make excellent progress on an outpatient basis with group psychotherapy as the main therapeutic modality and individual and family sessions taking a secondary role'. Progress was rated in the general area of physical symptoms, including weight. However, group members also reported improved mood, decreased irritability, more realistic body image, decreased preoccupation with food, and greater self-responsibility.

In concluding, *Huerta* [9, p. 118] states: 'Patients who do not do well in the group generally are those with borderline character structure, particularly that associated with the syndrome of bulimia.' She continues, saying that methods are being developed to identify group therapy-responsive and group therapy-resistant patients. This finding is consistent with that of *Lacey* [10] who found that patients with the syndrome of bulimia (now at normal or near normal weight) with a documented prior history of anorexia nervosa or with severe character problems also did not do well in group therapy (see chapter 16).

Report of Polivy

Polivy [11] reports her experience with two groups of anorectic patients. Overall her report is promising, however, certain qualifications and cautions are noted. She established two long-term groups with a maximum of 4 or 5 patients each. 11 of 14 patients started the group as inpatients, 5 patients dropped out in the first 4–12 weeks. The group was considered an adjunctive treatment; all patients were also involved in individual psychotherapy. Patients who were 'excessively competitive or regressed' [11, p. 280] were excluded.

The focus of the group was experiential and reeducative. Particular attention was paid to the relationship between emotions and eating behaviors. It should be noted, however, that certain supportive elements were included. Specifically, the exchange of information, correction of misinformation and encouragement for improvement. The curative factors are similar to those described by *Huerta* [9]. Four are particularly noted, universality, family reenactment, interpersonal feedback, and increase of self-esteem via the helping role.

Six of 14 patients remained in group therapy for more than 6 months. These 6 patients were distributed among the two groups. A genuine group process, with a strong commitment to the group, and a willingness to confront and accept confrontation is described. Among these members there seemed to be general improvement. The group appeared to facilitate insight into the emotional factors related to self-destructive eating behaviors. Improvements in social and occupational functioning were also noted. In view of the fact that these patients were in several forms of therapy, it was difficult, as *Polivy* [11] recognizes, to identify which treatment modality was responsible for these improvements.

Approximately one third (5 patients) of the original 14 members dropped out within 4–12 weeks. These patients were younger and physically closer to their families than the patients who stayed in the group.

In concluding *Polivy* [11] adds a word of caution noting that possible negative side effects may be encountered. The teaching of symptoms, extreme dependency on group members outside the group, and interruption of the relationship between the anorectic and her individual psychotherapist are considered to be potentially problematic.

The University of South Florida Eating Disorder Clinic Experience

An additional report on group therapy [previously unpublished] comes from the University of South Florida Eating Disorders Clinic (USF EDC). The author of this chapter and the co-editor of this volume *(Powers)* served as therapists for an insight-oriented therapy group, initially consisting of 12 anorectic patients. The group met weekly for 1.5 h for 9 months.

Characteristics of Group Members

All patients were female, aged 13–36 years. All were receiving additional psychiatric treatment. The duration of illness was 2–12 years. All patients had met the DMS III [5] criteria for anorexia nervosa, but none was more than 20% below ideal body weight when the group began. There was a predominance of certain psychological characteristics in the members. A tenuous, easily threatened sense of self-worth, a sense of very limited control over the external world, an excessive sense of responsibility and accompanying guilt for real and imagined inadequacies, and a sense of hopelessness and despair were common features. Indeed, a personality disorder as defined by DSM III or a borderline personality organization as defined by *Kernberg* [12] was present in 8 of 12 patients.

Group Method

The primary goal of this group was to address the psychological symptoms of anorexia nervosa. Weight gain, although a part of the overall treatment plan for some of the patients, was not a primary goal of this group.

The approach taken by the therapists changed somewhat after 8–10 meetings. Initially, the therapists' interventions were modeled on a traditional, insight-oriented psychoanalytic role. Group members were expected to take the responsibility for introducing and discussing topics. Interventions focused on labeling affects, identifying conflicting thoughts and feelings, and attempting to draw the group's attention to the ways in which conflicts were manifest in eating behaviors as well as other psychological symptoms. As problems with this approach became evident (see below under Group Process), supervision was arranged on a weekly basis and the therapists' interventions were modified to include some more directly supportive techniques.

Group Process

During the initial 5–7 meetings, the members were surprisingly open, talked directly to each other, asked personal questions and revealed personal information about themselves. The initial anxiety of meeting new people and revealing personal information gave way to a moderate cohesiveness and a general feeling of comfort. The early period may be characterized as mutual revealing of symptoms and identifying similar problems that these cause.

Unfortunately, major problems subsequently arose. This early phase was followed by a brief transitional phase of 2 or 3 sessions. During this time, the group looked more and more to the therapists for guidance. There was a sense that there was nothing else to say. Patients began to describe a feeling of emptiness. The previous optimism and high level of attendance changed markedly. The group then settled into a pattern which persisted, essentially, to termination.

This third phase was characterized by a sense of depression, despair, extreme isolation and sometimes paranoid hypersensitivity to even the mildest confrontation. The mere act of coming to the group emerged as terrible confirmation of the patient's inadequacy. Communication among group members diminished markedly. There was a great deal of competition for the attention of the therapists. Approximately half of the members dropped out, and 1 patient required hospitalization because of weight loss.

During the late part of the third month of the group, it became apparent to the group that the female therapist was pregnant. When the topic was not mentioned for several weeks, the female therapist finally mentioned that she was pregnant and told the group she would be taking a 6-week maternity leave, probably starting in the fifth month of the group. The discussion following this announcement was limited to brief polite comments with no apparent affect. The character of the group did not appear to change significantly in response to this information or during the therapist's absence, with the possible exception of 1 patient's need for hospitalization. When the therapist returned to the group, the members greeted her, but made virtually no other statement except in response to questions and at no time expressed the sadness, anger, fear or relief at her return that almost every other patient in her practice expressed.

There was an occasional glimmer of psychological insight during the group but this was shrouded by an oppressive feeling of depression. There were also occasional attempts by patients to offer each other some emotional support. Generally, however, these attempts were very limited, and in some respects, almost pathetic. These points are illustrated by the following example. One patient had a pre-school daughter who was cared for jointly by her and her mother. The patient became aware that her emotional availability and ability to express affection were directly related to her daughter coming to her rather than to her mother when upset. This initially pleased the patient. However, she then expressed great concern that her daughter might come to her too often and that she did not have a lot to give. Another patient, who seemed to be genuinely struggling to offer some support, suggested that if it was too much she could always have her mother take over again. Following this, there was a prevasive sense of depression, detachment, and withdrawal for the remainder of the session, as if to say: 'yes and if you ask for too much from the group, you will find the group as unable to respond to you as you are to your child'. This could indeed be seen as negative family reenactment.

Generally during this period, the dependence on the therapists increased considerably. The patients found themselves unable to obtain even the most limited emotional support from each other, and thus turned to the therapists to alleviate the emerging profound depression.

There was very little change as termination approached. Termination was rarely openly discussed by the group. The attitude of the group seemed to be that an unpleasant and possibly punitive experience was finally coming to an end.

Results

The therapists' general assessment of the group was that it provided limited, if any, benefit to the patients. While the psychological symptoms associated with anorexia nervosa did become clearer to the therapists and patients, this increased understanding apparently offered little benefit. The sense of depression and inadequacy that emerged was nearly overwhelming to therapists and patients alike. Indeed, there were significant symptomatic exacerbations during the life of the group. There was little sustained insight. One area where some change may have occurred is in the patients' acceptance of the seriousness of the illness. Indeed the high drop-out rate may represent a denial of this on the part of the patients who did not stay with the group.

Problems with this preliminary project include the high drop-out rate (only 6 patients attended 6 or more sessions), the high incidence of significant character pathology, lack of objective assessment measures and the brief duration (9 months) of the group. The therapist's pregnancy may also be a unique confounding factor. However, the depression and despair had emerged and was clearly evident before the pregnancy was apparent. It appears that the pregnancy exacerbated, rather than initiated, the depression and despair.

In retrospect, it may have been somewhat unrealistic to have expected changes in the target psychodynamics during the relatively brief time period. The extreme depression, sense of inadequacy and the almost punitive feeling associated with attending the group were not fully anticipated. Earlier supervision may have been helpful in identifying and responding more effectively to these problems. As noted previously, it was only after problems developed that regular supervision was arranged. The supervision ultimately became an essential part of the process. The focus of supervision was primarily to assist the therapists in recognizing and coping with their feelings of profound fatigue as well as considerable anger and resentment at the extreme emotional demandingness and dependency of the group. The subjective experience of the therapists was very similar to that described in individual psychotherapy with borderline patients [12].

USF EDC Group: Discussion

Group Therapy for Other Serious Illnesses

In an attempt to understand the group process that occurred in this particular group of anorexia nervosa patients, we considered the results of group therapy for other serious illnesses. These include groups of patients with serious medical illnesses [1–3], severe psychopathology (especially schizophrenia) [13] and psychosomatic disorders [3]. In essence, the group described had all three features: they were medically ill (from the physiological consequences of semistarvation), had severe psychopathology (predominantly borderline character structures) and had a psychosomatic disorder (see chapter 8 for the psychosomatic concept of anorexia nervosa).

Group therapy for patients with severe medical illnesses has a long history and has been an effective adjunct to somatic treatments. Asthma has been particularly well-studied and is considered by many to be an example of a psychosomatic illness [14, 15]. Factors considered to be correlated with poor prognosis in group therapy were frequent hospital admissions, disturbed relationships with family, unemployment, concealing facts or lying in the group, and lack of introspection, 'especially when combined with resistance toward acceptance of a causal relationship between life situations and illness' [1, p. 199]. Positive prognostic factors have included youth, few hospitalizations, satisfactory relationships with family members, satisfactory work record, capacity to bring personal conflicts into the group, acknowledgement of the role of relationship conflicts and their handling as a possible cause of physical symptoms. Many of the poor prognostic factors were analogous to observations of the group described in this report. For example, most group members had had two or more hospitalizations, all had disturbed family relationships, most had unsatisfactory work records and it was rare for the patient to identify a connection between relationship problems and her symptoms.

The use of group psychotherapy in the treatment of severe psychopathology has been extensive [13, 16–18]. However, systematic research demonstrating the benefit of group psychotherapy in the treatment of the psychological symptoms of patients with severe psychopathology is extremely rare. *Yalom* [4] reports a group of patients with schizoid personalities who were treated with considerable benefit in a group which continued for 30 months. Reports of the treatment of personality disorders and schizophrenia in groups give some indication of the problems encountered [19, 20]. A strong regressive element, a tendency toward considerable paranoid projection, and an extreme dependence on the therapist are common features. These are generally controlled by utilizing various specifically structured approaches. Didactic groups, group pharmacotherapy, behavioral modification groups, socialization groups and other problem-solving or problem-focused groups have been described. These approaches all have in common a formal or informal structure, which tends to reduce rather than stimulate anxiety; that is, these groups emphasize a supportive orientation rather than an insight orientation. The structure allows patients to interact and consider their experiences and symptoms in an atmosphere where there are definite restraints and controls. These group characteristics appear to be helpful in reducing overt symptomatology and improving compliance with treatment. In our group of anorectics, there was extreme dependence on the therapists and a marked regressive element (e.g. patients might miss a few sessions but respond by attending a group session if one of the therapists called). Although there was a marked absence of overt criticism of the therapists, the therapists frequently felt that they were not helping enough and in fact were exhausted after group sessions.

In psychosomatic groups [1], the similarity of symptoms and their effects on patients' lives are a powerful factor which tends to draw the patients into a cohesive group. Likewise, in anorexia nervosa there appears to be an initial mutual identification of symptoms which facilitates some degree of cohesiveness. In a psychosomatic group, this cohesiveness is utilized in the process of developing insights into the relationship between emotional factors and physical symptoms. The preceding reports suggest that this process is inconsistent in the group therapy of anorexia nervosa and may not occur in the presence of a high proportion of patients with personality disorders.

Ineffectiveness of 'Curative' Factors

Although the 'curative' factors described by *Yalom* [4] and *Huerta* [9] were noted in our group, these were not necessarily therapeutic. There was an initial sense of moderate cohesiveness which promoted the feeling that this group was one to which the anorectic truly belonged, but this was a two-edged sword in that if confirmed the patient's belief that she was a terrible failure. The universality factor was evident early in the group and was illustrated by the patient who referred to the 'shameful secrets of anorexia' but, unfortunately, this did not result in a lessening of the sense of isolation experienced by the patients. The worsening depression experienced by members of the group may have been related to the fact that hope was not instilled. Finally, reenactment of family psychodynamics is postulated to have occurred, but in a dramatic and counterproductive fashion: not only did the female therapist mother figure become pregnant (i.e. 'fat') but she left physically and emotionally. If the family model of group process is accurate, then the pregnancy of the therapist mother figure may have meant what it means in any family – i.e. that the other children must take an additional developmental step toward emancipation. In a group of women unable to recognize the connection between their emotions and their disturbed eating behavior and who possess meager ego strengths, this challenge to further emancipation may have seemed impossible and may have had profound negative implications for the group.

Discrepancies among Group Therapy Reports

There are apparent differences in the three reports of group psychotherapy discussed. There appears to be a continuum of optimism with *Huerta's* [9] report the most optimistic, the USF EDC's report the least optimistic and *Polivy's* [11] report somewhere in between. It is not clear what accounts for these differences. However, several factors may be important: the therapists' approach, the structure of the group and the particular patient population may be important differences.

There also appears to be a continuum of most structured and supportive to least structured and supportive which correlates with the reported benefit of the group. *Huerta's* [9] group appears most highly structured and her results appear most optimistic; the USF EDC group appears least structured and the results least optimistic, and *Polivy's* [11] group appears intermediate in both respects. It may be that the emergence of the profound depression and despair encountered in the USF EDC group can be controlled in a more highly structured group. A highly structured group would, however, be expected to place certain limits on the therapeutic potential of the group particularly with regard to changes in personality traits.

The patient population found in each of the groups described varies considerably. *Huerta* [9] reports that patients with borderline character structure did not do well in the group. *Polivy* [11] notes that patients who did well in the group were less likely to have borderline, hysterical, or other personality disorders; furthermore, she excluded patients who were 'excessively competitive or regressed'. The incidence of personality disorder in the USF EDC group was 75%. This data is certainly consistent with the conclusion that group psychotherapy can be used most effectively in anorectics who do not have personality disorders. However, the high incidence of personality disorder in patients with anorexia nervosa would considerably limit the proportion of anorectics who would benefit from group therapy.

Yalom's [4] discussion on homogeneity in groups may shed some light on the above phenomena. He notes the advantage of 'heterogeneity for conflict areas, and homogeneity for ego strength' [4, p. 262]. It appears that there was a homogeneity of ego strength in each of the three reports. However, *Huerta* [9] and *Polivy* [11] report a somewhat higher level of ego strength and seem to have obtained better results. The psychodynamics of anorexia nervosa (see chapter 6) suggest that there is also a homogeneity for conflict area. This would be expected to present similar difficulties for any group consisting entirely of anorectics.

Conclusion

Considering the limited number of reports as well as the relative lack of systematic assessment on the use of group psychotherapy in the treatment of anorexia nervosa, it is not possible to draw definite conclusions regarding its effects. However, some patterns have emerged which both clarify the questions which need to be addressed and suggest certain conclusions. As with any treatment modality, there are risks to be considered. Our experience illustrates some of the risks to which *Polivy* [11] alludes. The data suggest that the stress of group therapy may precipitate symptomatic exacerbations with weight loss serious enough to require hospitalization.

At present, the possible benefits of group psychotherapy appear to be limited to a subgroup of anorectics who do not suffer from a personality disorder. The subgroup of anorectics that do seem to benefit from group therapy apparently have greater ego strength, suffer from less severe developmental psychopathology, and have greater physical separation from their families. The benefits in this subgroup may include improvement in personality traits as well as in overt symptomatology.

Several important questions have emerged from these studies. Can a subgroup of anorectics who are more likely to benefit from group therapy be more clearly defined? Can the apparent benefits from group therapy be objectively documented with systematic assessment measures? Can the effects of other concurrent therapies be distinguished from the effects of group therapy? Is there a subgroup of anorectics, possibly with more severe psychopathology, who are at unusually high risk for the potential countertherapeutic effects of group psychotherapy?

In closing, it is the author's opinion that the place of group psychotherapy in the overall treatment of anorexia nervosa is not well defined. A moderately to highly structured psychotherapy group which utilizes insight, but also provides considerable support, may be used as an adjunctive treatment with benefit in a subgroup of anorectics. However, at present, it should remain an experimental procedure undertaken in an appropriate research context.

References

1 Groen, J.; Pelser, H.: Experiences with, and results of, group psychotherapy in patients with bronchial asthma. J. psychosom. Res. *4:* 191–205 (1960).
2 Hill, O.: The psychological management of psychosomatic diseases. Br. J. Psychiat. *131:* 113–136 (1977).

3 Rad, M.; Ruppell, A.: Combined inpatient and outpatient group psychotherapy: a therapeutic model for psychosomatics. Psychother. Psychosom. *26:* 237–243 (1979).

4 Yalom, I.: The theory and practice of group psychotherapy; 2nd ed. (Basic Books, New York 1975).

5 Diagnostic and Statistical Manual of Mental Disorders (DSM III); 3rd ed. (Am. Psychiatric Ass., Washington 1980).

6 Feighner, J.; Robins, E.; Guze, S.; Woodruff, R.; Winokur, G.; Munoz, R.: Diagnostic criteria for use in psychiatric research. Archs gen. Psychiat. *26:* 57–63 (1972).

7 Rockwell, W.; Ellinwood, E.; Doughterty, G.; Brodie, H.: Anorexia nervosa: review of current treatment practices. Sth. med. J., Nashville *75:* 1101–1106 (1982).

8 Powers, P.: Obesity: the regulation of weight (Williams & Wilkins, Baltimore 1980).

9 Huerta, E.: Group therapy for anorexia nervosa patients; in Gross, Anorexia nervosa: a comprehensive approach, pp. 111–118 (D.C. Health, Lexington 1982).

10 Lacey, J.: Bulimia nervosa, binge eating, and psychogenic vomiting: a controlled treatment study and long-term outcome. Br. med. J. *286:* 1609–1613 (1983).

11 Polivy, J.: Group therapy as an adjunctive treatment for anorexia nervosa. J. psychiat. Treat. Eval. *3:* 279–283 (1981).

12 Kernberg, O.: Borderline conditions and pathological narcissism (Aronson, New York 1975).

13 Fenn, H.; Dinaburg, D.: Didactic group psychotherapy with chronic schizophrenics. Int. J. grp Psychother. *31:* 443–451 (1981).

14 Alexander, F.: Psychosomatic medicine: its principles and application (Norton, New York 1950).

15 Minuchin, S.; Rosman, B.; Baker, L.: Psychosomatic families (Harvard University Press, Cambridge 1977).

16 Battegay, R.; Marshall, R. von: Results of a long-term group psychotherapy with schizophrenics. Compreh. Psychiat. *19:* 349–353 (1978).

17 Claghorn, J.; Johnstone, E.; Cook, T.; Itschner, L.: Group therapy and maintenance treatment of schizophrenics. Archs gen. Psychiat. *31:* 361–365 (1974).

18 Herz, M.; Spitzer, R.; Gibbon, M.; Greenspan, K.; Reibel, S.: Individual versus group aftercare treatment. Am. J. Psychiat. *131:* 808–812 (1974).

19 Bion, W.: Experiences in groups (Basic Books, New York 1961).

20 Freud, S.: Group psychology and the analysis of the ego. The complete psychological works of Sigmund Freud; standard ed., pp. 69–143 (Hogarth Press, London 1955).

16 Group Therapy of Bulimia

Robert C. Fernandez

Introduction

There is currently much interest in the possible uses of group therapy for the treatment of bulimia. This interest ranges from the use of groups as one aspect of a multidimensional treatment program to their use as the primary therapy vehicle. This interest appears to be the result of a number of factors. The first is the apparently epidemic nature of the problem, and the flood of requests for help. This has been highlighted by the attention given to the eating disorders in general, and specifically to bulimia in a number of articles in the lay literature and on television 'talk' shows. Each such article, or show, results in another torrent of referrals. Second, the limited number of resources available to provide adequate evaluation and treatment further complicates this problem. Third, the difficulties encountered in attempting to treat patients with eating disorders in individual psychotherapy, especially the cognitive and perceptual difficulties (see chapters 2, 4, 7), have also stimulated interest in the use of other treatment methods. The usefulness of incorporating behavioral and educational approaches as a part of the treatment of eating disorders has been well established. Such approaches have lent themselves well to presentation in a group format in the treatment of other psychiatric conditions. Fourth, the perceived benefits of self-help groups to patients with eating disorders, and to their families and friends, have also increased interest in group therapy approaches. The fifth and most significant factor is the appearance of a number of positive reports of group treatment of bulimic patients.

In this chapter we will review the reports on the use of group treatment of bulimia, and describe our experience with group therapy in the University of South Florida Eating Disorders Clinic (USF EDC). We will conclude with our recommendations and principles for the use of group therapy in the treatment of bulimia.

Reports on the Use of Group Treatment

Report of Boskind-Lodahl and White

The earliest report on the use of group treatment that we are aware of is that of *Boskind-Lodahl and White* [1] in 1978. For purposes of the study, bulimarexia was operationally defined, utilizing the following three criteria. First, the female patient is locked into cyclic eating behavior, in which she experiences an uncontrollable desire for food, consumes vast quantities and subsequently purges via forced vomiting, fasting, dieting, laxative, or amphetamine abuse. Second, she exhibits a distorted body image, complaining of being too fat though not perceived as such by the therapist or significant others. Third, she complains of low self-esteem, feelings of inadequacy, helplessness and despair. She is often isolated, fears men, distrusts women and expresses great shame regarding such behaviors. 58 women who responded to an advertisement in the university newspaper were screened. 26 met the above criteria. They were 19–26 years of age, mean age of onset of symptoms being 15, and all reported having symptoms for several years. The severity of their symptoms was not described. The first 13 were assigned to the treatment group, and the next 13 were assigned to a waiting list control group.

The treatment group met weekly for 11 2-hour sessions plus a 6-hour marathon session at the midway point. It was conducted by a female therapist utilizing a very strong feminist orientation [2]. Techniques employed included daily journals to record feelings and precipitating factors directly preceding binges, weekly short-term goal contracting, role play of feared situations, assertiveness training, sensory awareness and guided fantasy exercises. Of the 12 patients who completed the treatment group, 10 reported a decrease in bingeing and purging behavior, with 4 stopping completely. The other 6 reported that binges were less frequent and shorter, and that they could consistently stop themselves in the middle of a binge, which they were unable to do prior to treatment.

Report of Dixon and Kiecolt-Glaser

Dixon and Kiecolt-Glaser [3] reported promising results from a multidimensional therapy approach. 36 women who met DSM III criteria for bulimia were offered group therapy over the course of a 1-year period. Their mean age was 24.4 years (range 14–42 years). All were Caucasian, and all were from middle or upper socioeconomic classes. No prior commitment to the group was required, and patients were advised to attend one group session to help them decide if group would be beneficial. 6 patients attended less than 2 sessions. 19 patients attended 2 or more sessions, but either did not attend over a 10-week period (16 of 19 patients) or failed to return their questionnaire (3 of 19 patients). The treatment group was compared to 2 control groups of 8 women each, all of whom met DSM III criteria, and completed questionnaires at 6- to 10-month intervals. Between surveys, 1 control group had received no treatment and the other group had received at least 4 months of individual treatment in the previous 6 months.

Their approach utilized: (1) behavioral techniques, including use of food diaries, self-reports in group of the number of 'free days' (i.e. days with no bingeing or purging), discouraging fasting or severe dieting, reinforcing sensible meal patterns and a physical fitness program, identifying behavioral chains, setting goals and priorities for change, and developing specific behavioral interventions; (2) cognitive restructuring; (3) assertion and relaxation training; (4) introduction to biofeedback; and (5) insight-oriented discussions, which included as common themes the need for approval by others, use of food as an irresponsible escape from otherwise overly responsible lives, fear of success (misidentified as fear of failure), use of the eating disorder as revenge against parents or significant others, conflictual relationships with men and parents, a 'fat' identity (even though at normal weight or underweight), feeling out of control of their lives and perfectionistic attitudes.

They reported that at the end of 10 weeks of treatment, all 11 patients who completed the treatment had some improvement, with 3 binge-free, and 4 reduced to a frequency of 1–2 binges per week. At 5–10 months follow-up, 9 of 11 patients continued to improve, and 7 rated themselves even more improved than at the end of group treatment with a total of 5 binge-free. Their improvement far exceeded that of the no-treatment control group, and of the individual therapy-only control group. They also noted that patients with past or present excessive use of alcohol were either early drop-outs, or did not improve.

Report from the UCLA Eating Disorders Clinic

The experience of the UCLA Eating Disorders Clinic [4] is extensively described by *Yager* (chapter 4).

Report of Lacey

One of the most promising reports on the use of group therapy for patients with bulimia is that of *Lacey* [5] from St. George's Hospital Medical School in London, England. The program was developed in response to the awareness of large numbers of patients, and of the need for local treatment with limited specialized resources. The criteria for inclusion in the treatment study were: (1) that the patients met the diagnostic criteria for bulimia, as specified by DSM III and by *Russell* [6]; (2) that the patients were over 17 and under 45 years of age; (3) that the patients were clinically suitable for outpatient treatment (e.g. not suicidal), and (4) that the patients agreed in advance to the demands of the program. The sample consisted of 30 consecutive acceptors, with 7 other women having been screened who either did not meet the criteria, or decided against treatment. After a physical and psychiatric preassessment period lasting 2 weeks, they were alternately assigned to a 10-week treatment program or a 10-week nontreatment control program followed by a 2-week postassessment period. Following this postassessment period, the control group then went through the 10-week treatment program and another 2-week postassessment period. Follow-up consisted of an assessment by a psychiatrist, using a standard symptom checklist in formal follow-up clinics at 1 and 3 months following the treatment period, and every 3 months thereafter for up to 2 years.

The 30 patients were from 21 to 37 years of age, with histories of bingeing and vomiting of from 3 to 18 years. They had a mean frequency of bingeing and vomiting of over 3 times per day, and a mean presenting weight 3.2% greater than that of a matched general population sample. 5 of the 30 also had histories of previous anorexia nervosa diagnosed on the criteria established by *Feighner* et al. [7] and *Crisp* [8], but had recovered to normal body weight. Only 5 of the patients were married, and none had children.

The objectives of the treatment program were to remove all symptoms without the development of a weight disorder, and to provide enough psychiatric assistance so that the patients could deal with their emotional and relationship difficulties independently or, at worst, seek help from the general psychiatric treatment services for these difficulties without the presence of an eating disorder. The patients were divided into groups of 5, each of which contained 1 of the patients diagnosed as recovered from anorexia nervosa. The program was carried out on a half-day-per-week basis for 10 consecutive weeks. Each group was led by two therapists (both medical and nonmedical) who were described as having knowledge of psychiatric patients and psychiatric methods, and as being familiar with group work, but without special training in group techniques. Each patient met with one of the two therapists for a 30-min individual session. Later the same day, all 5 patients met with the two therapists for a 90-min group session. The group sessions were insight-oriented throughout. The individual sessions initially utilized simple behavioral and counseling techniques, and gradually shifted to insight-oriented psychotherapy. The patients were assisted in recognizing and delineating emotional and social factors associated with, or generated by, their symptoms. They were encouraged, particularly within the support provided by the group, to experiment with new ways of dealing with feelings and interpersonal difficulties.

The treatment program employed a rigid structure, including the development of a written contract between the patient and therapist during each individual session. Before treatment began, the patient agreed to attend the 10 individual sessions and groups, maintain her present weight throughout the 10 weeks and eat the prescribed diet. The patient was encouraged to first decrease and then stop bingeing and vomiting, with each stage being included in the weekly contract. If bingeing occurred, she was encouraged, and then contracted, not to vomit. Most importantly, the patient contracted to eat the next prescribed meal, regardless of its relationship to the last binge. The patient would write down the contract in her dietary diary, and the therapist would make a copy in his/her notes. The patient was instructed to carry the diary with her everywhere, and record all food and drink consumed, all episodes of bingeing, vomiting and laxative abuse, and her feelings and thoughts at the time. The diary was turned in each week, and a new one was issued. A diet sheet was provided weekly, describing a prescribed diet structured into three meals to be eaten at specific times. The amount of carbohydrates the patient agreed to eat was spelled out, but she had a choice as to the variety and quantity of other foods eaten. However, she was instructed not to change her diet without talking to the therapist. The patient was weighed weekly on the same scales by the individual therapist.

The control program revealed no demonstrable effect on bingeing or vomiting. The treatment program resulted in very significant changes. The mean incidence of total episodes of bingeing for the 30 patients during the 14-day assessment period pretreatment was 46.6, and post-treatment incidence was 2.36; for vomiting, these respective figures were 53 and 2.17. 24 of the 30 patients had stopped bingeing and vomiting entirely by the end of 10 weeks of treatment, and 4 more had stopped entirely by the 1 month follow-up. All 30 patients had reduced the frequency of bingeing and vomiting. Mean body weight of the sample, as compared to a matched general population sample, was 3.2% higher pretreatment, 3.6% higher at 10 weeks and 2.8% higher at 1-year follow-up, and no patients developed anorexia nervosa or progressively decompensating obesity. Follow-up of 28 patients (1 refused follow-up and 1 was hospitalized soon after treatment ended) revealed two patterns. 20 patients had no episodes of bingeing and vomiting, although all reported intermittent episodes of feeling emotionally disturbed. 6 considered further psychotherapy, but only 1 followed through and entered individual psychotherapy. The other 8 patients had occasional bulimic episodes on a mean of 3 times per year. 3 of this latter group requested further psychotherapy, and 2 began such treatment.

A history of alcohol abuse was associated with poorer outcome. The patient who refused follow-up and 4 of the 8 patients with occasional bulimic episodes during follow-up had such a history, whereas only 1 of the 20 patients with no bingeing and vomiting had a mild history of alcohol abuse. Of the 6 patients with previous histories of anorexia nervosa, 1 was completely free of bingeing and vomiting, 1 was the patient who required hospitalization at the end of treatment and the other 4 were among the 8 who had occasional episodes of bingeing and vomiting during follow-up.

The University of South Florida Eating Disorders Clinic Experience

Introduction

Based on some early reports of successful group approaches for the treatment of eating disorders, a pilot group for bulimic patients was conducted in the University of South Florida Eating Disorders Clinic (USF EDC). This group was co-led by the two editors of this text. The patients were chosen from consecutive patients evaluated in the USF EDC who met the DSM III criteria for bulimia, were suitable for outpatient treatment and were willing to participate in the group treatment program outlined for them, including agreeing to attend all 12 sessions. The program was presented as time-limited, aimed at helping reduce or eliminate their eating symptoms, increasing understanding of themselves and their emotional problems and adjunctive to their individual therapy and/or other efforts to help themselves. Those who were not in individual therapy were given a referral to an individual therapist, but compliance with the referral was not required. A fixed fee for the entire group treatment, payable in advance, was charged. This fee was roughly consistent with the local professional charges for 12 psychiatrically led group sessions. In addition, the members were asked to purchase two $25.00 gift certificates at a local department store. One of these certificates would be returned to the patients, contingent on their attendance at all group sessions, and the other would be returned, contingent on their maintaining their present weight within an acceptable range (to be negotiated with the therapists during the 1st group session). Any of the gift certificates not returned to the patients would be donated to a local charity.

USF EDC Group: Patient Selection

The 6 patients in the group (2 others met the criteria, but declined to participate, citing financial problems and hesitancy to be in a group setting as reasons) ranged from 16 to 43 years of age, with a mean age of 26.6 years. They had a mean duration of eating symptoms of 8 years, with a range of 1–20 years. In addition to the diagnosis of bulimia, 2 of the group members had previously met all the DSM III criteria for anorexia nervosa, except for percentage of weight loss, and also met the DSM III criteria for borderline personality disorder. 1 member had a significant problem with alcohol abuse, and 2 were significantly depressed.

The group met for 12 sessions of 90 min each scheduled in advance over a 14-week period. All the sessions after the initial one (during which permission was obtained) were videotaped, and were reviewed by the therapists between sessions. The group time was equally divided among behavioral, educative-cognitive, and traditional short-term dynamic group therapy approaches.

USF EDC Group: Behavioral Approaches

A dietary diary was provided in booklet form, in a $4\frac{1}{4} \times 7$ inch (10.8×17.8 cm) size (table I). The patients were instructed to carry the diary with them at all times, and to record the time and quantity of any food and drink consumed, what was going on immediately prior to and following the consumption, whether and when vomiting, laxative use, amphetamine use, or exercise occurred.

Initially, they were told to ignore the two columns labeled ‘F’. After they became familiar with keeping the diaries, and after the group began to discuss the relationship between feelings and the fast-binge-purge cycle and the relapse process, they were then instructed to utilize the ‘F’ column to code in their feelings/emotional states both pre- and post-eating, utilizing a simple code letter which they would describe in full at the bottom of the diary page.

Group attendance and maintaining weight within a target range were to be reinforced by the return of the gift certificates. A target weight and a range around that weight, within which the patient would agree to maintain weight during the entire treatment period, were negotiated during the 1st group ses-

Table I

Diet diary

Day of week ______________ Date ______________

Time	Food	Serv. size (calories)	F	Pre-events	F	Post-events	Purge follow?	Time

Individual goal: ______________

Was it met? ______________ If yes, what did you do? ______________

sion. Patients were instructed to weigh themselves weekly on the same scale prior to the group.

From the 3rd group session on, each patient was asked to develop a goal, with input from both patients and therapists, that they would attempt to achieve during the following week. Initially, these goals related to decreasing eating symptoms, and to changing conditions that increased the likelihood of bingeing and vomiting (e.g. not taking large quantities of food to work for a patient who would binge and vomit during breaks). Later, these goals included attempting to break the fast-binge-purge cycle by eating 3 planned meals, or by not purging after the binge had occurred. The patients were instructed to write down their goals in their diary. Progress on goals was reported at the beginning of the next meeting, and the group provided much support and encouragement for any successes reported, and for descriptions of difficulties encountered in attempting to meet goals. From the 5th group session on, the patients were instructed to develop and to write in their diaries rewards that they would provide themselves for successfully meeting their goals.

USF EDC Group: Educative-Cognitive Approaches

Handouts were distributed within the group and used as a guide for mini-lectures, group discussions and 'homework assignments'. Some of the most useful are described below. These handouts were modifications of those provided to us by *Judith Knight,* PhD, Decatur Hospital, Atlanta, Ga. For example, handout 1 (table II) was used to facilitate a discussion of the relapse process. This handout and the discussion drew heavily from the work of *Marlatt and Gordon* [9] on relapse prevention.

Then handout 2 (identical to handout 1, with certain points in the process highlighted) was utilized to discuss various points in the relapse process where the patients might attempt to interrupt the process. The patients were then given handout 3 (table III) for use as a homework assignment to be completed prior to the next session.

The completed handouts were then utilized for group discussion, which resulted in examples of high-risk situations being identified. Handout 4 (table IV) was then used for a homework assignment, and for future group discussions.

Particular attention was paid in the group sessions to highlighting the use of cognitive distortions (e.g. all-or-nothing thinking) as identified in discussions of the process of relapse, and in the patients' descriptions of their own relapses. The importance of cognitive disturbances and their management is

Table II

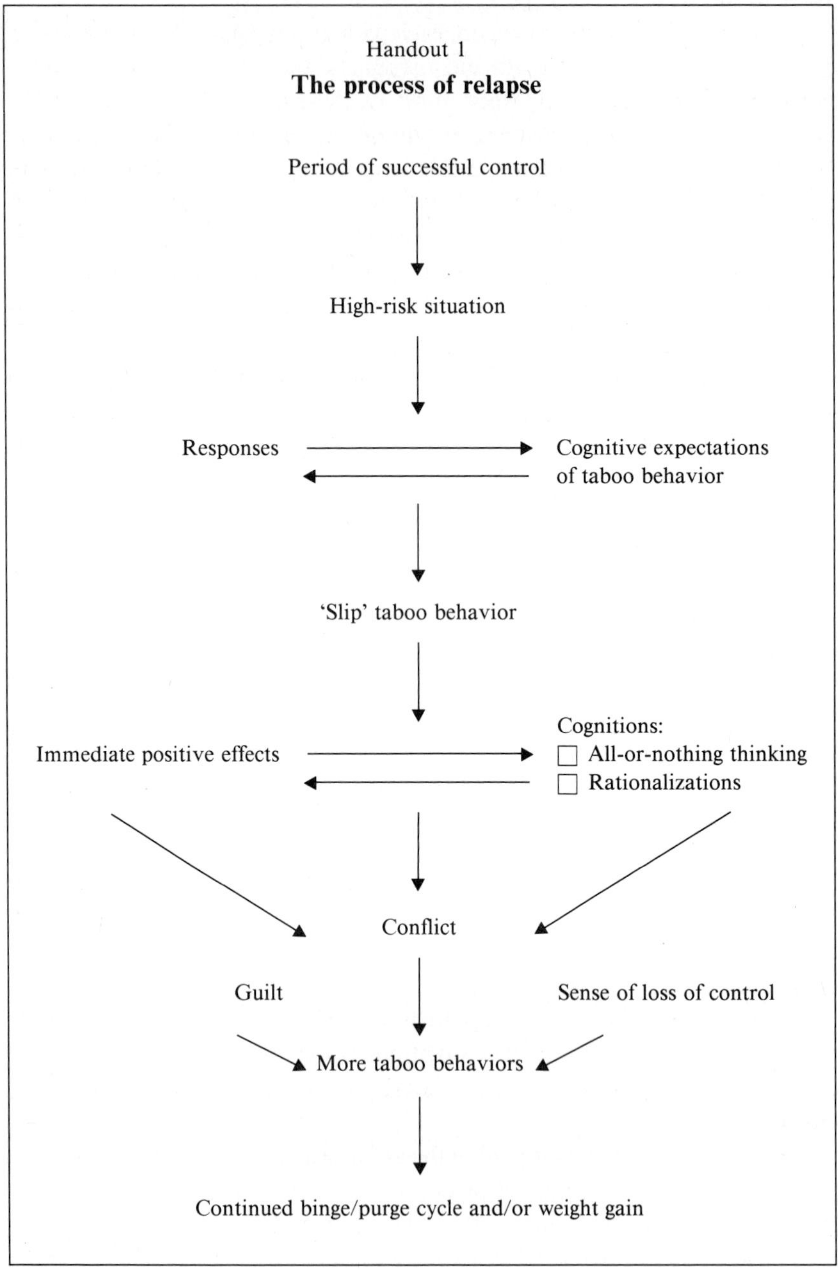
Handout 1
The process of relapse
Period of successful control
High-risk situation
Responses
Cognitive expectations of taboo behavior
'Slip' taboo behavior
Immediate positive effects
Cognitions:
All-or-nothing thinking
Rationalizations
Conflict
Guilt
Sense of loss of control
More taboo behaviors
Continued binge/purge cycle and/or weight gain

Table III

Handout 3

Your last relapse

A relapse is the resumption of a pattern of uncontrolled eating, with purging or fasting, *after* a period of successful control. That is, for a while you were able to maintain a reasonable weight without bingeing and purging, but then you started back with these behaviors. In this homework you will start to describe your most recent relapse.

1. When did your last relapse start, that is, when did you resume bingeing-purging or fasting after a period of control?

---

2. How long did the period of *control* (before the relapse) last?

---

3. How long did the period of *relapse* last? (If it is still going on, how long has it lasted as of now?)

The rest of the questions deal with the very beginning of this relapse – the first 'slip' – when you first strayed away from your period of control.

4. As best you can remember, what were the *behaviors* that changed when you first 'slipped'? (e.g. eating lots of sweets or other 'illegal' foods, stocking up on bingeing foods, purging (*vomiting or using laxatives,* etc.). Please be specific.

---

5. Where were you when the 'slip' occurred?

---

6. Who were you with?

---

7. How did you feel immediately before the 'slip'?

---

8. What were you thinking immediately before the 'slip'?

---

9. What were you doing when the slip occurred?

---

10. In general, what had changed in your life before the 'slip' occurred?

Table IV

Handout 4

Identifying your high-risk situations

This week we will ask you to try to determine the *high-risk situations* that pose the greatest threat to maintaining your weight control program.

In the space below, list those specific situations that give you most trouble (you may wish to review your eating diaries, descriptions of last relapse, etc.). Please be specific.

Feelings (for example, feeling depressed): __________

People: __________

Time of day: __________

Seasons: __________

Events (including social situations, types of dealings with people, etc.): __________

Places: __________

Day of week: __________

Day of month: __________

discussed in chapter 7. The patients became aware initially of other group members distortions and, later, of their own use of such cognitive distortions. They made appropriate comments as a part of group discussions. Nutrition information was provided via a nutritional review with the USF EDC nutritionist, as part of the patients' initial evaluations and the therapists would periodically review pertinent nutritional information, particularly when it was apparent that incorrect or distorted nutritional assumptions were being utilized by group members. For example, 1 of the members had combined her own private list of 'taboo' foods with the nutritional recommendations she had received from Weight Watchers, Int. She then spoke as if her taboo list had been provided by Weight Watchers.

USF EDC Group: Short-Term Dynamic Group Therapy Approaches

Group process comments, reflections and interpretations were utilized by the therapists. These were particularly effective for increasing the patients' awareness of their difficulties in interpersonal relationships with significant others. The process of termination, which quickly became important because of the time-limited nature of the group, had to be worked through in some detail. Particular attention was given to addressing the feelings of rejection and abandonment, their relationship to past events in the patients' lives, and the projection of anger onto the therapists (particularly the male therapist) that resulted.

USF EDC Group: Results

The group members developed a high degree of cohesion, extended their relationships outside the group via phone calls, and seemed to obtain a strong sense of relief, support and hope from learning that others shared their problems and feelings. All members attended all sessions. The patients were quite punctual, except for 1 patient who was habitually late especially as termination approached. From virtually the first session, they actively supported and reinforced efforts toward control of eating symptoms. It was much more difficult initially for the group members to offer such support and encouragement for each others' efforts regarding difficulties in interpersonal relationships. This was especially so where strong dysphoric affects, or any potential for confrontation was involved. There was an initial group collusion to avoid attaching any significance to emotional difficulties other than those directly related to bulimia. However, this was gradually replaced by an ability to label such significant emotional difficulties in others, and eventually in themselves. Also, the patients had great difficulty with cooperating in any way

Table V. General principles for the use of group therapy in bulimia

Multidimensional approach, including behavioral, educative-cognitive, and insight-oriented methods
Significant structure, especially in early phases
Concomitant alcohol abuse lowers effectiveness
History of anorexia nervosa and/or major character pathology pose special problems; percentage in any group should be limited

with the concepts of rewards. For example, not a single group member 'remembered' to buy the gift certificates, even after repeated reminders by the therapists. Similarly, when we discussed their developing self-rewards for attaining their weekly goals, only 1 member could 'think' of any reward she could provide herself. When, with much assistance, they were able to do so, they would consistently forget what it was, or forget to give it to themselves.

There was a marked decrease in bingeing and purging in all patients by the 4th to 6th group session. However, this was accompanied by an increase in dysphoric symptoms which, in 3 of the patients, were in the range of frank depression, with 1 patient making a suicide attempt (this was handled primarily by the patient's individual therapist, who was not one of the group therapists, and hospitalization was not necessary). The group, while shaken by this event, was able to offer much support and encouragement to the patient, and she was able to attend all group sessions. All but 1 of the patients appeared to handle the difficult termination process successfully. Information about a local self-help group was distributed for those interested, and a 6-month follow-up session was scheduled.

Recommendations

Based on our own experience, and that of others outlined above, we believe that group therapy approaches offer much promise in the treatment of patients with bulimia. Such approaches may be employed as the principle therapeutic tool, or as a significant adjunct to other treatment programs. They may also be very helpful to some patients in serving as a bridge to their acceptance of more intensive forms of therapy (e.g. hospitalization, intensive psychotherapy) that may have been previously unacceptable.

Attention to the principles highlighted in table V is appropriate, given the experience to date. First, a multidimensional approach utilizing behavioral, cognitive-educative and insight-oriented approaches appears to be of greatest utility. It is striking to note that therapists who began strongly emphasizing one of these approaches found themselves increasing the use of the others. Second, a fairly high degree of structure appears to be very helpful. This is especially true as regards attendance and other expectations of the patients, payment in advance, use of diaries and dietary prescriptions. This structure is quite helpful to patients especially in the early stages of treatment. Third, patients with a history of past or present excessive use of alcohol have a poor prognosis, both in being able to complete the treatment program, and in success in controlling or eliminating eating symptoms. Future group therapy efforts need to begin to address systematically how to meet better the needs of such patients. Fourth, patients with a past history of anorexia nervosa, and/or significant character pathology, also have a somewhat guarded prognosis, and additional knowledge about how to meet their needs is needed. The number of such patients in any given therapy group should be limited to a small percentage of the total membership.

References

1 Boskind-Lodahl, M.; White, W.: The definition and treatment of bulimarexia in college women – a pilot study. J. Am. Coll. Hlth Ass. *27:* 84–97 (1978).
2 Boskind-Lodahl, M.: Cinderella's stepsisters: a feminist perspective on anorexia nervosa and bulimia. Signs. J. Women Culture Soc. *2:* 342–356 (1976).
3 Dixon, K.; Kiecolt-Glaser, J.: An integrated group therapy approach to bulimia. Proc. 134th Annu. Meet. Am. Psychiat. Ass., New Orleans 1981.
4 Roy-Byrne, P.; Lee-Benner, K.; Yager, J.: Group therapy for bulimia: a year's experience. Int. J. Eating Disord. *2:* 97–116 (1984).
5 Lacey, J.: Bulimia nervosa, binge-eating, and psychogenic vomiting: a controlled treatment study and long-term outcome. Br. med. J. *286:* 1609–1613 (1983).
6 Russell, G.: Bulimia nervosa: an ominous variant of anorexia nervosa. Psychol. Med. *9:* 429–448 (1979).
7 Feighner, J.; Robins, E.; Guze, S.; Woodruff, R.; Winokur, G.; Munoz, R.: Diagnostic criteria for use in psychiatric research. Archs gen. Psychiat. *26:* 57–63 (1972).
8 Crisp, A.: Anorexia nervosa. Hosp. Med. *1:* 713–718 (1967).
9 Marlatt, G.; Gordon, J.: Relapse prevention (Guilford Press, New York 1983).

17 Support Groups for Eating Disorder Patients

Sharon Glick Miller, Henry P. Powers

Introduction

Until recently, the fabric of society was naturally replete with support groups to whom a troubled individual might turn. Advice, help, or support was found in the immediate family, the extended family, the leaders of the church, or the leaders of the neighborhood.

Support groups are still needed, and still exist. The difference is that while most former support groups were based on ethnicity or religion, most current support groups are organized around a common problem. There are support groups for the victim of a problem (e.g. medical, psychological or social), or for the family of the victim of a problem. *Stokes* [1] sees 'mutual aid support systems as the fastest growing means of providing human service in many countries'. He estimates that 5 million people in the USA alone belong to a support group for a particular psychological problem or health issue.

In this chapter we will review the use of support groups for individuals with anorexia nervosa and bulimia. The national associations which organize or authorize these groups will be reviewed and an ideal structure for a support group will be proposed. Issues for the therapist working with a member of a support group will also be identified.

Definition

The professional literature provides no working definition of a support group. One definition of a support system that is often cited is: 'Support system implies an enduring pattern of continuous or intermittent ties that play a significant part in maintaining the psychological and physical integrity of the individual over time' [2, p. 41].

We define a support group as the gathering of individuals who, sharing a common problem, work together towards increased understanding of the problem and its consequences, while offering each other empathy and help.

In the absence of any differential definition, we will use the terms 'support group' and 'self-help group' interchangeably.

To this date, we know of no citations in the literature about the role of the support group for the individual with anorexia nervosa or bulimia. References are made, however, to the national associations which sponsor the development of self-help groups for anorexia nervosa and bulimia. There has been no controlled study of those who seek out a support group and those who do not. *Lieberman and Borman* [3] suggest that those who attend support groups are generally those who also use professional services.

Impact of a Support Group

Many individuals with eating disorders not only face the problem of the disorder, but also their sense of failure at not meeting society's standards of normality. They may feel inadequate, guilty, unsure of who they are, angry and alone. Participation in a support group combats feelings of being alone with the problem. Further, it destigmatizes the label of 'anorectic' or 'bulimic'. The issue being detoxified for the group members, they will then often direct their energy to ensuring that the public or physicians are more informed about the illness.

By being involved in a support group, members may begin to feel that they are contributing something to the group. There are many activities in which they can participate which foster this feeling (e.g. developing a newsletter or participating on committees). Through this involvement, feelings of self-worth and independence are enhanced. Friendships formed within the group are often continued outside of it, still founded on mutual support and understanding. This increase in social connectedness is especially important for individuals with anorexia nervosa, many of whom come from enmeshed, socially isolated family systems.

Families: A Natural Support Group

Although today we tend to think of support groups as sponsored by an association or organization, it should be remembered that natural support groups still exist. Families are made up of individuals with a shared history, culture and affective involvement. In a well-functioning family, members can offer empathy, help in understanding a situation, or help in mastering a problem. When another member is seen to be grappling with a crisis they may encourage attempts to seek and accept appropriate help.

The potential of the family as a support system for the individual patient is worthy of consideration. Involvement of spouses in the treatment of individual patients with persistent psychiatric disorders has been suggested to be superior to individual therapy [4]. In a randomized controlled study, care involving the support of the family was seen as superior to individual supportive care in the management of schizophrenia [5]. Initial data from a program aimed at involving families in the management of their schizophrenic offspring also suggest the merit of such an approach [6].

The family can be mobilized to be more supportive if provided information about the patient's illness. As their understanding of the patient's symptoms and problems become more accurate, there will be a reduction in their own feelings of guilt over the possible cause of the condition, or anger at the patient for being unable to control the symptoms through the exercise of will. Further, the family can be guided in responding supportively, without attacking the patient. Patient and family may then be free to work together toward agreed upon goals. With dysfunctional families, a therapist may need to intervene to move the family away from a destructive mode to one that is more constructive, dealing perhaps with long-standing marital discord, or other issues that discourage individuation of the identified patient.

Associations which Organize Support Groups

This section will review seven local and national associations which organize support groups. The groups were chosen because of their well-publicized nature. Information was obtained by means of a structured interview by telephone, and addressed issues of definition, purpose, structure and leadership.

Associations Reviewed

The seven organizations contacted along with their addresses are listed in table I. Two organizations (AABA and ANAD) have a strong national base. The others are local or regional, but will send information to those interested in starting a group outside of their area.

Definition

There was a general absence of a clear definition of a support group. All use the term 'support group' and 'self-help group' interchangeably. All define a support group as an adjunct to psychological or psychiatric treatment.

These organizations all know what anorexia nervosa is. They know what bulimia is. They know how to organize groups, although one form may be favored over another. They know the value of therapy, of psychiatric, psychological or social work help. They have read extensively in the area of eating disorders. Therefore, it came as a surprise that not one of them has a working definition, in clear, concise and consistent terms, of what a support group is, such as the one we present earlier in this chapter. They tried to define a support group by what it *does,* rather than by what it *is.* Sample comments were: 'It is an ongoing process where people can come and go, to learn and demystify the illness'; 'Problems can be shared'; 'The causes and treatment of the illness are examined'; 'Anything that isn't a therapy group'.

Purpose

All saw referral to appropriate resources as a fundamental purpose of the group. One organization identified that as its only purpose, while another added motivating individuals to seek help. Education was cited as a purpose by four organizations; this referred to the dissemination of information to group members and/or the group's sponsorship of educational programs for the community. One organization also sponsored research. Only three defined their purpose as mutual support. It is interesting to note that another two, although seeing themselves as adjuncts to therapy, define their purpose in a way that sounds like therapeutic goals (e.g. 'peer confrontation', 'change thinking', 'working on relationships and social skills').

Table I

American Anorexia/Bulimia Association Inc. (AABA), 133 Cedar Lane, Teaneck, NJ 07666 (USA).
National Association of Anorexia Nervosa and Associated Disorders (ANAD), Box 271, Highland Park, IL 60035 (USA).
National Anorexic Aid Society (NAAS), PO Box 29461, Columbus, OH 43229 (USA).
Anorexia Nervosa and Related Eating Disorders (ANRED), PO Box 5102, Eugene, OR 97405 (USA).
Bulimia Anorexia Nervosa Foundation Association (BANFA), 3211 Nassau Street, Everett, WA 98201 (USA).
Anorexia Nervosa Aid Society (ANAS), Box 213, Lincoln Center, MA 01773 (USA).
Bulimia Anorexia Self Help (BASH), 621 S. New Ballas, Suite 6005, Tower B, St. Louis, MO 63141 (USA).

Group Structure

Generally, meetings are held weekly or every other week. While most groups consist of 10–15 members, some organizations have large meetings attended by 25–100 people. For the latter, the structure consists of a presentation to the large group, followed by discussion in smaller groups of 15–20.

Most do not charge any fee. One seeks voluntary donations, another charges an annual fee of $ 50.00 and another charges $ 100.00. Most organizations call those who direct groups 'facilitators'. These individuals are usually responsible for leading all groups, but their background and level of expertise in group process varies. Two organizations have leadership training workshops. The various organizations differ somewhat in their philosophies of leadership. Generally, they use some combination of professionals and recovered/recovering patients. However, some use only professionals while others exclude professionals.

The facilitators, both professional and non-professional, are usually screened and chosen by the leaders (i.e. founders or directors) of the organizations. Professionals are chosen for their knowledge of eating disorders, and for their willingness to volunteer their services; in some cases, they are employed by the organization. Non-professionals are chosen for their knowledge of eating disorders, but other factors are also considered. For example, one organization wants its patient facilitators to have had a minimum of 3 years in personal therapy. Another group considers the relationship capacity of potential facilitators, as well as how they have handled their own eating problems. One agency director interviews potential facilitators over lunch, in order to observe how they control their own eating behavior. Two organizations (BASH and ANAS) have training workshops for would-be facilitators.

Consultation

Most organizations use professionals as consultants who support and advise the group facilitator. They are usually unpaid. Some use their own more experienced leaders as consultants. Meetings between consultants and facilitators may take place weekly or twice monthly depending on the frequency of support group meetings. Professionals may also be used as consultants in a more general sense. For example, two national associations identify a professional in each chapter meeting who will have some input into policy decisions. Consultants may or may not be invited to group meetings, depending on the philosophy of each organization.

Dissemination of Information

The fundamental importance given to the dissemination of information is reflected in the fact that six of the associations publish a newsletter and one publishes a pamphlet. They provide information about meeting times and locations, new publications on the subject of eating disorders, new research findings and case histories or personal vignettes.

Most of the organizations are readily accessible by telephone and several have hotlines. They are conscientious about spending time with individuals with the illness, concerned friends or relatives and interested professionals. They also fill requests for information that are received by mail.

Regional and National Groups

Some groups have chosen to remain centered regionally, and others have chosen to expand nationally. BANFA, for example, is centered in Everett, Washington. NAAS is primarily contained in one center in Columbus, Ohio, but maintains a national directory of support groups, and these are listed in their newsletter. AABA helps to organize support groups (ten, at this writing) in different parts of the country, and there is a highly organized central control factor in that an AABA representative visits these local groups periodically to monitor their progress. ANAD has groups in 40 states and Canada. Organizations such as NAAS and ANRED do not monitor or administer groups outside their central area but, instead, encourage the outlying groups to become autonomous.

Proposed Ideal Structure of a Support Group

The quality of support groups varies greatly from one group to another. We have identified nine factors which appear to be important determinants (table II).

A support group is not a therapy group and as such, it would be inappropriate for a therapist to lead it. This does not mean, however, that it would be inappropriate to have a trained facilitator as the group leader. There is more to facilitating group process than initially apparent. One becomes keenly appreciative of the skill when observing one group led by a trained facilitator and another led by a well-intentioned, but untrained, individual. The trained facilitator promotes group cohesion, points out the common ground among members and seeks out empathic help. When appropriate, a weak message is amplified or a strong reaction is diffused. The facilitator also

Table II. Proposed ideal structure of a support group

1	The group is led by a facilitator with some expertise in leading groups
2	The purpose of the group is clearly stated
3	The facilitator receives consultation from a professional with experience in treating eating disorders
4	The group is an adjunct to therapy
5	Confidentiality is observed
6	The group promotes mutual aid
7	The group is concerned with issues of dissemination of information and education
8	A regular opportunity is provided for group members to provide feedback on the effectiveness and direction of the group
9	The group maintains a good relationship with the treatment facilities in its area

deals with obstacles to the group's purpose, and gently, but effectively, contains the member who is monopolizing or disrupting the group.

There are several resources for finding a trained facilitator who will not lead a support group as a therapy group, or have a conflict of interest with respect to private practice. For example, mental health counselors affiliated with a community agency are appropriately skilled and are often interested in such a task.

The role of the facilitator is clearly defined as being neutral and having no vested interests. He or she is there solely to facilitate group process and help the group work toward its goals. Should an individual who has recovered from the illness be used as a facilitator, the potential difficulty in objectivity needs to be carefully considered; for example, the facilitator may inappropriately feel responsible for showing others the way to recovery. Further, since the desire to facilitate the group may be a further attempt at mastery of the issues, the experience may prove too stressful (we have witnessed the relapse of one such facilitator). The use of co-facilitators (one recovered patient and one professional) may be considered as an alternative.

Attention must also be given to quality control. Those national self-help organizations which have representatives observing member groups from time to time are commended. Quality can be further enhanced by regular consultation from a professional with experience in treating eating disorders. The process of consultation encourages the facilitator to observe and think about the direction of the group. The consultant can answer questions specific to the eating disorders, and can ensure that the pathology of group members is not inadvertently being supported by the group process. Further, an evaluative component should exist, whereby feedback is sought from members about the effectiveness and direction of the group.

The self-help group should identify itself as an adjunct to therapy, and not a replacement for therapy. Any members who present with symptomatology, and who are also not in treatment, should be helped by the facilitator and the group to enter treatment. The facilitator and other group members can underline the prescribed role of the support group and the need for treatment, identify treatment resources, facilitate access to these resources and follow-up on the recommendation that treatment be sought.

The self-help group should have clearly stated goals. Again, because the group is not a treatment group, weigh-ins or behavioral charting would be inappropriate. One goal of the group is to promote mutual aid among members so that they do not feel alone with the problem. This is achieved through their empathic support of each other and their work together on common projects that will help them become better informed about the illness, and may result in the dissemination of information to those less informed, both lay and professional.

Finally, the effective liaison between the support group and the eating disorder treatment facilities in its area will facilitate the appropriate referral of patients to the group. Further, a mutual understanding and respect of the specific role each has to play will maximally benefit the eating disorder patient and prevent any inadvertent adversarial relationship.

Issues for the Therapist: When to Support a Support Group

Before referring a patient to a support group, the therapist must consider both the needs of the patient and the quality of the group. Most patients will benefit from the social support offered by the group. However, there are contraindications which are patient-specific. For example, some patients feel worse hearing others talk of their dilemma. Similarly, support groups are not of uniform quality. The therapist needs to be assured of the quality of the leadership, and the appropriateness of the group's goals. There should not be an inadvertent reinforcement of pathological issues. Sessions should not focus on weight or food, and should not foster an exchange of 'techniques'. The group should also not foster an antimedical or antitreatment stance, or the patient will be caught in a split between treatment and support facility.

The therapist of an eating disorder patient in a support group must remain vigilant to the potential split between group and therapist. The therapist must delicately handle the patient's presentation of information from the support group with which he or she disagrees. For example, one anorectic mentioned in her support group that she would begin to supplement her diet with Sustacal as a beginning attempt to deal with her severe weight loss. The group discouraged this, saying that it was a false solution, the real issue being to gain and maintain weight on 'real' food. Hearing this, the therapist had to bear in mind that the report may not have been an accurate representation of what occurred. The source of the issue (group or patient) was less important than dealing with the issue for the patient without creating a split between group and therapist. The therapist identified the 'all-or-none' thinking of both the support group and the patient (either one is eating entirely normally or one is still completely ill) that was now being raised around the issue of taking a food supplement. The therapist then helped the patient focus on her own reluctance to take intermediate steps forward.

Conclusion

Support groups can play an important role in the rehabilitation of eating disorder patients. They provide a place and an opportunity for anorectic and bulimic patients and their families to come together, not only to comfort each other and to demonstrate that they are not alone, but also to encourage and help the patients to seek psychotherapy. Support groups are not appropriate for all patients and are not of uniform quality. Therapists working with eating disorder patients should be knowledgeable of what is available locally and attend to the possibility of a split arising between therapist and support group. Several local and national organizations help by providing both didactic and statistical material, as well as specific referral resources.

References

1 Stokes, B.: Helping ourselves: local solutions to global problems (Norton, New York 1981).

2 Killilea, M.: Mutual help organizations: interpretations in the literature; in Caplan, Killilea, Support systems and mutual help: multidisciplinary explorations, pp. 37–93 (Grune & Stratton, New York 1976).

3 Lieberman, M.; Borman, L.: Self-help groups for coping with crisis (Jossey-Bass, San Francisco 1979).

4 Hafner, R.; Badenoch, A.; Fisher, J.; Swift, M.: Spouse aided individual therapy in persisting psychiatric disorders: a systemic comparison. Family Process *22:* 385–400 (1983).

5 Faloon, I.; Boyd, J.; McGill, C.; Razani, J.; Moss, H.; Gilderman, A.: Family management in the prevention of exacerbations of schizophrenia: a controlled study. New Engl. J. Med. *306:* 1437–1440 (1982).

6 Anderson, C.; Hagarty, G.; Reiss, D.: Family treatment of adult schizophrenic patients: a psycho-educational approach. Schizophrenic Bull. *6:* 490–505 (1980).

Appendix

EATING DISORDERS QUESTIONNAIRE

UNIVERSITY OF SOUTH FLORIDA
DEPARTMENT OF PSYCHIATRY AND BEHAVIORAL MEDICINE
COLLEGE OF MEDICINE

This questionnaire covers several eating problems that may or may not apply to you. You may find it difficult to answer some questions if your eating pattern is irregular or has changed recently. Please read each question carefully and choose the answer that BEST describes your situation MOST OF THE TIME.

Also, please feel free to write remarks in the margins or on the back of the questionnaire if this will clarify your answer. Please PRINT or WRITE LEGIBLY.

This information will be kept STRICTLY CONFIDENTIAL. Thank you for your cooperation.

IDENTIFYING DATA

Today's Date: ____________________

Name: ______________________________________
(last) (first) (initial)

Social Security #: ____________ Sex: ______ Age: ______ Date of Birth: ____________

Home Address: ______________________________________

Home Telephone: ____________________ Work Telephone ____________________

(FOR OFFICE USE ONLY) Date Sent Out: ____________ Date Received: ____________

Part I. WEIGHT HISTORY

1. Birth Weight: _________ lbs. _________ oz.

2. Current Weight: _________ lbs.

3. Height: _________ feet _________ inches

4. How would you describe your present weight? (check one)
   _____ Very underweight
   _____ Slightly underweight
   _____ About average
   _____ Slightly overweight
   _____ Very overweight

5. At what weight have you felt your best, or at what weight do you think you would feel your best?
   __________ lbs.

6. At the present time, I want to: (check one)
   _____ Lose weight
   _____ Gain weight
   _____ Maintain my current weight

7. How satisfied are you with the way you look at your present weight?
   _____ Completely satisfied
   _____ Moderately satisfied
   _____ Neutral
   _____ Moderately dissatisfied
   _____ Very dissatisfied

8. At your present height, what is your *lowest* weight ever?
   __________ lbs.

9. At your present height, what is your *greatest* weight ever?
   __________ lbs.

10. Have you had a time at your current height when you lost weight?
    _____ No If no, please skip to Item 14
    _____ Yes
    If yes, how much weight was lost?
    From __________ lbs. to __________ lbs.

    Did you then gain weight?
    _____ No
    _____ Yes If "yes", how many pounds?
    __________ lbs.

11. Did you lose weight again?
______ No If "no", please skip to Item #14.
______ Yes If "yes", at what age?
______ years

How much weight was lost?
From __________ lbs. to __________ lbs.

Did you then gain weight?
______ No
______ Yes If "yes", how many pounds?
__________ lbs.

13. Have there been additional episodes of weight loss?
______ No
______ Yes

14. Over the last six months, I have (check ONE):
______ Lost 10 or more pounds
______ Gained 10 or more pounds
______ Both of the above
______ Neither of the above

15. Did you try to diet the first time you lost weight?
______ No
______ Yes If "yes", what led you to diet? (check ONE)
______ It was a voluntary decision.
______ Encouragement from family members
______ Insults or negative pressure from family members
______ Encouragement from friends
______ Negative pressure from friends
______ Other reason (specify): ____________________

16. Do you try to diet now?
______ No
______ Yes

17. My appetite is (check ONE):
______ Poor
______ Good
______ Good, but I am afraid of losing control.

18. What do you estimate your daily caloric intake to be?
__________ calories per day

19. Please complete the following Weight Record, being as specific as possible.

AGE RANGE	WEIGHT	WERE YOU . . . 1=Underweight 2=Normal Weight 3=Overweight (Circle one)			DURING THIS PERIOD, DID YOU TRY TO LOSE WEIGHT? (Circle one)		BELOW, PLEASE LIST ANY SIGNIFICANT EVENTS IN YOUR LIFE THAT YOU THINK WERE RELEVANT TO YOUR WEIGHT AT THAT TIME
0-1	______	1	2	3	No	Yes	______
1-2	______	1	2	3	No	Yes	______
3-5	______	1	2	3	No	Yes	______
6-9	______	1	2	3	No	Yes	______
10-15	______	1	2	3	No	Yes	______
16-20	______	1	2	3	No	Yes	______
20-25	______	1	2	3	No	Yes	______
25-30	______	1	2	3	No	Yes	______
30-40	______	1	2	3	No	Yes	______
40-50	______	1	2	3	No	Yes	______
50-60	______	1	2	3	No	Yes	______
60+	______	1	2	3	No	Yes	______

20. On the chart below, please describe a typical day's food intake. Be as specific as possible. Include all meals and snacks. Use the back if you need more room. For example:

7:30 a.m.	Breakfast	1 bowl cereal 1 8-oz. glass whole milk 2 slices bacon 1 cup black coffee

Approximate Time of Day	Which Meal?	Foods Eaten and Portion Sizes
______	______	______ ______ ______
______	______	______ ______ ______
______	______	______ ______ ______
______	______	______ ______ ______

21. How does your weight affect your daily activities?
    ______ It has no effect.
    ______ It has some effect.
    ______ It often interferes.
    ______ It has an extreme effect.

22. How physically active are you?
    ______ Very active
    ______ Active
    ______ Average
    ______ Inactive
    ______ Very inactive

23. What do you do for physical exercise and how often do you do it? (Check ALL that apply)

	1 hour/week or Less	Between 2 & 6 hours/week	7 hours/week or More
Jogging/Running	______	______	______
Swimming	______	______	______
Dancing/Aerobics	______	______	______
Walking	______	______	______
Calisthenics (situps, kneebends)	______	______	______
Other Sports (specify: ______________)	______	______	______

Most of the questions below relate to food or eating, although some other types of questions have been included. Please place an (x) under the column which best applies to each statement. Please answer each question carefully.

	Always	Very often	Often	Sometimes	Rarely	Never	
24.	( )	( )	( )	( )	( )	( )	Like eating with other people.
25.	( )	( )	( )	( )	( )	( )	Prepare food for others, but do not eat what cook.
26.	( )	( )	( )	( )	( )	( )	Become anxious prior to eating.
27.	( )	( )	( )	( )	( )	( )	Am terrified about being overweight.
28.	( )	( )	( )	( )	( )	( )	Avoid eating when I am hungry.
29.	( )	( )	( )	( )	( )	( )	Find myself preoccupied with food.
30.	( )	( )	( )	( )	( )	( )	Have gone on eating binges where I feel that I may not be able to stop.
31.	( )	( )	( )	( )	( )	( )	Cut my food into small pieces.
32.	( )	( )	( )	( )	( )	( )	Am aware of the calorie content of the foods that I eat.
33.	( )	( )	( )	( )	( )	( )	Particularly avoid foods with a high carbohydrate content (bread, potatoes, rice, etc.).
34.	( )	( )	( )	( )	( )	( )	Feel bloated after meals.
35.	( )	( )	( )	( )	( )	( )	Feel that others would prefer if I ate more.
36.	( )	( )	( )	( )	( )	( )	Vomit after I have eaten.
37.	( )	( )	( )	( )	( )	( )	Feel extremely guilty after eating.
38.	( )	( )	( )	( )	( )	( )	Am preoccupied with a desire to be thinner.
39.	( )	( )	( )	( )	( )	( )	Exercise strenuously to burn off calories.
40.	( )	( )	( )	( )	( )	( )	Weigh myself several times a day.
41.	( )	( )	( )	( )	( )	( )	Like my clothes to fit tightly.
42.	( )	( )	( )	( )	( )	( )	Enjoy eating meat.
43.	( )	( )	( )	( )	( )	( )	Wake up early in the morning.
44.	( )	( )	( )	( )	( )	( )	Eat the same foods day after day.
45.	( )	( )	( )	( )	( )	( )	Think about burning up calories when I exercise.
46.	( )	( )	( )	( )	( )	( )	Have regular menstrual periods. (Males SKIP.)
47.	( )	( )	( )	( )	( )	( )	Other people think that I am too thin.
48.	( )	( )	( )	( )	( )	( )	Am too preoccupied with the thought of having fat on my body.
49.	( )	( )	( )	( )	( )	( )	Take longer than others to eat my meals.
50.	( )	( )	( )	( )	( )	( )	Enjoy eating at restaurants.
51.	( )	( )	( )	( )	( )	( )	Take laxatives.
52.	( )	( )	( )	( )	( )	( )	Avoid foods with sugar in them.
53.	( )	( )	( )	( )	( )	( )	Eat diet foods.
54.	( )	( )	( )	( )	( )	( )	Feel that food controls my life.
55.	( )	( )	( )	( )	( )	( )	Display self-control around food.
56.	( )	( )	( )	( )	( )	( )	Feel that others pressure me to eat.
57.	( )	( )	( )	( )	( )	( )	Give too much time and thought to food.
58.	( )	( )	( )	( )	( )	( )	Suffer from constipation.
59.	( )	( )	( )	( )	( )	( )	Feel uncomfortable after eating sweets.
60.	( )	( )	( )	( )	( )	( )	Engage in dieting behavior.
61.	( )	( )	( )	( )	( )	( )	Like for my stomach to be empty.
62.	( )	( )	( )	( )	( )	( )	Enjoy trying new rich foods.
63.	( )	( )	( )	( )	( )	( )	Have the impulse to vomit after meals.
64.	( )	( )	( )	( )	( )	( )	Am very active and industrious.
65.	( )	( )	( )	( )	( )	( )	Sleep very well.
66.	( )	( )	( )	( )	( )	( )	Pretend to eat food that I have hidden or thrown away.
67.	( )	( )	( )	( )	( )	( )	Take diuretics.

Questions 24-64 are the Eating Attitudes Test (EAT) designed by Garner and Garfinkel and used by permission. Garner DM, Garfinkel PE: The Eating Attitudes Test: An Index of the Symptoms of Anorexia Nervosa. Psychol Med 9:273-279, 1979.

Part II. BINGE EATING

1. Do you ever have "eating binges"—that is, episodes of impulsively eating large amounts of food within a short period of time?
   _____ Yes
   _____ Yes, in the past, but not now
   _____ No, never
   If "no", skip to Part III, MEDICAL HISTORY

2. When did you have your last binge?
   ____

3. During your last binge, what did you eat? Please be as specific as possible, including approximate amounts.
   ____
   ____
   ____
   ____

4. About how long did this binge last?
   Specify number of _____ hours or _____ minutes.

5. What do you think triggered this binge?
   ____
   ____
   ____
   ____

6. How often do your binges occur?
   _____ Several times a day
   _____ Once a day
   _____ At least once a week
   _____ A few times a month
   _____ Once a month or less

7. How long does a typical binge last?
   Specify number of _____ hours or _____ minutes.

Please answer the next three questions by circling the number that best describes your binges:

(1) ALWAYS (2) OFTEN (3) SOMETIMES (4) RARELY (0) NEVER

8.	1	2	3	4	0	During a binge, I eat a large amount of food.
9.	1	2	3	4	0	During a binge, I eat very rapidly.
10.	1	2	3	4	0	During a binge, I feel I can't stop—out of control.

11. A variety of foods are listed below. For each type of food, please circle the number that best describes your eating patterns.

BINGE	NON-BINGE	BOTH	TYPE OF FOOD
1	2	3	Bread, cereal, pasta
1	2	3	Cheese, milk, yogurt
1	2	3	Fruit and fruit juices
1	2	3	Meat, fish, poultry, eggs
1	2	3	Salty snack foods
1	2	3	Sweets or "desserts"
1	2	3	Vegetables
1	2	3	Soft drinks
1	2	3	Restaurant "fast foods" (Burger King, MacDonalds, Dairy Queen, etc.)
1	2	3	"Formula" drinks (protein powders, Instant Breakfast, etc.)

12. About how many calories do you consume in a typical binge?
_________ calories

13. About how much money would you estimate that you spend on the food that is consumed in a typical binge?
$_________

14. How old were you when you first started binge eating?
_________ years

15. How long have you had a problem with binge eating?
Specify number of _____ years, _____ months, or _____ weeks

16. What times are you most likely to binge? (Check ALL THAT APPLY)
_____ Morning (7:00 am. till 12:00 noon)
_____ Afternoon (12:00 noon till 5:00 p.m.)
_____ Evening (5:00 p.m. till 10:00 p.m.)
_____ Night (after 10:00 p.m.)
_____ Weekends
_____ Varies

17. Which one of the following statements best applies to your binge eating?
_____ I eat until I have had enough to satisfy me.
_____ I eat until my stomach feels full.
_____ I eat until my stomach hurts.
_____ I eat until I can't eat any more.

18. How concerned are you about your binge eating?
_____ I am not bothered at all.
_____ It bothers me a little.
_____ I am moderately concerned about it.
_____ It is one of my major concerns.

19. Which one of the following statements best applies to your binge eating?
_____ I am always alone when I binge.
_____ Sometimes I am alone and sometimes I am with others when I binge.
_____ I only binge with others.

The following questions describe a variety of feelings that some people experience during a binge or after a binge. Please answer by circling the answer that best describes your feelings:

20. DURING a binge, I feel. . .

Calm	YES	NO
Helpless	YES	NO
Stimulated	YES	NO
Excited	YES	NO
Angry	YES	NO
"Spaced Out", Dazed	YES	NO
Disgusted	YES	NO
Energized	YES	NO
Secure	YES	NO
Panicked	YES	NO
Relieved	YES	NO
Guilty	YES	NO
Ashamed	YES	NO
Afraid	YES	NO
Euphoric or "High"	YES	NO
Lonely	YES	NO
Depressed	YES	NO

Any other feelings: ______________

____

21. AFTER a binge, I feel. . .

Calm	YES	NO
Helpless	YES	NO
Stimulated	YES	NO
Excited	YES	NO
Angry	YES	NO
"Spaced Out", Dazed	YES	NO
Disgusted	YES	NO
Energized	YES	NO
Secure	YES	NO
Panicked	YES	NO
Relieved	YES	NO
Guilty	YES	NO
Ashamed	YES	NO
Afraid	YES	NO
Euphoric or "High"	YES	NO
Lonely	YES	NO
Depressed	YES	NO

Any other feelings: ______________

____

22. What kinds of feelings or events might start a binge episode? Have you noticed any pattern to your binge eating?

____

____

____

____

23. What makes you stop the binge?

____

____

____

____

24. Why do you think you started binge-eating in the first place?

____

____

____

____

Part IIB. PURGING

25. Have you ever induced yourself to vomit, or have you ever thrown up after a binge?
______ Yes, I used to, but I don't now
______ Yes, I do now
______ No, never

If you answered "yes" above, answer Question #25a.
If you answered "no", go to Question #25b.

25a. When was the first time you induced vomiting?
Specify number of ______ months, ______ weeks, or ______ days ago
. . . then skip to Question #26.

25b. Have you ever been tempted to induce vomiting?
______ Yes, very much so
______ Yes, somewhat
______ No, never
. . . then skip to Question #34.

26. How often do you induce vomiting?
______ More than once a day
______ Daily
______ At least once a week
______ A few times a month
______ Once a month or less

27. How old were you when you induced vomiting for the first time?
______ years old

28. How long have you been vomiting in this way?
Specify number of ______ years, ______ months, or ______ weeks

29. How do you usually get yourself to throw up?

____

____

30. Since you first began inducing vomiting, has it become harder or easier?
______ Harder
______ Easier
______ No real change

31. Do you remember why you did this originally? Please explain.

____

____

32. How concerned are you about your vomiting?
    ______ I am not bothered at all.
    ______ It bothers me a little.
    ______ I am moderately concerned about it.
    ______ It is one of my major concerns.

33. Please check ALL of the following choices that describe how you feel AFTER you have purged, by vomiting, for weight control:

    ______ Calm
    ______ Helpless
    ______ Stimulated
    ______ Excited
    ______ Angry
    ______ "Spaced Out" or Dazed
    ______ Disgusted
    ______ Energized
    ______ Secure
    ______ Panicked
    ______ Relieved
    ______ Guilty
    ______ Ashamed
    ______ Afraid
    ______ Euphoric or "High"
    ______ Lonely
    ______ Depressed
    Other: ______________________________

34. Have you ever used laxatives to control your weight or "get rid of food"?
    ______ Yes, I used to, but I don't now.
    ______ Yes, I do now.
    ______ No, never.

If you answered "yes" above, answer Question **#34a**.
If you answered "no", go to Question #34b.

34a. When was the last time you took laxatives for weight control?
Specify number of ______ months, ______ weeks, or ______ days ago
. . .then skip to Question #35.

34b. Have you ever been tempted to use laxatives for weight control?
    ______ Yes, very much so
    ______ Yes, somewhat
    ______ No, never
If "no", please skip to Part III, "MEDICAL HISTORY".

35. How often do you use laxatives for weight control?
    ______ More than once a day
    ______ Daily
    ______ At least once a week
    ______ A few times a month
    ______ Once a month or less

36. How old were you when you first took laxatives for weight control?
    ______ years old

37. How long have you been using laxatives in this way?
Specify number of ______ years, ______ months, or ______ weeks

38. What kind(s) of laxatives do you use?

BRAND NAME: ______________________ DOSAGE: ______________________
BRAND NAME: ______________________ DOSAGE: ______________________
BRAND NAME: ______________________ DOSAGE: ______________________
BRAND NAME: ______________________ DOSAGE: ______________________

39. Do you remember why you first started using laxatives for weight control? Please explain:

____

____

40. How concerned are you about your use of laxatives for this purpose?
_____ I am not bothered at all.
_____ It bothers me a little.
_____ I am moderately concerned about it.
_____ It is one of my major concerns.

41. Check ALL of the following choices that describe how you feel AFTER you have purged, by using laxatives, for weight control:

_____ Calm
_____ Helpless
_____ Stimulated
_____ Excited
_____ Angry
_____ "Spaced Out" or Dazed
_____ Disgusted
_____ Energized
_____ Secure
_____ Panicked
_____ Relieved
_____ Guilty
_____ Ashamed
_____ Afraid
_____ Euphoric or "High"
_____ Lonely
_____ Depressed
Other: ______________________

Questions in Part II adapted from Eating Problems Questionnaire by Stuckey M, Lewis L, Jacobs, B, Johnson, C and Schwartz, D, 1981, and used by permission.

Part III. MEDICAL HISTORY

1. What are your present medical problems?

____

____

2. What medication or drugs are you taking? Please list names and amounts, including any for weight control, and including birth control pills.

	NAME OF MEDICATION OR DRUG	AMOUNT	HOW OFTEN
a.	______	______	______
b.	______	______	______
c.	______	______	______
d.	______	______	______

3. Are you allergic to any medication, drugs, or foods?
   ______ No
   ______ Yes   If "yes", please list:
   ____

4. When did you last have a complete physical exam?
   Date (Month, Day, Year): _____/_____/_____

5. Who is your current doctor? ____

6. How much alcohol do you usually drink?
   ______ One or more drink daily
   ______ Two or more drinks a week
   ______ One drink a week
   ______ One drink a month
   ______ Less than one drink a month, OR None

7. How many cigarettes do you smoke daily?
   ______ Three packs or more
   ______ Between one and three packs
   ______ Less than one pack
   ______ None

8. How many cups of coffee do you drink daily?
   ______ Six cups or more
   ______ Three or five cups
   ______ One or two cups
   ______ None

9. How many hours of sleep do you need to feel your best?
   ______ Ten hours or more
   ______ Eight to ten hours
   ______ Six to eight hours
   ______ Less than six hours

10. Check one:
_____ I get enough sleep.
_____ I do not get enough sleep.
_____ I sleep too much.

11. How would you describe your overall physical health? (check one)
_____ Excellent
_____ Better than average
_____ Average
_____ Worse than average
_____ Poor

12. How old were you when your first menstrual period began?
_____ years
OR _____ Not Applicable (for females who have never menstruated)
_____ Not Applicable (for males)
If "not applicable", skip to Question #20.

13. How much did you weigh when your first menstrual period began?
_____ lbs.

14. How many times have you missed your menstrual period for 3 consecutives months or more (excluding pregnancy)
_____ times
OR _____ Never
If "never", skip to Question #19.

15. Please complete the following for each time your menstrual period stopped:

	MOST RECENTLY	PREVIOUS TIME	PREVIOUS TIME	PREVIOUS TIME
Date periods stopped	_____	_____	_____	_____
Weight when periods stopped	_____	_____	_____	_____
Date periods resumed	_____	_____	_____	_____
Weight when periods resumed	_____	_____	_____	_____

16. Have your periods ever stopped because of a major weight loss?
_____ Yes
_____ No
If "no", please skip to Question #18.

17. When did your menstrual periods stop in relation to your first major weight loss?
_____ Periods stopped before weight loss (about _____ months before loss)
_____ Periods stopped at the beginning of the weight loss
_____ Periods stopped after the weight loss began

18. Have your periods ever stopped because of a major weight gain?
_____ Yes
_____ No

19. EXCEPT for any times when your periods may have stopped because of a major weight loss or gain, what is the approximate regularity of your periods?
_____ Fairly regular (same number of days, not more than 3 days early/late)
_____ Somewhat irregular (within 4 to 10 days early or late)
_____ Very irregular (more than 10 days early or late)

20. NOT COUNTING ANY HOSPITALIZATION FOR WEIGHT PROBLEMS OR CHILDBIRTH, please list all hospitalizations, indicating your age and the reason for each admission:

	AGE	REASON FOR HOSPITALIZATION
a.	_____	_____
b.	_____	_____
c.	_____	_____

21. Please list any serious illnesses you have had which DID NOT REQUIRE HOSPITALIZATION:

	AGE	ILLNESS
a.	_____	_____
b.	_____	_____
c.	_____	_____

22. Please complete the following information for any hospitalizations you have had SPECIFICALLY FOR TREATMENT OF YOUR WEIGHT PROBLEM:

	MOST RECENT ADMISSION	PREVIOUS ADMISSION	PREVIOUS ADMISSION	PREVIOUS ADMISSION
Date admitted	_____	_____	_____	_____
Date discharged	_____	_____	_____	_____
Age at admission	_____	_____	_____	_____
Weight at admission	_____	_____	_____	_____
Weight at discharge	_____	_____	_____	_____

Treatment received (check all that apply in each of the 4 columns):

Medication	_____	_____	_____	_____
Intravaneous (IV) Fluids	_____	_____	_____	_____
Psychotherapy	_____	_____	_____	_____
Behavior Modification	_____	_____	_____	_____
Family Therapy	_____	_____	_____	_____
Other: _____	_____	_____	_____	_____

23. Briefly describe your feelings about the hospitalization(s) for treatment of your weight problem:

____

____

____

____

____

24. Have you ever received psychiatric counseling, or are you now receiving psychiatric counseling? (FOR ANY REASON— NOT JUST FOR WEIGHT PROBLEMS)

____ No, never

If "no", skip to Part IV, "Social History".

____ Yes, in the past

____ Yes, at the present

25. Please complete the section below regarding your psychiatric counseling.

AGE	REASON FOR CONTACT	TYPE OF COUNSELING RECEIVED	LENGTH OF TREATMENT
________	____________	________________	________
________	____________	________________	________
________	____________	________________	________
________	____________	________________	________

26. Please complete the following information for any prior *outpatient* treatment that you have received for anorexia nervosa or bulimia.

	MOST RECENT TREATMENT	PREVIOUS TREATMENT	PREVIOUS TREATMENT
Date series of treatment began	_____	_____	_____
Date series of treatment ended	_____	_____	_____
Your age during treatment	_____	_____	_____
Weight at beginning of treatment	_____	_____	_____
Weight at end of treatment	_____	_____	_____
Initial reason for seeking treatment (check one box in each of the three columns):			
Weight loss	_____	_____	_____
Other medical problem: _____	_____	_____	_____
Other reason: _____	_____	_____	_____
Treatment received (check all that apply in each of the three columns):			
Medication	_____	_____	_____
Family therapy	_____	_____	_____
Behavior modification	_____	_____	_____
Psychotherapy	_____	_____	_____

Below, please describe your feelings about this treatment that you have received in the past. (Which type seemed most effective? etc.)

____

____

____

____

____

____

____

____

Part IV. SOCIAL HISTORY

1. Race (check one):
   ______ American Indian or Alaskan Native
   ______ Asian
   ______ Black
   ______ White

2. Hispanic origin (check one):
   ______ No
   ______ Yes

3. Please *circle* the last year of school that you have completed:

1 2 3 4 5 6 7 8	9 10 11 12	13 14 15 16	17 18	19 20 21
Grade School	High School	College	Master's	Doctorate

4. My grades in school were/are:
   ______ Excellent
   ______ Above average
   ______ About average
   ______ Below average

5. Did you ever leave home to attend school?
   ______ No
   ______ Yes
   If "yes", at what age? ______

6. Are you employed?
   ______ No
   If "no", please skip to Question #10.
   ______ Yes (includes "student" and "homemaker")

7. Briefly describe the kind of work you do.

8. How long have you done this kind of work?
   ______ years

9. There are some jobs that most people would like, and others that few would like. On a scale from 0-10, with "0" being a job that few would want and with "10" being a job most people would want, *circle* the number that describes your work.

   0---1---2---3---4---5---6---7---8---9---10
   Few People Would Want The Job — Most People Would Want The Job

10. What is the total annual income of your family? (check ONE)
    ______ Under $8,000
    ______ Between $8,000 and $12,000
    ______ Between $12,000 and $18,000
    ______ Between $18,000 and $30,000
    ______ Between $30,000 and $45,000
    ______ Over $45,000

11. What is your usual living arrangement?
    ______ Living alone
    ______ Living with a roommate
    ______ Living with a spouse and/or family
    ______ Living with others (specify): ______________________
    ______ Living in an institution (specify): ______________________

12. What is your present marital status?
    ______ Married
    ______ Separated
    ______ Divorced
    ______ Widowed
    ______ Never married
    If "never married", skip to Question #18.

13. Please provide the following information for each marriage:

DATE OF MARRIAGE		DATE OF TERMINATION	REASON FOR TERMINATION (Death, Divorce, etc.)	NUMBER OF CHILDREN FROM THIS MARRIAGE
______	to	______	______	______
______	to	______	______	______
______	to	______	______	______

If not currently married, skip to Question #18.

14. Is your spouse employed?
    ______ No
    ______ Yes

15. When employed, what kind of work does your spouse do?

    ____

16. Please circle the last year of school that your spouse has completed:

1 2 3 4 5 6 7 8	9 10 11 12	13 14 15 16	17 18 19	20 21
Grade School	High School	College	Master's	Doctorate

17. On a scale from 0-10, with "0" being a job that few would want and with "10" being a job most people would want, *circle* the number that describes your spouse's work.

0---1---2---3---4---5---6---7---8---9---10

Few People Would Want The Job — Most People Would Want The Job

18. Is your father living?
_____ No If "no", year of death: _____
If "no", cause of death: _____
_____ Yes If "yes", how old is he now? _____

19. Is your mother living?
_____ No If "no", year of death: _____
If "no", cause of death: _____
_____ Yes If "yes", how old is she now? _____

20. Describe your father's occupation: _____

21. Circle the last year of school that your father completed:

1 2 3 4 5 6 7 8	9 10 11 12	13 14 15 16	17 18	19 20 21
Grade School	High School	College	Master's	Doctorate

22. Describe your mother's occupation: _____

23. Circle the last year of school that your mother completed:

1 2 3 4 5 6 7 8	9 10 11 12	13 14 15 16	17 18	19 20 21
Grade School	High School	College	Master's	Doctorate

24. How would describe your father's weight while you were growing up?
_____ Very overweight
_____ Slightly overweight
_____ About average
_____ Slightly underweight
_____ Very underweight

25. How would you describe your mother's weight while you were growing up?
_____ Very overweight
_____ Slightly overweight
_____ About average
_____ Slightly underweight
_____ Very underweight

26. How would you describe your family's attitudes toward food and eating when you were growing up?
_____
_____
_____
_____

27. Were your parents ever separated or divorced?
 ______ No
 ______ Yes   If "yes", how old were you at the time?
 ______ years

28. Who raised you as a child?
 ____

29. How would you describe your relationship with your father when you were growing up?
 ______ Excellent
 ______ Good
 ______ Average
 ______ Below Average
 ______ Poor

30. How would you describe your relationship with your father now?
 ______ Excellent
 ______ Good
 ______ Average
 ______ Below Average
 ______ Poor

31. How would you describe your relationship with your mother when you were growing up?
 ______ Excellent
 ______ Good
 ______ Average
 ______ Below Average
 ______ Poor

32. How would you describe your relationship with your mother now?
 ______ Excellent
 ______ Good
 ______ Average
 ______ Below Average
 ______ Poor

33. Was there anything unusual about your first two years of life? (For example: Were you separated from your parents? Were you adopted? Were your parents separated or divorced? Did anyone in your family die? Did anyone in your family get sick? Did your family move around, etc.)
 ______ No
 ______ Yes
 If "yes", explain:
 ____
 ____

34. Please check one:
 ______ I was bottle fed.
 ______ I was breastfed.
 ______ Don't know

35. How many brothers and sisters do you have?
 ______ brothers and ______ sisters

Part V. WEIGHT PROFILE

1. Briefly describe your weight problem as you see it.

____

____

____

____

2. Briefly describe your weight problem as others see it (How do other people feel about your weight? Do they react to your weight? etc.).

____

____

____

3. How does your weight problem affect your relationships with others?

____

____

____

4. Listed below are various people who might have attitudes about your weight problem and your desire to change your weight. Please circle the number that best describes each person's attitude, as you see it.

NEGATIVE	INDIFFERENT	POSITIVE	
1	2	3	Your Spouse
1	2	3	Your Children
1	2	3	Your Mother
1	2	3	Your Father
1	2	3	Your Employer
1	2	3	Your Friends
1	2	3	Other: __________

5. How do the attitudes/behavior of your family affect your weight loss or gain? (Both in day-to-day situations and when on a weight program)

____

____

____

____

6. In the space below, please provide the information requested on each of your brothers and sisters. If you have no siblings, skip to Question #7.

1=Very overweight
2=Slightly overweight
3=About average
4=Slightly underweight
5=Very underweight

SIBLING #	FIRST NAME	AGE	SEX	WEIGHT	HEIGHT	DESCRIPTION (Circle ONE)				
Sibling 1	______	__	__	_____	_____	1	2	3	4	5
Sibling 2	______	__	__	_____	_____	1	2	3	4	5
Sibling 3	______	__	__	_____	_____	1	2	3	4	5
Sibling 4	______	__	__	_____	_____	1	2	3	4	5
Sibling 5	______	__	__	_____	_____	1	2	3	4	5
Sibling 6	______	__	__	_____	_____	1	2	3	4	5
Sibling 7	______	__	__	_____	_____	1	2	3	4	5
Sibling 8	______	__	__	_____	_____	1	2	3	4	5

7. How many children do you have (including children from previous marriages whether they are living with you or not)?
_____ sons and _____ daughters

8. Please provide the information requested for your children. If you have no children, please skip to Question 9.

1=Very overweight
2=Slightly overweight
3=About average
4=Slightly underweight
5=Very underweight

SIBLING #	FIRST NAME	AGE	SEX	WEIGHT	HEIGHT	DESCRIPTION (Circle ONE)				
1st Child	______	__	__	_____	_____	1	2	3	4	5
2nd Child	______	__	__	_____	_____	1	2	3	4	5
3rd Child	______	__	__	_____	_____	1	2	3	4	5
4th Child	______	__	__	_____	_____	1	2	3	4	5
5th Child	______	__	__	_____	_____	1	2	3	4	5
6th Child	______	__	__	_____	_____	1	2	3	4	5
7th Child	______	__	__	_____	_____	1	2	3	4	5
8th Child	______	__	__	_____	_____	1	2	3	4	5

9. How were you referred to the Eating Disorders Clinic?

_____ Family member (relationship): ______________________
_____ Physician (name): ______________________
_____ Family member: ______________________
_____ Therapist (specify): ______________________
_____ Friend
_____ Clergy
_____ Other (specify): ______________________

10. Below, briefly state your expectations concerning the Eating Disorders Clinic.

Please write a brief autobiography including those aspects of your life that you consider significant. This information should not be limited to your weight problem, but it should include the role that your weight has played in your current situation. Please include anything that you expect to happen in the near future. Please limit your remarks to the two pages that are attached.

Thank you for your cooperation in completing this questionnaire.

AUTOBIOGRAPHY

Subject Index